ADVANCEMENTS IN TUMOR IMMUNOTHERAPY AND CANCER VACCINES

Edited by **Hilal Arnouk**

Advancements in Tumor Immunotherapy and Cancer Vaccines
Edited by Hilal Arnouk

Published by InTech

Janeza Trdine 9, 51000 Rijeka, Croatia

Publishing Process Manager Petra Nenadic

Technical Editor Teodora Smiljanic

Cover Designer InTech Design Team

Additional hard copies can be obtained from orders@intechopen.com

Advancements in Tumor Immunotherapy and Cancer Vaccines, Edited by Hilal Arnouk
p. cm.
ISBN: 978-953-307-998-1

For EU product safety concerns:
IN TECH d.o.o., Prolaz Marije Krucifikse Kozulić 3, 51000 Rijeka, Croatia,
info@intechopen.com or visit our website at intechopen.com.

Meet the editor

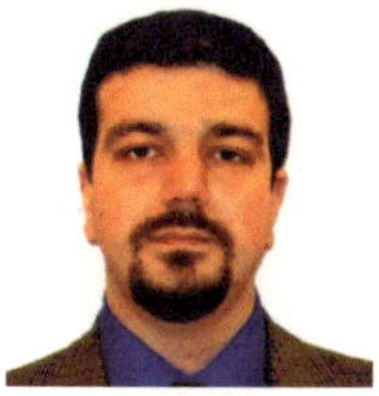

Hilalal Arnouk, MD, PhD, is the Director of Research and Development at Cell Constructs, Inc. affiliated with Georgia State University. Dr Arnouk received his education and post-doctorate training at Roswell Park Cancer Institute, Medical College of Georgia and University of Alabama in Birmingham, AL. His major areas of expertise include Cancer Immunotherapy, Biomarker Discovery and Regenerative Medicine.

Contents

Preface

..Suddenly we heard a voice crying, "This is the sea. This is the deep sea. This is the vast and mighty sea." And when we reached the voice it was a man whose back was turned to the sea, and at his ear he held a shell, listening to its murmur"

Khalil Gibran – The Madman

For decades we have been learning about the interplay between tumors and the immune system. Our knowledge seemed somewhat incomplete and indirect, like listening to the ocean waves through a shell. Only recently, cancer immunotherapy has started to become a reality, with Provenge (Dendreon Corporation, WA), an autologous antigen-presenting cell preparation, earning the approval of United States Food and Drug Administration (FDA) for the treatment of advanced prostate cancer in 2010.

This book provides an excellent review of the field of cancer immunotherapy, with special focus on prostate cancer, one of the most common cancers and a leading cause of cancer deaths in industrialized countries. The directions of immunotherapy of melanomas are also dicsussed in some detail within this book. Several chapters are dedicated to novel immunotherapeutic approaches utilizing the immunostimulatory functions of cell-based and protein-based vaccines, Toll-like receptors, Glycosphingolipids, Stress molecules, Type III Interferons, Interleukin 12 and biological plant-based compounds such as Triterpenes.

I would like to thank the people who helped with this publication, especially Ms Petra Nenadic. Finally, I dedicate this book to my family, my mentors and mentees throughout my career.

Hilal Arnouk, MD, PhD
Director of Research and Development,
Cell Constructs, Inc.,
Affiliated with Georgia State University,
Atlanta, GA,
USA

1

Immunotherapy in Urologic Malignancies: The Evolution and Future of Pattern Recognition Receptors

Jane Lee and Arnold I. Chin
University of California, Los Angeles, USA

1. Introduction

Urologic malignancies, including prostate, bladder, and kidney cancer, have been in the forefront in the use of immunotherapies. However, the tight link between inflammation and cancer can lead to both pro-tumorigenic and anti-tumorigenic effects. Elucidating the crosstalk between immune and cancer cells of the tumor microenvironment will enhance our ability to manipulate the immune system towards generation of an anti-tumor response. Over the last decade, the discovery of pattern recognition receptors of innate immunity has revolutionized the understanding of host-pathogen interactions and shed new light on the mechanisms of existing immunotherapies. In this chapter, we will discuss the role of inflammation in cancer, highlight the current status of immunotherapies in urologic malignancies, review the evolution of pattern recognition receptors, and discuss strategies in harnessing pattern recognition receptors to develop novel therapies.

2. Dual nature of inflammation in cancer

The initial observation associating leukocytes with tumor cells by Rudolf Virchow in 1863 marked the link between inflammation and cancer. Since then, inflammation has been shown to play distinct roles during tumor initiation, promotion, and metastasis. While growing evidence demonstrates the ability of chronic inflammation to initiate tumors, other examples support a role of tumor immune surveillance in cancer elimination. Perhaps the role of inflammation in cancer is analogous to a balance, with scales on opposite sides tightly interdependent. The challenge remains in skewing these inflammatory responses to tip the balance towards an anti-tumor response (Figure 1).

Arguably the cornerstone of anti-tumor immunity rests on the concept of immune surveillance, proposed by Sir Macfarlane Burnet and Lewis Thomas in 1957, whereby the immune system surveys, recognizes, and eliminates developing tumors. Tumor surveillance necessitates recognition of tumor antigens or "altered" self-antigens, and gained acceptance as new models emerged in the field of immunology. This included pre-clinical studies demonstrating tumor sensitivity to IFNγ treatment *in vivo* and increased carcinogen-induced tumor formation in perforin-deficient mice (Dighe et al., 1994; Russell and Ley, 2002). With the development of mice deficient in recombination activating gene 2 (Rag2), a gene essential in rearrangement and recombination of immunoglobulins and the T cell receptor, more convincing evidence revealed increased spontaneous development of tumors (Shankaran et al., 2001). Indeed, immunocompromised humans have increased risks of developing cancers including those of the bladder, kidney, colon, lung, non-Hodgkin's lymphoma, and melanoma (Dunn et al., 2002). More recently, the concept of tumor surveillance has been modified to incorporate a broader context of immunoediting, which not only encompasses the ability to recognize and eliminate tumors, but also suggests that immunogenicity of tumors can be shaped during tumor development, requiring constant interaction and modulation with the immune system. This was based on studies showing that tumors formed in an immunodeficient host were more immunogenic than tumors from an immunocompotent host. In these series of experiments, increased rejection of tumors generated from Rag2-deficient mice occurred when transplanted into immunocompetent hosts, but not Rag2-deficient hosts, while tumors derived from immunocompetent hosts grew similarly both in immunocompetent and Rag2-deficient hosts (Shankaran et al., 2001).

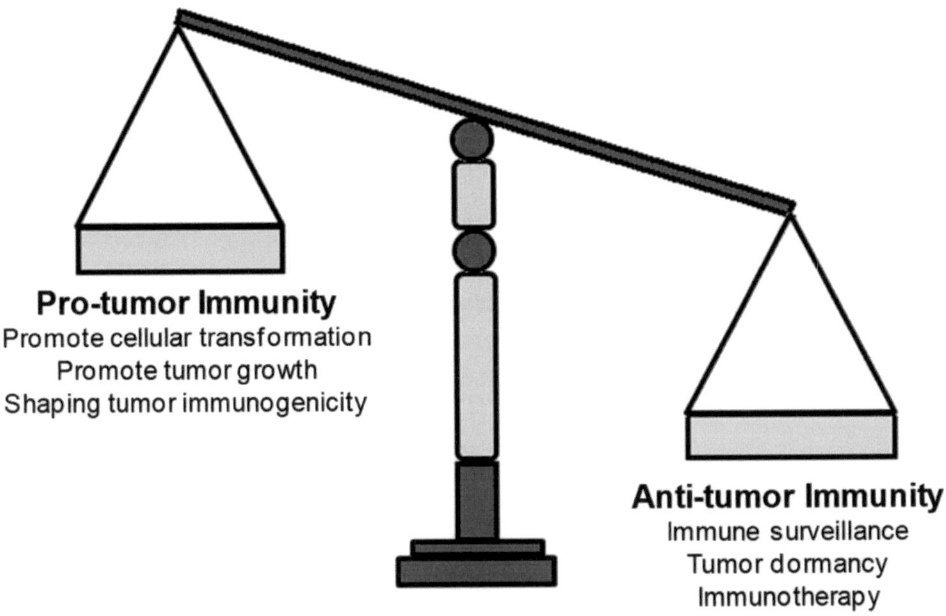

Fig. 1. Balance of Inflammatory Responses.

Interestingly, activation of the immune system to treat cancer predates the understanding of modern immunology and tumor surveillance. Together with reports since the 17th century describing regression of tumors following attacks of erysipelas, the origins of immunotherapy stems from the work of Freidrich Fehleisen in the late 1800's, who inoculated patients with sarcoma using the bacteria causing erysipelas, *Streptococcus pyogenes*. William Coley, the "father of immunotherapy," began treating cancer patients with inoculation combining *Streptococcus pyogenes* and *Serratia marcesens*. In many instances, injection of the live bacteria induced complete regression of tumors. The use of Coley's toxin continued from 1893 to 1963, largely until the advent of radiotherapy and chemotherapy. In 1943, isolation of lipopolysaccharide as the active component of Coley's toxin and more recently, identification of Toll-like receptor (TLR) 4 as the receptor for lipopolysaccharide, defined the molecular basis for this cancer regression. These findings marked the resurgence in the use of pathogens and pathogen-based components in cancer therapy (Rakoff-Nahoum and Medzhitov, 2009).

However, certain types of inflammation can promote deleterious effects. Although the typical immune response is self-limiting, persistent activation of the immune system may lead to a condition of chronic inflammation (Naugler et al., 2007). Loss of epithelial barrier function with resulting tissue destruction allows the entrance of pathogens and the recruitment of inflammatory cells and mediators. Combined with the persistence of inflammatory signals and the absence of factors that normally mediate resolution of the acute response, it is postulated that chronic inflammation ensues. Chronic inflammation defines many human conditions including chronic gastritis, hepatitis, and atherosclerosis. An epidemiologic association exists between several inflammatory diseases and an increased risk for malignant transformation. Furthermore, infection with a specific pathogen predisposes to the inflammatory disease, suggesting a causative link from pathogen to chronic inflammation to the initiation of cancer. The most clearly defined example is infection with *Helicobacter pylori* resulting in chronic gastritis, peptic ulcer disease, and ultimately gastric carcinoma. In addition, this association is found in the development of hepatitis, cirrhosis, and hepatocellular carcinoma following infection by the hepatitis B and C viruses, in Burkitt's lymphoma in parts of Africa and nasopharyngeal carcinoma in Southeast Asia with Epstein Barr virus, and in the development of cervical carcinoma following infection with certain types of the human papilloma virus. However, the majority of individuals infected with these pathogens do not develop clinical disease, much less the corresponding cancer.

In later stages of cancer, solid malignancies can develop necrotic centers as they outgrow their blood supply, releasing inflammatory mediators such as IL-1 and intracellular components such as heat shock proteins and high-mobility group protein B1 (HMG-B1) (Vakkila and Lotze, 2004). These factors activate recruitment of inflammatory cells such as tumor associated macrophages (TAMs) and myeloid-derived suppressor cells (MDSCs) that facilitate angiogenesis to sustain tumor growth, leading to a cascade of cytokines and chemokines such as TGFβ. In some instances, these inflammatory responses may influence epithelial-to-mesenchymal transition and development of tumor invasion and metastases, while in others, inflammation associated with radiation or chemotherapy may augment anti-tumor immunity (Ghiringhelli et al., 2009; Grivennikov et al., 2010).

The dichotomy between anti- and pro-tumor inflammation may be dictated by the type, location, and timing of the inflammatory response. This may elucidate why certain patients respond to immunotherapy and others do not. Dissecting the composition of the cells within the tumor microenvironment, the cytokines and chemokines involved in autocrine and paracrine signaling cascades, and understanding its molecular mechanisms will be central in understanding the paradigm on how inflammation influences tumorigenesis. The discovery of Toll-like receptors has provided insight into a molecular basis for antigen recognition and modulation of innate and adaptive immunity, but as you will see, has only widened the dualistic understanding of inflammation and cancer.

3. Components of the tumor microenvironment

The tumor microenvironment consists of a complex milieu of stromal and inflammatory cells, soluble factors, and extracellular matrix, intertwined with tumor cells. Identifying and understanding the regulation of the tumor microenvironment will be critical in designing therapies to inhibit tumor growth and invasion.

3.1 Stroma

The stromal components of the tumor microenvironment include fibroblasts, endothelial cells, and pericytes. Cancer associated fibroblasts (CAFs) provide growth factors, chemokines, and metalloproteinases essential for cellular communication during cancer proliferation and invasion (Bhowmick et al., 2004; Sato et al., 2009). Endothelial cells and pericytes deliver nutrients and oxygen to the cancer cells, allowing their continued growth and survival. The stromal cells along with the extracellular matrix present not only a physical barrier for tumor invasion and metastases, but also a lymphatic and vascular barrier to cancer-specific antibodies preventing immunoconjugates from reaching tumor cells (Yasunaga et al., 2011).

3.2 Inflammatory cells

Tumor-associated macrophages (TAMs) constitute the majority of infiltrating cells in the microenvironment (Jinushi et al., 2011). TAMs are classified into M1 and M2 types similar to Th1 and Th2 $CD4^+$ T cells, with M1 macrophages favoring pathogen elimination and M2 macrophages associated with angiogenesis and tissue remodeling (Balkwill and Mantovani, 2001). The most potent of antigen-presenting cells, dentritic cells (DCs), process and present antigens on their surface in context with major histocompatibilty complex class I (MHC) and class II molecules, to interact with $CD8^+$ T lymphocytes and $CD4^+$ T helper cells respectively. These are divided into myeloid DCs and plasmacytoid DCs, characterized by production of type I interferons. Natural killer cells (NKs) of innate immunity eradicate cells by inducing cytotoxicity through the release of perforin and granzyme that target the cell to destruction by apoptosis, while NKT cells share similarities with T cells, with recognition of lipid and glycolipid antigens. A subset of early myeloid cells termed myeloid derived suppressor cells (MDSCs) has the ability to suppress NK, NKT, and T cell responses, marked by production of L-arginine and upregulation of nitric oxide synthase 2 (Dolcetti et al., 2008).

Tumor infiltrating lymphocytes (TILs) represent the adaptive arm of immunity and include cytotoxic $CD8^+$ T cells (CTLs), B lymphocytes, and $CD4^+$ T helper cells, including Th1, Th2, and Th17 cells typically associated with autoimmunity. T regulatory (Treg) cells, characterized by the expression of the forkhead box P3 transcription factor (Foxp3), along with MDSCs, may play an important role in immune tolerance, regulating the immunosuppressive environment of cancer and posing as a barrier to successful immunotherapy.

3.3 Cytokines and chemokines

Cytokines and chemokines provide autocrine and paracrine signaling and play a critical role in shaping the tumor microenvironment. These include cytokines that favor development of anti-tumor immunity include IL-12, IFNα, and IFNγ, and those that enhance immune suppression such as IL-10, IL-17, and TGFβ or tumor progression such as IL-1 or IL6 (Grivennikov et al., 2010). Chemokines of the CC and CXC family secreted by tumors and infiltrating leukocytes, recruit inflammatory cells to the tumor microenvironment. This network of cytokines and chemokines plays an active role in regulating communication between the tumor, stroma, and inflammatory cells. Together, they have shown to influence tumor survival, growth, and epithelial-to-mesenchymal transition (EMT).

4. Immunotherapy in urologic malignancies

The incidence of urologic malignancies with bladder, kidney, and prostate cancer comprise almost 40% of cancer in men and almost 23% of all cancers in the United States, according to statistics provided by the 2010 American Cancer Society. Remarkably, in each of these malignancies, a Food and Drug Administration (FDA) approved immunotherapy exists (Figure 2). The following section briefly discusses the approved therapies and the strategies utilized.

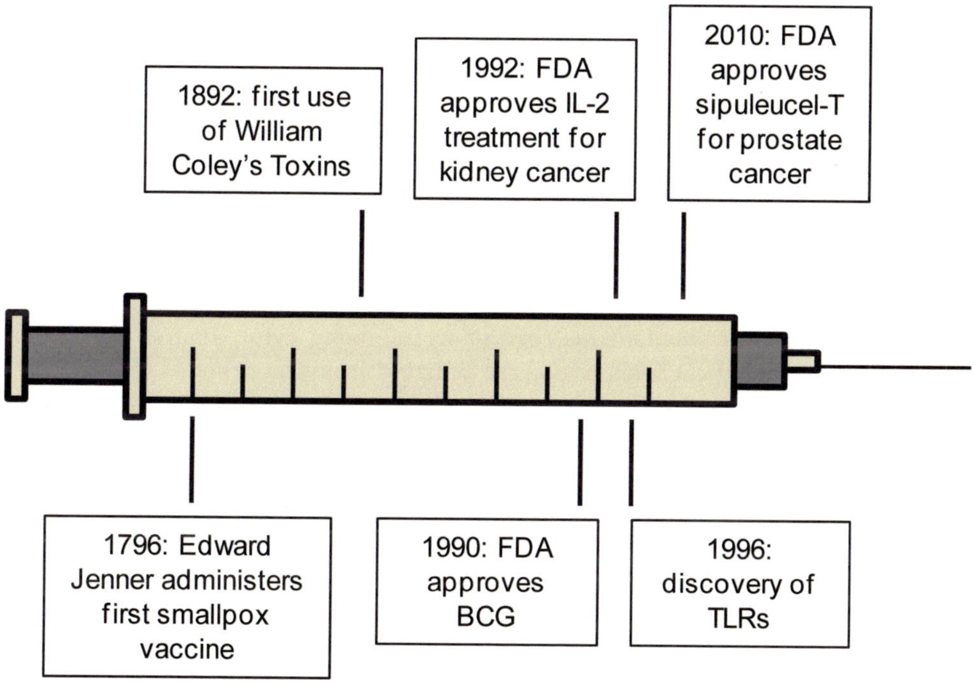

Fig. 2. Use of Immunotherapies in Bladder, Kidney, and Prostate Cancer.

4.1 Bladder cancer

Bladder cancer incidence ranks the 4th and 9th most prevalent in men and women, respectively, in the United States. Since its first therapeutic instillation in the bladder by Jean B. deKernion in 1975 for melanoma and later by Alvaro Morales for urothelial cancer, intravescical instillation of *bacillus calmette-guerin (BCG)*, an attenuated strain of *Mycobacterium bovis*, has demonstrated to be more effective than chemotherapy and is the standard intravesical treatment for non-muscle invasive bladder cancer and carcinoma *in situ*, garnering FDA approval in 1990. In the landmark trial, *BCG* administration in nine patients with a history of recurrent urothelial carcinomas reduced recurrences from a pre-treatment rate of 22 recurrences amongst the nine patients within 77 months, to just one during 41 months following therapy (Morales et al., 1976). *BCG* immunotherapy induces a local inflammatory response recruiting macrophages, DCs, T cells, NK cells, and neutrophils (Saint et al., 2001). Elevated cytokines including IL-6, IL-10, IL-12, IFNγ, and TNFα have been reported in patients following intravesical *BCG* (de Reijke et al., 1996). *BCG* can bind fibronectin on urothelial cells and more recently has been shown to mediate its effector functions through activation of TLR2 and TLR4 (Rakoff-Nahoum and Medzhitov, 2009; Ratliff, 1991; Tsuji et al., 2000).

BCG treatment can lead to significant morbidity including debilitating arthritis or sepsis. Efforts to increase its efficacy and decrease toxicity led to co-administration of *BCG* with IFNα, first recognized as an effective intravesical treatment in 1988 (Torti et al., 1988). Pre-clinical studies established a synergy between *BCG* and IFNα, with clinical trials demonstrating efficacy and safety using combinatorial administration of low-dose BCG and IFNα-2b with improved side effect profiles (Bazarbashi et al., 2011; Stricker et al., 1996; Torti et al., 1988). Currently, this combination has been used in *BCG* refractory patients with an additional 25% response rate (Gallagher et al., 2008).

4.2 Kidney cancer

As the 7th and 8th leading site of new cancer cases in men and women in the United States respectively, renal cell carcinoma (RCC) is relatively resistant to chemotherapy and radiotherapy. Reports of spontaneous regression following cytoreductive nephrectomy suggested an immunological basis of disease initiated from the primary tumor. The use of cytokine therapy has made important impacts in its treatment. This includes high dose IL-2, which garnered FDA approval in 1992 for metastatic RCC following a review of 225 patients in seven phase II trails, with complete responses occurring in 10%-20% of patients (Fyfe et al., 1995). IFNα, although currently not FDA approved for this indication, has shown efficacy for melanoma as well as for metastatic RCC. A landmark trial on the benefits of nephrectomy in 120 metastatic RCC patients undergoing IFNα -2b therapy revealed that IFNα with cytoreductive nephrectomy resulted in a median survival of 11.1 months over IFNα alone with a median survival of 8.1 months (Flanigan et al., 2001). IL-2 is a potent T cell activator, while IFNα induces T cell activation, upregulates MHC class I and II, and augments NK cells. In the age of targeted therapies to various tyrosine kinases, cytokine therapy remains the only curative therapy for metastatic RCC.

4.3 Prostate cancer

Prostate cancer remains the leading incidence of cancer in men, and the second highest cause of cancer death in men in the United States. Following hormone ablation for metastatic disease, patients inevitably develop castrate-resistant prostate cancer (CRPC), with options limited to systemic chemotherapy. The approval of the first in class cell-based vaccine for prostate cancer in 2010, sipuleucel-T, ended the search for an immunological treatment for prostate cancer that began decades earlier. Sipuleucel T combines *ex vivo* patient-derived DCs with a fusion of the tumor antigen prostatic-acid phosphatase and GM-CSF. In a phase III trial on 127 men with CRPC, median survival of those treated with sipuleucel-T was 25.9 months compared to 21.4 months for placebo, with generation of PAP-specific T cell immunity (Small et al., 2006).

5. Inflammation in urologic malignancies

An emerging theme in cancer is how the inflammatory composition of the tumor microenvironment influences cancer prognosis and overall patient survival. This has been demonstrated in breast cancer, where the ratio of $CD68^+$ macrophages to $CD8^+$ T cells, $CD4^+$ to $CD8^+$ T cells, or Th2 to Th1 $CD4^+$ T cells have all independently correlated with survival (Kohrt et al., 2005). In colon cancer, infiltration of $CD8^+$ T cells, CD45RO, and $Foxp3^+$ Tregs predicts overall survival better than grade and stage (Galon et al., 2006; Salama et al., 2009).

In human bladder cancer patients, elevated numbers of $CD8^+$ T cells in TILs have predicted greater disease-free and overall survival (Sharma et al., 2007). However, negative regulators have been linked with more aggressive cancers, including $CD4^+CD25^+Foxp3^+$ Tregs and cytokines important in their development such as TGFβ (Loskog et al., 2007). These suppressive effects may lead to T cell anergy and ineffective cytotoxic responses, questioning the functionality of infiltrating $CD8^+$ T cells. A similar observation exists in kidney and prostate cancer. In advanced renal cell carcinoma patients, elevated levels of Tregs are present in peripheral blood, with IFNα treatment resulting in inhibition of both $CD4^+$ T lymphocytes and Tregs (Tatsugami et al., 2010). Increased circulating $CD4^+$ and $CD8^+$ Tregs have been linked in human prostate cancer, while a murine model demonstrated tolerization of $CD8^+$ T cells (Anderson et al., 2007; Kiniwa et al., 2007; Miller et al., 2006; Sfanos et al., 2008).

The balance in TILs towards a suppressive state suggests a major role of antigen tolerance in tumorigenesis. Current strategies aimed at targeting these negative regulatory populations include monoclonal antibody therapies against the CD28 family of co-receptors CTLA-4 or PD-1, with an anti-CTLA-4 monoclonal antibody ipilimumab recently approved by the FDA in 2011 (Mangsbo et al., 2010; May et al., 2011). The signals that program the composition of the tumor microenvironment and the ability to alter individual components to favor a cell-mediated anti-tumor immunity will be an important future direction.

6. Pattern recognition receptors

Charles Janeway first proposed the idea of germline-encoded pattern recognition receptors (PRRs) of innate immunity that recognized conserved motifs of microbial origin termed pathogen-associated molecular patterns (PAMPs). These evolutionarily conserved receptors found throughout the animal kingdom activate the innate arm of immunity as well as direct adaptive immunity. Humans and microbes exist in direct interaction. In an environment with constant exposure to microbes, the host immune system is challenged to discern between benign flora and potential pathogens, and to initiate an appropriate immune response. The innate immune response initiated immediately upon pathogen entry mediates components such as macrophages, neutrophils, NK cells, alternative complement proteins, and other anti-microbial molecules. Recognition of pathogens in innate immunity utilizes germ line-encoded proteins, without the generation of lasting immunity. In addition to phagocytosis and killing of pathogens, innate immune cells synthesize and secrete a broad range of inflammatory mediators and cytokines that regulate systemic responses to infection, recruit additional white blood cells to sites of inflammation, and importantly, dictate the nature of the adaptive response. In contrast, the adaptive response, mediated by lymphocytes and their effector functions, requires several days to develop. Adaptive immunity has the ability to generate antigen-specific receptors in T cell receptors and immunoglobulins through somatic cell DNA rearrangement, and to elicit lasting immunity through development of memory cells.

The PRR superfamily now includes the family of Toll-like receptors (TLRs), cytosolic NOD-like receptors (NLRs) and RIG-I-like receptors, and membrane-bound C-type lectin receptors (CLRs) (Elinav et al., 2011; Kawai and Akira, 2011). In addition to host defense, PRRs may also play a major role in tissue repair and maintenance of tissue homeostasis, and emerging evidence suggests a role in cancer. In the following section, we will discuss the most well characterized family of Toll-like receptors and their role in tumor surveillance and cancer therapy.

6.1 Toll-like receptors signaling

TLRs are best defined in their host defense role through their ability to recognize PAMPs, leading to enhanced uptake of microorganisms, generation of reactive oxygen and nitrogen intermediates, and recruitment of leukocytes to the area of inflammation (Kawai and Akira, 2011; Modlin and Cheng, 2004). TLRs also shape the induction of adaptive immunity through activation of APCs by upregulation of co-stimulatory molecules CD80 and CD86. Currently, 10 human and 12 murine TLRs have been identified with PAMPs ranging from lipopolysaccharide (LPS) found in gram-negative bacterial walls recognized by TLR4, peptidoglycan and lipoprotein from gram-positive bacteria specific to TLR2 in conjunction with TLR1 or TLR6, double stranded RNA produced by many viruses for TLR3, single stranded RNA by TLR7 and TLR8, unmethylated CpG motifs with TLR9, and flagellin for TLR5 (Table 1). More recently, endogenous ligands termed danger-associated molecular patterns (DAMPs), including heat-shock proteins, the chromatin component HMG-B1, surfactant, protein A, fibronectin, heparan sulfate, fibrinogen, hyaluronan, and other components of injured cells, have also been identified suggesting a role for this receptor family in inflammatory responses resulting from tissue damage, such as lung injury or ischemic-reperfusion injury, or during tumor growth and necrosis (Rakoff-Nahoum and Medzhitov, 2009).

TLRs contain multiple leucine-rich repeats in the extracellular domain, and an intracellular Toll/IL-1R/Resistance (TIR) domain conserved in all TLRs (Kawai and Akira, 2011).

Proximally, the TIR interacts with other TIR domain adaptor proteins including recruitment of myeloid differentiation factor 88 (MyD88) and TIR domain-containing adaptor protein (TIRAP/Mal), which initiate a signaling cascade to the serine kinase IL-1R-associated kinase (IRAK) to tumor necrosis factor (TNF)-receptor-associated factor 6 (TRAF6), activating transforming growth factor-β-activated protein kinase 1 (TAK1). This results in activation of downstream transcription factors including NF-κB, MAP kinases, Jun N-terminal kinases, p38, ERK, and interferon regulator factors (Modlin and Cheng, 2004).

Toll-like receptor	Ligand(s)	Localization
TLR-1	Lipoprotein - bacteria	Membrane
TLR-2	Lipoprotein - bacteria; Heat-shock protein 70 - endogenous	Membrane
TLR-3	Double-stranded RNA - virus	Endosome
TLR-4	Lipopolysaccharide - gram-negative bacteria; Heat-shock protein 60/70 - endogenous	Membrane
TLR-5	Flagellin - bacteria	Membrane
TLR-6	Lipoprotein - bacteria	Membrane
TLR-7	Single-strand RNA - virus	Endosome
TLR-8	Single-strand RNA - virus	Endosome
TLR-9	CpG-containing DNA - bacteria and virus	Endosome
TLR-10	Unknown	Membrane
TLR-11	Urogenic bacteria	Membrane

Table 1. Human Toll-like Receptors and Known Ligands (So and Ouchi, 2010).

Although most TLRs utilize the MyD88 pathway, TLR3 and TLR4 interact with the adaptor protein TIR-domain-containing adapter-inducing interferon-β (TRIF) also known as Toll-like receptor adaptor molecule 1 (TICAM-1) to activate a MyD88-independent pathway leading to IRF3 activation and production of type I interferons. TLR3 has been implicated in NK cell activation, and while MyD88-dependent pathways largely regulate CTL induction, NK activation requires MyD88-independent pathways (Akazawa et al., 2007; Alexopoulou et al., 2001; Guerra et al., 2008).

6.2 Toll-like receptors in activation and regulation of inflammatory responses

Predominantly expressed on innate immune cells such as macrophages, DCs, and plasmacytoid DCs, recognition of PAMPS by TLRs leads to activation of transcription factors leading to production of inflammatory target genes such as cell cycle regulator genes c-myc and cyclin D1, cell survival genes bcl-xL, angiogenesis factors including VEGF, inflammatory cytokines such as IL-1, IL-6, and IL-8, type I interferons, chemokines, and T cell co-stimulatory molecules. These signals are crucial elements in the coordination of the host innate immune responses leading to recruitment of neutrophils, natural killer cells, and induction of antimicrobial peptides, resulting in killing of pathogens. Activation of TLRs ultimately dictate the nature of adaptive responses through dendritic cell maturation and the development of CTLs (Modlin and Cheng, 2004).

While stimulation of TLRs induces robust inflammatory pathways, negative regulatory mechanisms exist to balance immune activation to prevent chronic inflammation and autoimmunity. This includes decoy receptors, intracellular or transmembrane regulators, control of TLR expression, or caspase-dependent apoptosis of TLR-expressing cells (Kobayashi et al., 2002; Liew et al., 2005; Liu and Zhao, 2007). Activation of suppressor pathways through induction of cytokines IL-10, IL-27, and cells such as Tregs or MDSCs, may pose a significant barrier in antigen tolerance during tumor surveillance, reflected by increased numbers of suppressor cells in cancer patients (van Maren et al., 2008). Several lines of evidence support a critical role of TLRs in manipulating these suppressor cell populations. Multiple TLRs, including TLR2, TLR4, and TLR8 are expressed on the surface of Tregs, and may have a direct regulatory role with suppression of human prostate tumor infiltrating $CD8^+$ Treg cells following activation of TLR8 (Liu and Zhao, 2007). TLR9 activation has been shown to inhibit Tregs through IL-6 produced by DCs, although reports also show a TLR9-mediated induction of IL-10 and thus activation of Tregs (Jarnicki et al., 2008; Pasare and Medzhitov, 2003). In an autochthonous prostate cancer model, TLR3 activation increased infiltration of tumor infiltrating T and NK cells, and suppressed splenic Tregs, suggesting the ability of TLR activation to selectively modify the tumor microenvironment (Chin et al., 2010). The relationship between TLRs and MDSCs is less clear, but a recent study showed that TLR9 activation may inhibit MDSCs in a murine model (Ostrand-Rosenberg and Sinha, 2009; Peng et al., 2005; Zoglmeier et al., 2011). Collectively, these studies suggest that selective activation of TLRs may not only increase tumor infiltration of cytotoxic T and NK cells, but may also inhibit specific types of suppressor populations.

6.3 Toll-like receptors on tumor cells

In addition to immune cells, a broad variety of epithelial cells including colon, ovarian, bladder, kidney, and prostate express various TLRs. Although the endogenous role of TLRs on epithelial cells is unclear, it may stem from regulation of tissue growth and repair. Activation of TLRs in various tumor lines and models has shown both evidence of tumor reduction and cancer progression (Maruyama et al., 2011). In prostate and kidney cancer cell lines, TLR3 activation has been shown to induce apoptosis, while TLR9 has been shown to promote prostate cancer invasion, and IL-8 and TGFβ production *in vitro* (Di et al., 2009; Ilvesaro et al., 2007; Paone et al., 2008; Taura et al., 2010). In bladder cancer lines, elevated expression of TLR2-4, 5, 7, and 9 was detected in non-muscle invasive tumors, with decreased expression in muscle invasive tumors (Ayari et al., 2011).

The role of TLRs on epithelial cells needs to be clarified. What is the impact of TLR expression on epithelial cells during tumor initiation, growth, and response to immunotherapies? In human population studies, a sequence variant in a 3′-untranslated region of TLR4 as well as polymorphisms in the TLR gene cluster encoding TLR1, 6 and 10, and the downstream signaling mediator IRAK1 and IRAK4 confer increased prostate cancer risk (Lindstrom et al., 2010). However, the contribution of these TLR signaling components is unclear. In order to distinguish the role of TLRs on epithelial cells versus stromal or immune cells, tissue specific models will need to be examined.

6.4 Toll-like receptors in immune surveillance

The evidence of TLRs in mediating immune surveillance is based on tumor growth in knockout models of TLRs and their signaling adaptors, with studies supporting tumor promoting as well as suppressing effects. Exogenous administration of TLR ligands may not truly demonstrate a role of tumor surveillance and may enhance host immunity above physiologic levels. In support of a role of TLRs in tumor surveillance, mice deficient in TLR3 and TLR9 show increased growth of subcutaneously implanted prostate cancer, while deficiency in the negative regulatory adaptor molecule IRAK-M impairs growth of implanted tumor cells (Chin et al., 2010; Xie et al., 2007). Supporting a role in tumorigenesis, MyD88 mediates tumor initiation in a mouse model of spontaneous intestinal tumorigenesis and diethylnitrosamine-induced hepatocellular tumors (Naugler et al., 2007; Rakoff-Nahoum and Medzhitov, 2007; Xie et al., 2007). These opposing effects are confounded by the tumor origin, tumor model used, and potential contribution of TLRs on tumor cells, and further studies will need to explore this important issue.

7. Toll-like receptors in human immunotherapy

The role of TLRs in cancer therapy harnesses the exogenous use of synthetic TLR agonists to enhance host immunity. Despite pre-clinical evidence supporting anti-tumor responses as well as facilitating tumor promotion, the use of TLR agonists have a significant clinical importance and a promising future. Most clinical trial designs focus on the adjuvant properties of TLRs, predominantly by stimulating APCs through upregulation of co-stimulatory molecules such as CD80 and CD86 (Medzhitov et al., 1997). In addition to activation of adaptive immunity, effector functions include increase recruitment of innate immune cells such as NK, NKT, γδT cells, modulating the cytokine milieu, and direct cytotoxicity of tumor cells (Figure 3). Overcoming immune suppression is a major obstacle for successful immunotherapy and TLR activation may suppress Tregs and MDSCs to break antigen tolerance in conjunction with activation of adaptive immunity (Pasare and Medzhitov, 2003). More recently, strategies have adopted the use of TLR agonists with tumor antigens for the development of cancer vaccines.

Freund's complete adjuvant (FCA) has been the most common adjuvant for antibody production, produced in a water-in-oil emulsion containing heat-killed mycobacterial cells (Stewart-Tull, 1996). TLR2 and TLR4 play a crucial role in the recognition of FCA, which has increased antibody responses crucial for delayed-type hypersensitivity reactions over Freund's incomplete adjuvant lacking mycobacteria (Azuma and Seya, 2001). *BCG* has been used for over three decades as intravesical therapy in bladder cancer and mediates its function through TLR2 and 4 pathways as well. Recent trials utilizing components of mycobacterial cell walls rather than live bacteria may have similar efficacy while reducing toxicity (Chin et al., 1996). In fact, activation of TLRs using synthetic PAMPs reduces tumor growth in pre-clinical models in bladder and prostate cancer. With the impact of IFNα in kidney cancer patients, it is likely that TLR activation may play an important role in kidney cancer in particular with TLRs that activate type I interferons such as TLR3.

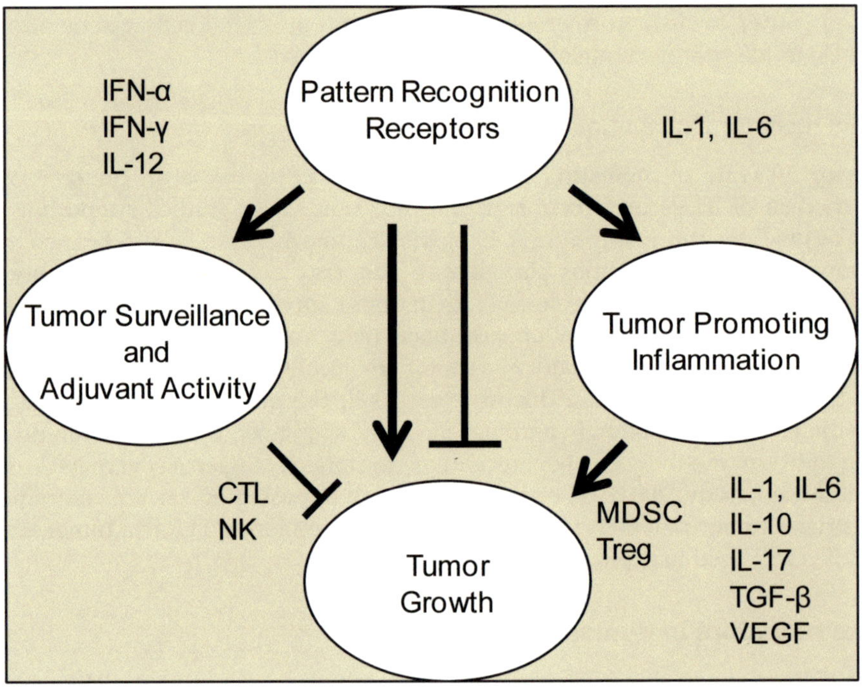

Fig. 3. The Direct and Indirect Influences of Pattern Recognition Receptors on Tumor Growth.

Although many TLRs share common signaling pathways, it is evident that ligation of different TLRs will induce unique gene expression profiles that translate to specific effector functions (Doyle et al., 2002). As supported by the wide variation in pre-clinical responses, the effector functions and resulting tumor response by TLR activation may change based on tumor type, location, dose, and timing. In the near future, perhaps activation of specific TLRs can be tailored to augment a desired tissue-specific effector function that partners with a particular vaccine.

To date, three TLR agonists have been used in clinical trials, all recognizing nucleic acids for receptors expressed on endosomal membrances. The only approved agonist, the single-stranded RNA analogue imiquimod specific for TLR7, showed activity in murine colon cancer and sarcoma models, inducing IFNγ and IL-12 to activate CTLs and myeloid DCs (Maruyama et al., 2011). Initially used clinically for actinic keratosis and genital warts, imiquimod has show activity against superficial basal cell carcinoma and received FDA approval in 2004.

Unmethylated CpG oligodeoxynucleotides (ODN) found in bacterial and viral DNA has been used in phase I-III trials against multiple malignancies including kidney, breast, melanoma, and lymphomas (Krieg, 2008). Ligands for TLR9 have been grouped into three different classes based on their roles in activating the immune system. A-class CpG ODN (CpG-A) stimulate type I interferon production by plasmacytoid dendritic cells, activating natural killer cells and IFNγ (Krug et al., 2001); B-Class CpG ODNs (CpG-B) induce B cell and monocyte maturation, leading to B cell proliferation with little pDC activation; and C-Class CpG ODNs (CpG-C) mediate signaling pathways of both CpG-A and CpG-B (Rothenfusser et al., 2004). Although pre-clinical trials demonstrate that TLR9 activation potently induces Th1 responses, NK activation, stimulation of cytokines TNFα, IL-12, and IFNγ, and induces a strong $CD8^+$ T-cell response, clinical trials have not yielded robust results (Valmori et al., 2003). This may be in part due to different expression of TLR9 in murine models with broad expression in myeloid DCs, plasmacytoid DCs, macrophages, and B cells, with expression limited to pDCs and B cells in humans.

To address this disparity, combinatorial strategies attempt to enhance the activity of CpG ODN, with the addition of alum, emulsigen, and polyphosphazenes (Malyala et al., 2009). Other strategies include inhibition of p38 that may enhance T cell activation or through blockade of CTLA-4 or PD-1 (Mangsbo et al., 2010; Takauji et al., 2002). These combinatorial strategies will be increasingly important in promoting synergic responses to augment host immunity, while unhinging negative regulatory factors.

TLR3 ligand polyriboinosinic:polyribocytidylic acid (poly(I:C)), a synthetic analog of double-stranded RNA, has demonstrated to be a promising adjuvant for immunotherapy. Studies have reported poly(I:C) as an effective inducer of inflammatory cytokines, dendritic cells, and macrophages, leading to subsequent activation of natural killer cells. While poly(I:C) has proven effective in inhibiting tumor metastasis and prolonging survival in animal models, the drawback exists in its inability to efficiently penetrate the cell membrane in order to bind to its cognate receptor. The development of stabilized compounds, including polyICLC, has been used in phase II studies against gliomas (Butowski et al., 2009). A recent phase I trial against multiple malignancies including advanced bladder cancer utilized a novel vaccine approach combining a human chorionic gonadotropin-β antigen fusion protein with adjuvants poly ICLC and the TLR7/8 agonist resiquimod (Morse et al., 2011). This orchestration of TLR-based adjuvant activation with tumor antigen stimulation is promising and utilizes the ability of TLRs for cross antigen presentation, allowing extracellular antigens to be processed and presented by class I MHC (Oh and Kedl, 2010).

8. Therapeutic design and conclusion

Urologic malignancies comprise 23% of all cancers in the United States, excluding basal skin cancer. Immunotherapeutic approaches in urologic malignancies broadly encompass cytokine-based, bacteria-mediated, and cell-based vaccine therapies. This demonstrates the immunological sensitivity of urologic malignancies and opens avenues to develop novel strategies. Clearly the composition of inflammation in the tumor microenvironment influences tumor growth, metastases, and overall survival. Toll-like receptors play important roles in host defense against pathogens, and tissue homeostasis and repair in response to tissue damage. Mounting evidence suggests that TLRs can recognize endogenous antigens released from tumors and mediate tumor immune surveillance. Furthermore, exogenous activation of TLRs can alter the tumor microenvironment and induce adaptive immunity, influencing the response not only to immunotherapies, but also potentially to radiation, chemotherapy, and targeted therapies.

Understanding the specificities of various TLRs will be critical, as will be determining the timing of agonist stimulation, dose, and tissue specificity. Exploring the potential of other PRR families in cancer is clearly an open field. Similarly, challenges in modulating immunity to prevent antigen tolerance or an inappropriate response will need to be addressed. By incorporating activation of distinct PRR and PRR signaling pathways, specific components of the tumor microenvironment may be modulated to augment cell-mediated immunity. Combining the ability of PRRs to regulate suppressor cells, novel vaccine strategies may overcome antigen tolerance. At the same time, caution needs to be exercised to understand direct PRR effects on tumors and development of pro-tumorigenic immunity.

9. References

Akazawa, T., Ebihara, T., Okuno, M., Okuda, Y., Shingai, M., Tsujimura, K., Takahashi, T., Ikawa, M., Okabe, M., Inoue, N., *et al.* (2007). Antitumor NK activation induced by the Toll-like receptor 3-TICAM-1 (TRIF) pathway in myeloid dendritic cells. Proc Natl Acad Sci U S A *104*, 252-257.

Alexopoulou, L., Holt, A. C., Medzhitov, R., and Flavell, R. A. (2001). Recognition of double-stranded RNA and activation of NF-kappaB by Toll-like receptor 3. Nature *413*, 732-738.

Anderson, M. J., Shafer-Weaver, K., Greenberg, N. M., and Hurwitz, A. A. (2007). Tolerization of tumor-specific T cells despite efficient initial priming in a primary murine model of prostate cancer. J Immunol *178*, 1268-1276.

Ayari, C., Bergeron, A., LaRue, H., Menard, C., and Fradet, Y. (2011). Toll-like receptors in normal and malignant human bladders. J Urol *185*, 1915-1921.

Azuma, I., and Seya, T. (2001). Development of immunoadjuvants for immunotherapy of cancer. Int Immunopharmacol *1*, 1249-1259.

Balkwill, F., and Mantovani, A. (2001). Inflammation and cancer: back to Virchow? Lancet *357*, 539-545.

Bazarbashi, S., Soudy, H., Abdelsalam, M., Al-Jubran, A., Akhtar, S., Memon, M., Aslam, M., Kattan, S., and Shoukri, M. (2011). Co-administration of intravesical bacillus Calmette-Guerin and interferon alpha-2B as first line in treating superficial transitional cell carcinoma of the urinary bladder(a). BJU Int.

Bhowmick, N. A., Chytil, A., Plieth, D., Gorska, A. E., Dumont, N., Shappell, S., Washington, M. K., Neilson, E. G., and Moses, H. L. (2004). TGF-beta signaling in fibroblasts modulates the oncogenic potential of adjacent epithelia. Science *303*, 848-851.

Butowski, N., Lamborn, K. R., Lee, B. L., Prados, M. D., Cloughesy, T., DeAngelis, L. M., Abrey, L., Fink, K., Lieberman, F., Mehta, M., *et al.* (2009). A North American brain tumor consortium phase II study of poly-ICLC for adult patients with recurrent anaplastic gliomas. J Neurooncol *91*, 183-189.

Chin, A. I., Miyahira, A. K., Covarrubias, A., Teague, J., Guo, B., Dempsey, P. W., and Cheng, G. (2010). Toll-like receptor 3-mediated suppression of TRAMP prostate cancer shows the critical role of type I interferons in tumor immune surveillance. Cancer Res *70*, 2595-2603.

Chin, J. L., Kadhim, S. A., Batislam, E., Karlik, S. J., Garcia, B. M., Nickel, J. C., and Morales, A. (1996). Mycobacterium cell wall: an alternative to intravesical bacillus Calmette Guerin (BCG) therapy in orthotopic murine bladder cancer. J Urol *156*, 1189-1193.

de Reijke, T. M., de Boer, E. C., Kurth, K. H., and Schamhart, D. H. (1996). Urinary cytokines during intravesical bacillus Calmette-Guerin therapy for superficial bladder cancer: processing, stability and prognostic value. J Urol *155*, 477-482.

Di, J. M., Pang, J., Pu, X. Y., Zhang, Y., Liu, X. P., Fang, Y. Q., Ruan, X. X., and Gao, X. (2009). Toll-like receptor 9 agonists promote IL-8 and TGF-beta1 production via activation of nuclear factor kappaB in PC-3 cells. Cancer Genet Cytogenet *192*, 60-67.

Dighe, A. S., Richards, E., Old, L. J., and Schreiber, R. D. (1994). Enhanced in vivo growth and resistance to rejection of tumor cells expressing dominant negative IFN gamma receptors. Immunity *1*, 447-456.

Dolcetti, L., Marigo, I., Mantelli, B., Peranzoni, E., Zanovello, P., and Bronte, V. (2008). Myeloid-derived suppressor cell role in tumor-related inflammation. Cancer Lett *267*, 216-225.

Doyle, S., Vaidya, S., O'Connell, R., Dadgostar, H., Dempsey, P., Wu, T., Rao, G., Sun, R., Haberland, M., Modlin, R., and Cheng, G. (2002). IRF3 mediates a TLR3/TLR4-specific antiviral gene program. Immunity *17*, 251-263.

Dunn, G. P., Bruce, A. T., Ikeda, H., Old, L. J., and Schreiber, R. D. (2002). Cancer immunoediting: from immunosurveillance to tumor escape. Nat Immunol *3*, 991-998.

Elinav, E., Strowig, T., Henao-Mejia, J., and Flavell, R. A. (2011). Regulation of the antimicrobial response by NLR proteins. Immunity *34*, 665-679.

Flanigan, R. C., Salmon, S. E., Blumenstein, B. A., Bearman, S. I., Roy, V., McGrath, P. C., Caton, J. R., Jr., Munshi, N., and Crawford, E. D. (2001). Nephrectomy followed by interferon alfa-2b compared with interferon alfa-2b alone for metastatic renal-cell cancer. N Engl J Med *345*, 1655-1659.

Fyfe, G., Fisher, R. I., Rosenberg, S. A., Sznol, M., Parkinson, D. R., and Louie, A. C. (1995). Results of treatment of 255 patients with metastatic renal cell carcinoma who received high-dose recombinant interleukin-2 therapy. J Clin Oncol *13*, 688-696.

Gallagher, B. L., Joudi, F. N., Maymi, J. L., and O'Donnell, M. A. (2008). Impact of previous bacille Calmette-Guerin failure pattern on subsequent response to bacille Calmette-Guerin plus interferon intravesical therapy. Urology *71*, 297-301.

Galon, J., Costes, A., Sanchez-Cabo, F., Kirilovsky, A., Mlecnik, B., Lagorce-Pages, C., Tosolini, M., Camus, M., Berger, A., Wind, P., *et al.* (2006). Type, density, and location of immune cells within human colorectal tumors predict clinical outcome. Science *313*, 1960-1964.

Ghiringhelli, F., Apetoh, L., Tesniere, A., Aymeric, L., Ma, Y., Ortiz, C., Vermaelen, K., Panaretakis, T., Mignot, G., Ullrich, E., *et al.* (2009). Activation of the NLRP3 inflammasome in dendritic cells induces IL-1beta-dependent adaptive immunity against tumors. Nat Med *15*, 1170-1178.

Grivennikov, S. I., Greten, F. R., and Karin, M. (2010). Immunity, inflammation, and cancer. Cell *140*, 883-899.

Guerra, N., Tan, Y. X., Joncker, N. T., Choy, A., Gallardo, F., Xiong, N., Knoblaugh, S., Cado, D., Greenberg, N. M., and Raulet, D. H. (2008). NKG2D-deficient mice are defective in tumor surveillance in models of spontaneous malignancy. Immunity *28*, 571-580.

Ilvesaro, J. M., Merrell, M. A., Swain, T. M., Davidson, J., Zayzafoon, M., Harris, K. W., and Selander, K. S. (2007). Toll like receptor-9 agonists stimulate prostate cancer invasion in vitro. Prostate *67*, 774-781.

Jarnicki, A. G., Conroy, H., Brereton, C., Donnelly, G., Toomey, D., Walsh, K., Sweeney, C., Leavy, O., Fletcher, J., Lavelle, E. C., *et al.* (2008). Attenuating regulatory T cell induction by TLR agonists through inhibition of p38 MAPK signaling in dendritic cells enhances their efficacy as vaccine adjuvants and cancer immunotherapeutics. J Immunol *180*, 3797-3806.

Jinushi, M., Chiba, S., Yoshiyama, H., Masutomi, K., Kinoshita, I., Dosaka-Akita, H., Yagita, H., Takaoka, A., and Tahara, H. (2011). Tumor-associated macrophages regulate tumorigenicity and anticancer drug responses of cancer stem/initiating cells. Proc Natl Acad Sci U S A.

Kawai, T., and Akira, S. (2011). Toll-like receptors and their crosstalk with other innate receptors in infection and immunity. Immunity *34*, 637-650.

Kiniwa, Y., Miyahara, Y., Wang, H. Y., Peng, W., Peng, G., Wheeler, T. M., Thompson, T. C., Old, L. J., and Wang, R. F. (2007). CD8+ Foxp3+ regulatory T cells mediate immunosuppression in prostate cancer. Clin Cancer Res *13*, 6947-6958.

Kobayashi, K., Hernandez, L. D., Galan, J. E., Janeway, C. A., Jr., Medzhitov, R., and Flavell, R. A. (2002). IRAK-M is a negative regulator of Toll-like receptor signaling. Cell *110*, 191-202.

Kohrt, H. E., Nouri, N., Nowels, K., Johnson, D., Holmes, S., and Lee, P. P. (2005). Profile of immune cells in axillary lymph nodes predicts disease-free survival in breast cancer. PLoS Med *2*, e284.

Krieg, A. M. (2008). Toll-like receptor 9 (TLR9) agonists in the treatment of cancer. Oncogene *27*, 161-167.

Krug, A., Rothenfusser, S., Hornung, V., Jahrsdorfer, B., Blackwell, S., Ballas, Z. K., Endres, S., Krieg, A. M., and Hartmann, G. (2001). Identification of CpG oligonucleotide sequences with high induction of IFN-alpha/beta in plasmacytoid dendritic cells. Eur J Immunol *31*, 2154-2163.

Liew, F. Y., Xu, D., Brint, E. K., and O'Neill, L. A. (2005). Negative regulation of toll-like receptor-mediated immune responses. Nat Rev Immunol *5*, 446-458.

Lindstrom, S., Hunter, D. J., Gronberg, H., Stattin, P., Wiklund, F., Xu, J., Chanock, S. J., Hayes, R., and Kraft, P. (2010). Sequence variants in the TLR4 and TLR6-1-10 genes and prostate cancer risk. Results based on pooled analysis from three independent studies. Cancer Epidemiol Biomarkers Prev *19*, 873-876.

Liu, G., and Zhao, Y. (2007). Toll-like receptors and immune regulation: their direct and indirect modulation on regulatory CD4+ CD25+ T cells. Immunology *122*, 149-156.

Loskog, A., Ninalga, C., Paul-Wetterberg, G., de la Torre, M., Malmstrom, P. U., and Totterman, T. H. (2007). Human bladder carcinoma is dominated by T-regulatory cells and Th1 inhibitory cytokines. J Urol *177*, 353-358.

Malyala, P., O'Hagan, D. T., and Singh, M. (2009). Enhancing the therapeutic efficacy of CpG oligonucleotides using biodegradable microparticles. Adv Drug Deliv Rev *61*, 218-225.

Mangsbo, S. M., Sandin, L. C., Anger, K., Korman, A. J., Loskog, A., and Totterman, T. H. (2010). Enhanced tumor eradication by combining CTLA-4 or PD-1 blockade with CpG therapy. J Immunother *33*, 225-235.

Maruyama, K., Selmani, Z., Ishii, H., and Yamaguchi, K. (2011). Innate immunity and cancer therapy. Int Immunopharmacol *11*, 350-357.

May, K. F., Jr., Gulley, J. L., Drake, C. G., Dranoff, G., and Kantoff, P. W. (2011). Prostate Cancer Immunotherapy. Clin Cancer Res.

Medzhitov, R., Preston-Hurlburt, P., and Janeway, C. A., Jr. (1997). A human homologue of the Drosophila Toll protein signals activation of adaptive immunity. Nature *388*, 394-397.

Miller, A. M., Lundberg, K., Ozenci, V., Banham, A. H., Hellstrom, M., Egevad, L., and Pisa, P. (2006). CD4+CD25high T cells are enriched in the tumor and peripheral blood of prostate cancer patients. J Immunol *177*, 7398-7405.

Modlin, R. L., and Cheng, G. (2004). From plankton to pathogen recognition. Nat Med *10*, 1173-1174.

Morales, A., Eidinger, D., and Bruce, A. W. (1976). Intracavitary Bacillus Calmette-Guerin in the treatment of superficial bladder tumors. J Urol *116*, 180-183.

Morse, M. A., Chapman, R., Powderly, J., Blackwell, K., Keler, T., Green, J., Riggs, R., He, L. Z., Ramakrishna, V., Vitale, L., *et al.* (2011). Phase I Study Utilizing a Novel Antigen-Presenting Cell-Targeted Vaccine with Toll-like Receptor Stimulation to Induce Immunity to Self-antigens in Cancer Patients. Clin Cancer Res *17*, 4844-4853.

Naugler, W. E., Sakurai, T., Kim, S., Maeda, S., Kim, K., Elsharkawy, A. M., and Karin, M. (2007). Gender disparity in liver cancer due to sex differences in MyD88-dependent IL-6 production. Science *317*, 121-124.

Oh, J. Z., and Kedl, R. M. (2010). The capacity to induce cross-presentation dictates the success of a TLR7 agonist-conjugate vaccine for eliciting cellular immunity. J Immunol *185*, 4602-4608.

Ostrand-Rosenberg, S., and Sinha, P. (2009). Myeloid-derived suppressor cells: linking inflammation and cancer. J Immunol *182*, 4499-4506.

Paone, A., Starace, D., Galli, R., Padula, F., De Cesaris, P., Filippini, A., Ziparo, E., and Riccioli, A. (2008). Toll-like receptor 3 triggers apoptosis of human prostate cancer cells through a PKC-alpha-dependent mechanism. Carcinogenesis *29*, 1334-1342.

Pasare, C., and Medzhitov, R. (2003). Toll pathway-dependent blockade of CD4+CD25+ T cell-mediated suppression by dendritic cells. Science *299*, 1033-1036.

Peng, G., Guo, Z., Kiniwa, Y., Voo, K. S., Peng, W., Fu, T., Wang, D. Y., Li, Y., Wang, H. Y., and Wang, R. F. (2005). Toll-like receptor 8-mediated reversal of CD4+ regulatory T cell function. Science *309*, 1380-1384.

Rakoff-Nahoum, S., and Medzhitov, R. (2007). Regulation of spontaneous intestinal tumorigenesis through the adaptor protein MyD88. Science *317*, 124-127.

Rakoff-Nahoum, S., and Medzhitov, R. (2009). Toll-like receptors and cancer. Nat Rev Cancer *9*, 57-63.

Ratliff, T. L. (1991). Bacillus Calmette-Guerin (BCG): mechanism of action in superficial bladder cancer. Urology *37*, 8-11.

Rothenfusser, S., Hornung, V., Ayyoub, M., Britsch, S., Towarowski, A., Krug, A., Sarris, A., Lubenow, N., Speiser, D., Endres, S., and Hartmann, G. (2004). CpG-A and CpG-B oligonucleotides differentially enhance human peptide-specific primary and memory CD8+ T-cell responses in vitro. Blood *103*, 2162-2169.

Russell, J. H., and Ley, T. J. (2002). Lymphocyte-mediated cytotoxicity. Annu Rev Immunol *20*, 323-370.

Saint, F., Patard, J. J., Groux Muscatelli, B., Lefrere Belda, M. A., Gil Diez de Medina, S., Abbou, C. C., and Chopin, D. K. (2001). Evaluation of cellular tumour rejection mechanisms in the peritumoral bladder wall after bacillus Calmette-Guerin treatment. BJU Int *88*, 602-610.

Salama, P., Phillips, M., Grieu, F., Morris, M., Zeps, N., Joseph, D., Platell, C., and Iacopetta, B. (2009). Tumor-infiltrating FOXP3+ T regulatory cells show strong prognostic significance in colorectal cancer. J Clin Oncol *27*, 186-192.

Sato, Y., Goto, Y., Narita, N., and Hoon, D. S. (2009). Cancer Cells Expressing Toll-like Receptors and the Tumor Microenvironment. Cancer Microenviron *2 Suppl 1*, 205-214.

Sfanos, K. S., Bruno, T. C., Maris, C. H., Xu, L., Thoburn, C. J., DeMarzo, A. M., Meeker, A. K., Isaacs, W. B., and Drake, C. G. (2008). Phenotypic analysis of prostate-infiltrating lymphocytes reveals TH17 and Treg skewing. Clin Cancer Res *14*, 3254-3261.

Shankaran, V., Ikeda, H., Bruce, A. T., White, J. M., Swanson, P. E., Old, L. J., and Schreiber, R. D. (2001). IFNgamma and lymphocytes prevent primary tumour development and shape tumour immunogenicity. Nature *410*, 1107-1111.

Sharma, P., Shen, Y., Wen, S., Yamada, S., Jungbluth, A. A., Gnjatic, S., Bajorin, D. F., Reuter, V. E., Herr, H., Old, L. J., and Sato, E. (2007). CD8 tumor-infiltrating lymphocytes are predictive of survival in muscle-invasive urothelial carcinoma. Proc Natl Acad Sci U S A *104*, 3967-3972.

Small, E. J., Schellhammer, P. F., Higano, C. S., Redfern, C. H., Nemunaitis, J. J., Valone, F. H., Verjee, S. S., Jones, L. A., and Hershberg, R. M. (2006). Placebo-controlled phase III trial of immunologic therapy with sipuleucel-T (APC8015) in patients with metastatic, asymptomatic hormone refractory prostate cancer. J Clin Oncol *24*, 3089-3094.

So, E. Y., and Ouchi, T. (2010). The application of Toll like receptors for cancer therapy. Int J Biol Sci *6*, 675-681.

Stewart-Tull, D. E. (1996). The Use of Adjuvants in Experimental Vaccines : II. Water-in-Oil Emulsions: Freund's Complete and lncomplete Adjuvants. Methods Mol Med *4*, 141-145.

Stricker, P., Pryor, K., Nicholson, T., Goldstein, D., Golovsky, D., Ferguson, R., Nash, P., Ehsman, S., Rumma, J., Mammen, G., and Penny, R. (1996). Bacillus Calmette-Guerin plus intravesical interferon alpha-2b in patients with superficial bladder cancer. Urology *48*, 957-961; discussion 961-952.

Takauji, R., Iho, S., Takatsuka, H., Yamamoto, S., Takahashi, T., Kitagawa, H., Iwasaki, H., Iida, R., Yokochi, T., and Matsuki, T. (2002). CpG-DNA-induced IFN-alpha production involves p38 MAPK-dependent STAT1 phosphorylation in human plasmacytoid dendritic cell precursors. J Leukoc Biol *72*, 1011-1019.

Tatsugami, K., Eto, M., and Naito, S. (2010). Influence of immunotherapy with interferon-alpha on regulatory T cells in renal cell carcinoma patients. J Interferon Cytokine Res *30*, 43-48.

Taura, M., Fukuda, R., Suico, M. A., Eguma, A., Koga, T., Shuto, T., Sato, T., Morino-Koga, S., and Kai, H. (2010). TLR3 induction by anticancer drugs potentiates poly I:C-induced tumor cell apoptosis. Cancer Sci *101*, 1610-1617.

Torti, F. M., Shortliffe, L. D., Williams, R. D., Pitts, W. C., Kempson, R. L., Ross, J. C., Palmer, J., Meyers, F., Ferrari, M., Hannigan, J., and et al. (1988). Alpha-interferon in superficial bladder cancer: a Northern California Oncology Group Study. J Clin Oncol *6*, 476-483.

Tsuji, S., Matsumoto, M., Takeuchi, O., Akira, S., Azuma, I., Hayashi, A., Toyoshima, K., and Seya, T. (2000). Maturation of human dendritic cells by cell wall skeleton of Mycobacterium bovis bacillus Calmette-Guerin: involvement of toll-like receptors. Infect Immun *68*, 6883-6890.

Vakkila, J., and Lotze, M. T. (2004). Inflammation and necrosis promote tumour growth. Nat Rev Immunol *4*, 641-648.

Valmori, D., Dutoit, V., Ayyoub, M., Rimoldi, D., Guillaume, P., Lienard, D., Lejeune, F., Cerottini, J. C., Romero, P., and Speiser, D. E. (2003). Simultaneous CD8+ T cell responses to multiple tumor antigen epitopes in a multipeptide melanoma vaccine. Cancer Immun *3*, 15.

van Maren, W. W., Jacobs, J. F., de Vries, I. J., Nierkens, S., and Adema, G. J. (2008). Toll-like receptor signalling on Tregs: to suppress or not to suppress? Immunology *124*, 445-452.

Xie, Q., Gan, L., Wang, J., Wilson, I., and Li, L. (2007). Loss of the innate immunity negative regulator IRAK-M leads to enhanced host immune defense against tumor growth. Mol Immunol *44*, 3453-3461.

Yasunaga, M., Manabe, S., Tarin, D., and Matsumura, Y. (2011). Cancer-stroma targeting therapy by cytotoxic immunoconjugate bound to the collagen 4 network in the tumor tissue. Bioconjug Chem.

Zoglmeier, C., Bauer, H., Norenberg, D., Wedekind, G., Bittner, P., Sandholzer, N., Rapp, M., Anz, D., Endres, S., and Bourquin, C. (2011). CpG blocks immunosuppression by myeloid-derived suppressor cells in tumor-bearing mice. Clin Cancer Res *17,* 1765-1775.

2

Vaccine and Cancer Therapy for Genitourinary Tumors

Robert J. Amato and Mika Stepankiw
University of Texas Health Science Center at Houston/ Memorial Hermann Cancer Center, USA

1. Introduction

Immunotherapy for human cancer has remained in the experimental stage for more than a century. This lengthy duration reflects as much the scope of failures in the area as it does the continuous and remarkable expansion of understanding of immune responses and host-tumor interaction. Immunotherapy for human cancer has largely focused on immunization with peptides or whole antigens, intact tumor cells, or dendritic cells pulsed with antigenic peptides isolated from cancers; adoptive transfer of T-cells or immunomodulatory strategies such as the use of blocking antibody to cytotoxic T-lymphocyte antigen-4.

Currently, cytokines have been described and there is much more knowledge of how the immune system functions, in particular, how cellular immune responses are generated and how peptides can be presented by class I or II molecules. This knowledge has led to the peptide approach to tumor immunotherapy. Dendritic cells have emerged and have been shown to play an essential role in generating immune responses in patients with cancer. Various other methods have also applied for the generation of cell-free vaccines. In addition, there are several methods of measuring cellular immunity—cytotoxic T-lymphocytes, T-cell proliferation, flow cytometry, ELISPOT, and major histocompatibility complex class I/class II tetramers to follow immune activation. Currently, there are two vaccines approved for genitourinary cancers (Table 1) with a few others in late stage clinical trials. This chapter reviews the development of vaccine cancer immunotherapy in genitourinary cancers.

Cancer	Drug	Interaction	Status
Renal Cell Carcinoma	Vitespen	Heat shock proteins from autologous cells	Approved by Russia in 2008, on U.S. fast track for approval
Prostate	Sipuleucel-T	Dendritic Cells	Approved in 2010
Prostate	PROSTVAC	Prostate-specific antigen	Seeking FDA approval
Bladder	OncoTice	Bacille Calmette-Guerin	Approved

Table 1. Approved Genitourinary Cancer Vaccines

2. Prostate cancer

As the most common noncutaneous malignancy to affect men and the second leading cause of cancer-related deaths in men in the United States, prostate cancer is expected to afflict approximately one in six men during their lifetime (Waeckerle-Men, Allmen, Fopp, et al., 2009). Prostatectomy and radiation therapy has been successful in approximately 80% of patients who are diagnosed to be in the early stages of prostate cancer. If a patient fails these early stage therapies or has advanced stages of prostate cancer, he undergoes hormonal therapies. Unfortunately, not all hormonal therapy is effective in eliminating malignant cells, and eventually all patients reach castration-resistant prostate cancer levels. For these patients, there are a limited number of successful treatment options, and all of these treatments are considered palliative with a median survival of less than two years (Waeckerle-Men, Allmen, Fopp, et al., 2009). The approval of docetaxel by the Food and Drug Administration in 2004 was able to extend the life expectancy of these patients by two months (Thomas-Kaskel, Zeiser, Jochim, et al., 2006). However, docetaxel is cell-cycle specific, which means that it is cytotoxic to all dividing cells and not just tumor cells. Patients who take docetaxel are likely to experience neutropenia, anemia, neuropathy, alopecia, and nail damage. Docetaxel-based therapy is not a cure as some patients fail therapy. Because of this, therapeutic strategies that offer a more favorable toxicity profile while providing more effective treatments are needed for the management of disease progression. Prostate cancer vaccines have the ability to target tumor-specific antigens while leaving healthy cells intact (Vieweg, Dannul, 2005). Currently one vaccine is approved for the treatment of prostate cancer, and a second vaccine is in the process of seeking Food and Drug Administration approval.

2.1 Peptides and proteins

One vaccine approach is to use peptides and proteins with or without adjuvant treatment to stimulate T cell activation. Many peptide and protein vaccines focus on human leukocyte antigen class I-binding prostate-specific antigens or prostate-specific membrane antigens. Often a multi-epitope, broad spectrum approach is used. Prostate-specific antigens are the most characterized antigen and thus currently the best antigen for the creation of a prostate cancer vaccine. Several trials have demonstrated prostate-specific antigen vaccines as producing an immunological response. However, the problem with prostate-specific antigen vaccines is that this antigen is a secreted protein so it is expressed on healthy cells as well as malignant cells.

Prostate stem cell antigen is expressed on more than 85% of prostate cancer specimens with these expression levels increasing with the higher Gleason scores and androgen independence (Thomas-Kaskel, Zeiser, Jochim, et al., 2006). One phase I/II study involving 12 patients receiving four vaccinations bi-weekly examined the safety of prostate stem cell antigen vaccines. No adverse reactions were observed, and six patients achieved stable disease, and median survival achieved was 22 months.

Currently, PROSTVAC is in the final stages of clinical development, seeking Food and Drug Administration approval. PROSTVAC uses a prostate-specific antigen in combination with two poxviruses and three immune enhancing molecules. One randomized, controlled, and blinded (2:1 ratio) phase II trial involving 125 patients with minimally systematic castration-resistant metastatic prostate cancer evaluated PROSTVAC for safety, progression free survival, and overall survival. No association to progression free survival was found in the patients receiving PROSTVAC, yet a strong association was found between overall survival and those patients receiving PROSTVAC (Kantoff, Schuetz, Blumenstein, et al., 2010). Research supports that peptide and protein vaccines may be a viable option for treating castration-resistant prostate cancer.

2.2 Dendritic cell vaccines

Dendritic cells have been identified as having a critical role in the induction of antitumor response as dendritic cells help present tumor-associated antigens to T lymphocytes. Researchers have become interested in dendritic cells because all class I or class II-restricted protein antigens must be processed by dendritic cells in order to activate the body's immune response (Banchereau, & Steinman, 1998) and to prime and activate CD4+ and CD8+ cells. Dendritic cell vaccines have no significant adverse reactions, and an immune response against prostate-specific membrane antigen, prostate-specific antigen, prostatic acid phosphatase, and telomerase reverse transcriptase has been found in patients receiving the vaccine. More recent dendritic cell vaccine trials have adopted a multi-epitope approach to overcome malignant cells from evading the body's immune system.

Some vaccines focus on prostatic acid phosphatase antigen, an enzyme produced by the prostate that is typically only expressed on normal and malignant prostate cells (McNeel, Dunphy, Davies, et al., 2009). Preclinical murine studies using vaccines that target prostatic acid phosphatase have demonstrated an immunological response as evidenced by CD8+ activation (Johnson, Frye, Chinnasamy, et al., 2007). One phase I/IIa trial using a prostatic acid phosphatase vaccine found an increase in prostate-specific antigen doubling time and CD4+ and CD8+ proliferation with no evidence of significant adverse events cells (McNeel, Dunphy, Davies, et al., 2009).

The only prostate cancer vaccine currently holding Food and Drug Administration approval is sipuleucel-T (Provenge), which utilizes autologous dendritic cells activated with the proteins PA2024 and prostatic acid phosphatase-linked granulocyte-macrophage colony stimulating factor. One randomized trial of sipuleucel-T studied 225 patients with castration resistant prostate cancer. Patients received three intravenous infusions approximately two weeks apart, and those who received the sipuleucel-T vaccine versus the placebo demonstrated a 33% reduction in the risk of death. Overall toxicity profile was favorable and consisted mainly of grade 1 or 2 asthenia, chills, dyspnea, headache, pyrexia, vomiting, and tremor (Higano, Schellhammer, Small, 2009).

Multi-epitope dendritic cell vaccines have been under focus as a feasible approach that may generate efficient cellular antitumor response. In a phase I/II trial, six patients received a total of six dendritic cell vaccines pulsed with prostate stem cell antigen, prostatic acid phosphatase, prostate-specific membrane antigen, and prostate-specific antigen biweekly followed by a monthly booster injection. Two patients were removed to the study due to conflicting treatments or severe pyelonephritis. In the remaining patients, three showed evidence of significant antitumor response. With no side effects, this study demonstrated that using a multi-epitope approach on a dendritic cell vaccine can elicit a broad T cell response (Waeckerle-Men, Allmen, Fopp, et al., 2009).

Another multi-epitope dendritic cell vaccine phase I/II randomized, single center trial studied 19 human leukocyte antigen-A2 positive patients. Patients received six vaccinations, and an immune response was found in eight of the patients with and improved prostate-specific antigen doubling time in four of those patients (Feyerabend, Stevanovic, Gouttefangeas, et al., 2009). A second dendritic vaccine trial focusing on human leukocyte antigen-positive patients used a dendritic cell vaccine in combination with prostate-specific antigens, prostate-specific membrane antigen, survivn, and prostein. Eight patients received four vaccinations bi-weekly demonstrated evidence of prostate-specific antigen response and CD8+ T cell activation against prostein, survivn, and prostate-specific membrane antigen with no side effects outside of local skin irritation (Fuessel, Meye, Schmitz, et al., 2006). Evidence from various research trials suggests that multi-epitope vaccines are a promising treatment option for advanced prostate cancer.

2.3 Viral-based immunotherapy

Using highly immunogenic viruses to express all of the cytotoxic proteins increases the visibility of malignant cells to the immune system, and T cells are able to target cancer-specific antigens. Finding the most beneficial tumor-associated antigens to target has been difficult for the development of effective cancer vaccines. However, by using viruses, tumor-associated antigen vaccines are able to help the immune system recognize malignant cells, which eliminates the need to isolate antigens. Virus-based vaccines deliver recombinant DNA in a mutated virus that is designed to contain the target antigen within their genome. These mutated virus vaccines have been shown to be more potent in stimulating an immune response in comparison to proteins and peptides (Pardoll, 2002).

In prostate cancer vaccines that utilize viruses for the delivery of treatment, research has focused on the use of modified vaccinia Arkara virus. TroVax is a current treatment that uses vaccinia Arkara, and it is currently in phase II trials. TroVax uses the human oncofetal antigen 5T4, which is expressed in high levels on the placenta and on a wide range of cancers (including both renal and prostate) but rarely is expressed in healthy tissues (Amato, Drur, Naylor, et al., 2008). A phase 2 trial using TroVax involved 27 patients with castration-resistant prostate cancer. Of these 27 patients, 14 were treated with TroVax alone and 13 received a combination of TroVax and granulocyte macrophage colony-stimulating factor. Of the 24 evaluable patients, all achieved a 5T4-specific antibody response. No grade 3 or 4 toxicities were observed, and minor incidences of myalgia, bone discomfort, low-grade temperature elevation, and injection site irritation were experienced by patients. TroVax was shown to be effective and safe when administered alone or in combination with granulocyte macrophage colony-stimulating factor; however, no additional benefit seemed to be achieved through the addition of granulocyte macrophage colony-stimulating factor (Amato, Drur, Naylor, et al., 2008).

One study has found that patients who previously received cancer vaccines may respond for longer to docetaxel in comparison to a historical control of patients receiving docetaxel alone (Arlen, Gulley, Parker, et al., 2006). An active multi-center trial is evaluating progression-free survival in 80 patients with metastatic castration-resistant prostate cancer receiving 10 cycles of docetaxel with or without TroVax (Oxford BioMedica & MedSource). This trial is expected to conclude in 2016.

More recently in pre-clinical murine models, a vaccine has been developed that destroys prostate cancer in by producing antigens that attack the prostate tumor cells. By inserting a healthy prostate tissue into a mutated vesicular stomatitis virus, researchers are able to stimulate T cells to attack malignant cells. Researchers found that T cells only attacked the malignant cells and left the healthy tissue unaffected, and no trace of auto-immune disease was found in the mice that received the vaccine. Clinical trials in humans for this approach are expected to begin within two years.

3. Renal cell carcinoma

Early stage renal cell carcinoma is treated with nephrectomy; however, 20-30% of patients continue to develop metastatic lesions (Godley & Taylor, 2001). Once metastatic lesions have developed, or if distant metastases are already present in nephrectomized renal cell carcinoma patients, patients' prognosis is poor with a median survival of 7 to 11 months. In patients at high risk for progression, adjuvant therapy fails to be effective, and in patients with advanced renal cell carcinoma, cytotoxic chemotherapy and radiotherapy are ineffective while interleukin-2 or interferon-alpha only elicit minimal responses (10-15% of patients) (Amato, 2000, Bukowski, 2001). The low effectiveness and high toxicity profiles associated with current therapies for advanced renal cell carcinoma creates the need for more effective, yet safer, treatment options. Vaccine development for renal cell carcinoma proves to be promising with currently one vaccine obtaining Food and Drug Administration approval to date and a few other drugs entering phase II/III trials. Current vaccine treatments for renal cell carcinoma focus on heat shock proteins, viral vector-based immunotherapy, dendritic cells, and other tumor cells in combination with lysates.

3.1 Heat shock proteins

Heat shock proteins are a set of proteins that are expressed when the cells are exposed to higher temperatures. The genes that encode heat shock proteins were inadvertently identified in fruit flies exposed to high temperatures, but these genes, and the proteins that encode them, are present in all cells in all forms of life and in a variety of intracellular locations. Heat shock proteins have two properties of interest. First, they chaperone peptides, and second, they interact with antigen presenting cells in such a manner that leads to the presentation of heat shock protein-chaperoned peptides by the major histocompatibility complex class I molecules of antigen presenting cells. This has brought researchers to the following conclusions: (1) heat shock proteins chaperoning peptides is an essential part of the mechanism through which major histocompatibility complex class I molecules are charged, (2) heat shock protein-peptide complexes, rather than intact antigens, are responsible for antigens transfer during cross-presentation or cross-priming, and (3) heat shock protein-peptide complexes provide a distinct antigenic fingerprint for specific cancer tissues, which can be utilized in the development of cancer therapies. Most research focuses on GP96 (GRP94) and calreticulin, which are found in the endoplasmic reticulum, and the cystolic proteins HSP70 and HSP90.

Human heat shock protein–peptide complexes purified from tumor cells or reconstituted in vitro have shown effectiveness in mediating antigen-specific re-presentation of heat shock protein-chaperoned peptides and subsequent stimulation of CD4+ and CD8+ T cells. The first human clinical study with autologous heat shock proteins was conducted by Janetzki et al. in 16 patients with advanced malignancies. Each patient received 25µg subcutaneous injection of tumor-derived HSPPC-96 (vitespen) once weekly for four weeks (Janetzki, Palla, Rosenhauer, et al., 2000). Blood samples recovered from patients revealed the CD8+ restrictor response against autologous tumor in six out of 12 patients whose responses could be tested. Post-vaccination stabilization of disease for three to seven months was observed in four patients. One patient with hepatocellular carcinoma was observed to have necrosis of over 50% of the tumor coincident with vaccination. Interestingly, this patient had synchronous liver metastasis of a different primary tumor that did not respond to the vaccine prepared from her primary liver tumor. No evidence of significant toxicity associated with heat shock protein vaccine administration was observed in any patient in the study. The authors concluded there were signs of clinical responses and showed that a T-cell reaction could be generated in a fraction of patients.

A phase I study evaluated renal cell carcinoma patients treated with vitespen (Amato, Murray, Wood, et al., 1999). Patients received 2.5 µg, 25 µg, or 100 µg dose of autologous tumor-derived GP96 vaccine weekly for four weeks with a follow up dose at 12 or 20 weeks if the tumors showed stabilization or regression. Of the 16 patients in the 25 µg cohort, one patient achieved complete response, three patients achieved partial response, and three patients achieved prolonged stabilization of disease (≥52 weeks). A second phase II study confirmed the results (Assikis, Dallani, Pagliaro, et al., 2003). Sixty metastatic renal cell cancer patients received 25 µg of HSPPC-96 weekly for four weeks and then biweekly until progression. A median of 18 weeks for progression free survival in combination with no serious adverse events observed makes HSPPC-96 a promising agent for disease stability.

Another study evaluated time to progression and response rate of autologous vitespen administered with or without interleukin 2 in metastatic renal cell carcinoma patients (Jonasch, Wood, Tamboli, et al., 2008). Patients received treatments weekly for four weeks after surgery followed by two injections biweekly. Of the 60 evaluable patients, two demonstrated complete response, two achieved partial response, seven achieved stable response, and 33 had disease progression. Two of the patients who were treated with the vaccine alone achieved disease stabilization when interleukin 2 was added to the treatment regimen. Most patients experienced no discernable benefit from treatment that included vitespen; however, use of vitespen in combination with immunoregulatory agents may have enhance the efficacy.

As a result of these findings, a randomized, multicenter phase III trial in renal cell carcinoma patients comparing adjuvant vaccination with vitespen was conducted (Wood, Srivastava, Bukowski, et al., 2008). After a median follow up of 1.9 years in the intent to treat population, recurrence was reported in 37.7% patients in the vaccine group and 39.8% of patients in the observation group indicating that recurrence-free survival was not significantly improved with the vaccine. Further research is now being done to explore whether vitespen improves recurrence-free survival in patients with earlier stage disease. Vitespan was approved in 2008 in Russian as an adjuvant therapy to treat renal cell carcinoma, and it's currently on the U.S. Food and Drug Administration's fast track for approval.

3.2 Viral vector-based immunotherapy

Treatment options for advanced metastatic disease, particularly in renal cancer, are highly toxic with few clinical benefits. Researchers are focusing on new options that produce therapeutic potential while providing a favorable toxicity profile. The use of viral vectors has been explored to promote an immune response against target antigens. The primary focus of viral vectors is identifying optimal tumor-associated antigens and finding a suitable delivery system. Optimal tumor-associated antigens would show minimal expression in normal tissues but homogenous, high-level expression on tumors. Additional, optimal tumor-associated antigens would not only attack tumors but also actively interfere with tumorigenesis.

MVA-5T4 represents a compelling therapeutic option for certain types of advanced disease. More than 700 doses of MVA-5T4 have been given to humans, eliciting potent, sustained immune responses in 95% of the more than 200 patients tested (Amato, Karediy, Cao, et al., 2007). All studies have shown that MVA-5T4 has been safe and well-tolerated, resulting only in minor flu-like symptoms and mild reactions at the injection site. Researchers are studying the use of MVA-5T4 on metastasized cancers that have proved unresponsive to conventional systemic cytotoxic chemotherapy.

MVA-5T4 has been assessed in conjunction with both high-dose and low-dose interleukin 2 therapy. In a high-dose study in which patients received MVA-5T4 injections at three-week intervals along with 600,000IU/kg interleukin 2 at weeks three, six, nine, and 12 (Kaufman, Taback, Sherman, et al., 2009). The results attributed a large number of adverse events to high-dose interleukin 2, but only two events (grade I fevers) to MVA-5T4, indicating that the regimen is safe and well tolerated in this population of patients. All patients developed 5T4-specific antibody responses and 13 patients had an increase in 5T4-specific T cell responses. The baseline frequency of T regulatory cells was elevated in all patients, those with stable disease showed a trend toward increased effector CD8+ T cells and a decrease in T regulatory cells. Although vaccination with MVA-5T4 did not improve the objective response rates of interleukin 2 therapy but did result in stable disease associated with an increase in the ratio of 5T4-specific effector to regulatory T cells in selected patients.

The low-dose studies further validate the efficacy of MVA-5T4 in combination with low-dose interleukin 2 and indicate that clear-cell renal cell carcinoma patients appear more likely to respond to combination therapy. To validate the efficacy of MVA-5T4 in combination with low-dose interleukin 2 in addition to determine the safety, immunological and clinical efficacy has been completed (Amato, Shingler, Naylor, et al., 2008). Twenty-five patients with metastatic renal cell carcinoma were treated with MVA-5T4 plus low-dose interleukin 2. MVA-5T4 was well-tolerated with no serious adverse events attributed to vaccination. Of 25 intent-to-treat patients, 21 (84%) mounted 5T4-specific antibody responses. Two patients showed a complete response for ≥36 months and one a partial response for 12 months. Six patients had disease stabilization from six to 21 months. Median progression free survival and overall survival were 3.37 months (range 1.50–24.76) and 12.87 months (range 1.9–≥24.76), respectively. A statistically significant relationship was detected between the magnitude of the 5T4-specific antibody responses and progression free survival and overall survival. The authors had concluded that MVA-5T4 in combination with interleukin 2 was safe and well-tolerated in all patients. The high frequency of 5T4-specific immune responses and good clinical response rate were encouraging, and support the continued testing of MVA-5T4 vaccine in renal cancer patients.

Another approach in vaccine development for metastatic renal cell carcinoma is MVA-5T4 in combination with interferon-alpha. In one trial, 28 patients with metastatic renal cell carcinoma were treated with MVA-5T4 alone and in combination with interferon-alpha for the purpose of determining safety, immunological, and clinical efficacy (Amato, Shingler, Goonedwardena, 2009). The vaccine was well-tolerated with no serious adverse events. Of the 23 evaluable patients, 22 mounted 5T4-specific antibody and/or cellular responses. One patient treated with MVA-5T4 plus interferon-alpha showed a partial response for 12 months, whereas an additional 14 patients (seven receiving MVA-5T4 plus interferon-alpha and seven receiving MVA-5T4 alone) showed periods of disease stabilization ranging from 1.73 to 9.60 months. Median progression free survival and overall survival for all intent-to-treat patients was 3.8 months (range 1–11.47) and 12.1 months (range 1–27), respectively. MVA-5T4 administered alone or in combination with interferon-alpha was well tolerated in all patients. Despite the high frequency of 5T4-specific immune responses, it is not possible to conclude that patients were receiving clinical benefit. The immunological results were encouraging and the authors warrant further investigation. An open-label phase I/II trial administered TroVax alongside interferon-alpha to 11 patients with metastatic renal cell carcinoma. Treatment was well tolerated with no serious adverse events, and all patients demonstrated 5T4-specific antibody response. Overall median time to progression was longer than interferon-alpha when administered alone (Hawkins, Macdermott, Shablak, et al., 2009).

The TroVax renal immunotherapy survival trial (TRIST) was a randomized, placebo-controlled phase III study that investigated MVA-5T4 added to first-line standard of care to evaluate survival of patients with metastatic clear-cell renal cell carcinoma . Seven hundred thirty-three patients were recruited, and received a median of eight MVA-5T4 vaccinations (Amato, Hawkins, Kaufman, et al., 2010). The standard of care consisted of interleukin 2 in 24%, interferon-alpha in 51%, and sunitinib in 25% in each treatment arm. Results demonstrated that MVA-5T4 was well-tolerated and administered alongside IL-2, IFN-a, and sunitinib. No significant differences in overall survival were observed in the two treatment arms. Exploratory analyses found patients received significant benefit from this vaccine based on certain pretreatment hematologic factors.

As a result of the TRIST trial, a surrogate for 5T4 response was constructed (immune response surrogate). Out of 733 patients, 590 were assessed for immune response. Patients with 5T4 antibody response had an associated longer survival within the MVA-5T4 treated group. The immune response surrogate was constructed and shown to be a significant predictor of treatment benefit. The derivation of the immune response surrogate initiated an exploratory, retrospective analysis, which could have important implications for the development and use of MVA-5T4 vaccine (Harrop, Shingler, McDonald, et al., 2011).

3.3 Dendritic cells

Dendritic cell vaccines are a promising option for cancer vaccine development. Dendritic cell vaccines have been evaluated in several clinical studies of patients with advanced renal cell carcinoma.

In one study by the University of Innsbruck in Austria, isolated dendritic cells and administered three consecutive monthly intravenous infusions in seven patients. Results demonstrated that the treatment was well-tolerated with moderate fever as the only side effect. Immunological response was achieved, but only one patient achieved a partial clinical response (Höltl, Rieser, Papesh, et al., 1999, Rieser, Ramoner, Holtl, et al., 2000).

A second study used a hybrid vaccine of allogeneic dendritic cells and irradiated autologous tumor cells in 17 patients with renal cell carcinoma. Patients received the vaccine by injection followed by a second injection six weeks later. Patients who demonstrated no evidence of disease progression received further booster injections every three months. The vaccine was well tolerated with mild to moderate fever and tumor pain as the only adverse events observed. After 13 months, four patients had rejected all metastatic tumor lesions, and an additional two patients demonstrated a mass reduction of more than 50% (Kugler, Stuhler, Walden, et al., 2006). Of interest, the dendritic cell hybrid vaccine induced cytotoxic T cells reactive with mucin1 tumor-associated antigen—these results need to be further confirmed in larger, randomized trials.

Tumor-associated antigens can also be applied to the surface of cell-sized microspheres and then used as an immunogen. In a phase I/II study, a vaccine consisting of tumor cell membrane protein attached to 10 million microspheres was administered to patients following palliative resection of metastatic renal cell carcinoma or melanoma (Okazaki, Mescher, Curtsinger, et al., 2002). The vaccine was given alone, in combination with cyclophosphamide, or in combination with cyclophosphamide and interleukin 2. Two doses of vaccine were administered at four-week intervals. Cyclophosphamide was given one week before the first vaccine dose in order to decrease T regulatory cells, whereas interleukin 2 was administered for one week starting five days after each vaccination in order to increase immunogenicity. The first 13 patients in the study included four with metastatic renal cell carcinoma. One patient with resected metastatic renal cell carcinoma who was treated with the vaccine plus cyclophosphamide and interleukin 2 remained free of disease at six months after therapy.

Another study used a vaccine that contained electrofused allogeneic dendritic cells and autologous tumor-derived cells in patients with metastatic renal cell carcinoma. The tumors were processed into a single-cell suspension and cryopreserved. Dendritic Cells were generated from peripheral blood mononuclear cells isolated from volunteers and cultured with granulocyte macrophage colony-stimulating factor, interleukin 4, and tumor necrosis factor-alpha. Dendritic cells were then fused to the patient-derived renal cell carcinoma with serial electrical pulses. The patients received up to three vaccinations. Twenty-four patients underwent this approach. There was no evidence of toxicity related to the vaccine. Two patients demonstrated a partial response. Forty-eight percent of the patients demonstrated an immunological response with an increase in CD4 and/or CD8+ T-cell expression. The authors concluded that this approach was feasible and tolerable. Further development is under way in combination with granulocyte macrophage colony-stimulating factor (Avigan, Vasir, George, et al., 2007).

4. Bladder cancer

Approximately 70% to 80% of patients diagnosed with bladder cancer present with superficial, noninvasive malignancies, which can often be cured. Deeply invasive malignancies can sometimes be cured by surgery, radiation therapy, or a combination that includes chemotherapy. Patients with invasive tumors confined to bladder muscles after cystectomy experience a 75% five-year progression-free survival rate. Patents with deeply invasive tumors experience a 30% to 50% 5-year survival rate following cystectomy (Quek, Stein, Nichols, et al., 2005).

4.1 Vaccine approaches

Less attention has been paid on the development of a bladder cancer vaccine. Most treatment for bladder cancer has focused on the use of Bacille Calmette-Guerin following resection. Multiple studies have established that treating bladder cancer with a complete transurethral resection or fulguration of superficial disease followed by Bacille Calmette-Guerin prophylaxis significantly reduces recurrence and prolongs disease-free progression in comparison to transurethral resection alone (Lamm, 1992). Recurrence is reduced by 7% to 65% (Krege, Giani, Meyer, et al., 1996). One study of patients with T1 lesions who were treated with Bacille Calmette-Guerin following transurethral resection found that 91% of patients were free of tumor recurrence for a mean follow up of 59 months. Sixty-nine percent of these remained free of disease after the initial therapy, and another 22% underwent an additional transurethral resection followed by Bacille Calmette-Guerin before becoming disease free (Cookson & Sarosday, 1992). Bacille Calmette-Guerin following transurethral resection has proved to be effective in treating bladder cancer.

Additional studies are currently underway to determine alternative treatments for patients who fail resection and Bacille Calmette-Guerin. In preclinical studies, a conformulation of interleukin-12 with chitosan was well tolerated and efficient at curing mice with superficial bladder cancer, and an antitumor response was generated in mice receiving this conformulation, providing complete protection against intravesical tumor rechallenge (Zaharoff, Hoffman, Hooper, et al., 2009).

Two active studies are expected to near completion within the next two years. One phase II study by Iwate Medical University is examining the use of peptides in bladder vaccinations following surgery (Iwate Medical University). The investigators are focusing on human leukocyte antigen-A*2402 restricted epitope peptides, which when stimulated were found to produce a strong interferon-g production. The study will determine feasibility, cytotoxic T cell response, CD8+ population, the change in level of regulatory T cells, and overall survival. The study is expected to conclude in November 2011. Another active study (phase I/II) is focusing on developing a vaccine for metastatic bladder cancer to induce a cellular immune response involving both CD4+ and CD8+ T cell populations (Vaxil Therapeutics Ltd.). The study will determine the feasibility and safety of administering ImMucin peptide combined with human chorionic gonadotropin-colony stimulating factor as well as the efficacy of treatment. The study is expected to conclude in September 2012.

An active study is using CDX-1307, which stimulates an immune response against a protein called human chorionic gonadotropin-beta, on patients with muscle invasive bladder cancer given before or after cystectomy (Celldex Therapeutics.). This protein, which is made by several types of cancers including bladder cancer, has been associated with shorter times to development of metastases and reduced survival in bladder cancer. The vaccine in this study is expected to cause the immune system to attack human chorionic gonadotropin-beta-producing bladder cancer cells to kill or terminate metastasis. This study is expected to conclude in October 2017.

5. Conclusion

The key to making vaccine therapy a viable option for the treatment of cancer is in identifying the subject of patients for which a specific vaccine therapy would be most beneficial. Patients who have minimal disease or are in high-risk adjuvant settings are most likely to benefit from vaccine therapy as they are least likely to increase tumor suppression of the immune system. Patients with advanced disease who are more likely to have significant tumor immune suppression will probably benefit more from the use of vaccines in combination with other forms of treatment. Additionally, the use of vaccines in combination with other forms of immunotherapy may prove to be more effective in treating genitourinary cancers. One such form of immunotherapy is sunitinib, which preliminary data has shown the potential in decreasing T regulatory cells.

Cancer vaccines are promising for the treatment of genitourinary cancers, including prostate, renal cell carcinoma, and bladder. They offer immunogenic response with a low toxicity profile, making them attractive options for patients with advanced stages of cancer. In renal cell carcinoma, heat shock protein-based vaccines have demonstrated effectiveness in earlier stage renal cell carcinoma patients, but manufacturing the vaccine is time-consuming. MVA-5T4 has high potential as a viable vaccine therapy for metastatic renal cell carcinoma, and it is well tolerated in combination with other therapies. However, more information about tumor-associated antigens for renal cell carcinoma is needed before taking the next step forward into making viral-based vaccine therapy a viable option. The TRIST trial on TroVax helped form an exploratory analysis, which has the potential to make significant advances in the development and use of MVA-5T4 vaccines.

In prostate cancer vaccines, the identification of specific tumor-associated antigens and research into related immunogenic treatments is bringing us closer to developing effective tumor-specific vaccines that are only cytotoxic to malignant cells. However, further research on the molecular and cellular mechanism that regulate antitumor immunity and the malignant process will allow for further development of vaccines using more potent prostate specific antigens and new protocols to use as vaccines alone or in combination with adjuvant therapies.

Future studies for genitourinary cancer vaccines will need to be refined by optimizing patient selection and using tumor-response criteria that are specific to trials of immunotherapy. Currently, vitespen is on a fast track for Food and Drug Administration-approval in the treatment for renal cell carcinoma vaccine with further research being conducted in advanced phase clinical trials. One prostate cancer vaccine has already been approved by the Food and Drug Administration, and two more prostate cancer vaccines (TroVax and PROSTVAC) are in advanced stage trials with PROSTVAC currently seeking Food and Drug Administration approval. No vaccine currently is approved for the treatment of bladder cancer. Further research needs to be conducted in the way of bladder cancer vaccines although bladder cancer is less common and has better prognosis using current treatment methods.

6. References

Amato RJ. (2000). Chemotherapy for renal cell carcinoma. Seminars in Oncology, Vol. 27, No. 2 (April 2000), pp. 177-86

Amato R.J., Drury N., Naylor S., Jac J., Saxena S., Cao A., Hernandez-McClain J., & Harrop R. (2008). Vaccination of prostate cancer patients with modified vaccinia Ankara delivering the tumor antigen 5t4 (TroVax). *Journal of Immunotherapy*, Vol. 31, No. 60, (August 2008), pp. 577-585.

Amato R., Hawkins R., Kaufman H., Thompson J., Tomczak P., Szczylik C., McDonald M., Eastty S., Shingler W., de Belin J., Goonewardena M., Naylor S., & Harrop R. (2010). Vaccination of Metastatic Renal Cancer Patients with MVA-5T4: A randomized, double blind, placebo-controlled phase III study. *Clinical Cancer Research*, Vol. 16, No. 22, (November 2010), pp. 5539-47

Amato R., Karediy M., Cao A., et al., (2007). Phase II trial to assess the activity of MVA 5T4 (TroVax) alone versus MVA 5T4 plus granulocyte macrophage colony-stimulating factor in patients with progressive hormone refractory prostate cancer, *Journal of Clinical Oncology*, Proceedings of the 2007 ASCO Annual Meeting, 2007;25:241s

Amato R., Murray L., Wood L., Savary C., Tomasovic S., & Reitsma D. (1999). Active specific immunotherapy in patients with renal cell carcinoma (RCC) using autologous tumor derived heat shock protein-peptide complex-96 (HSPP-96) vaccine, *Proceedings of American Society of Clinical Oncology*, 18:322a

Amato R., Shingler W., Goonedwardena M., de Belin J., Naylor S., Jac J., Willis J., Saxena S., Hernandez-McClain J., & Harrop R. (2009). Vaccination of Renal Cell Cancer Patients with Modified Vaccinia Ankara Delivering the Tumor Antigen 5T4 (TroVax) Alone or Administered in Combination with Interferon-α (IFN-α): A Phase 2 Trial, *Journal of Immunotherapy*, Vol. 32, No. 7, (September 2009), pp. 765–72

Amato R., Shingler W., Naylor S., Jac J., Willis J., Saxena S., Hernandez-McClain J., & Harrop R. (2008). Vaccination of Renal Cell Cancer Patients with Modified Vaccinia Ankara Delivering Tumor Antigen 5T4 (TroVax) Administered with Interleukin 2: A Phase II Trial, *Clinical Cancer Research*, Vol. 14, No. 22, (November 2008), pp. 7504-10

Arlen, P.M., Gulley, J.L., Parker, C., Skarupa L., Pazud M., Panicali, D., Beetham, P., Tsang K. Y., Grosenbach D.W., Feldman J., Steinberg S.M., Jones E., Chen C., Marte J., Schlow J., & Dahut W. (2006). A randomized phase II study of concurrent docetaxel plus vaccine versus vaccine alone in metastatic androgen independent prostate cancer. *Clin Cancer Research*, Vol. 12, No. 4, (February 2006), pp. 1260-1269

Assikis V.J., Dallani D., Pagliaro L., Wood, C., Perez C., Logothetis C., Papandreou C., Hawkins E.S., & Srivastava P.K. (2003). Phase II study of an autologous tumor derived heat shock protein-peptide complex vaccine (HSPPC-96) for patients with metastatic renal cell carcinoma (mRCC), Proceedings of American Society of Clinical Oncology, 2003;22:386

Avigan D.E., Vasir B., George D.J., Oh W.K., Atkins M.B., McDermott D.F., Kantoff P.W., Figlin R.A., Vasconcelles M.J., Xu Y., Kufe D., & Bukowski R.M. (2007). Phase I/II study of vaccination with electrofused allogeneic dendritic cells/autologous tumor-derived cells in patients with stage IV renal cell carcinoma, *Journal of Immunotherapy*, Vol. 30, No. 7, (October 2007), pp. 749–61

Banchereau, J., & Steinman, R.M. (1998). Dendritic cells and the control of immunity. *Nature,* Vol. 392, No. 6673, (March 1998), pp. 245-252

Bukowski RM. (2001). Cytokine therapy for metastatic renal cell carcinoma. *Seminars in Urologic Oncology,* Vol. 19, No. 2 (May 2001), pp. 148-54

Celldex Therapeutics. A phase II, open-label study of the CDX-1307 vaccine regimen as neoadjuvant and adjuvant therapy in patients with newly diagnosed muscle-invasive bladder cancer expressing hCG-β. In: ClinicalTrials.gov [Internet]. Bethesda (MD): National Library of Medicine (US). 2000- [cited July 2011]. Available from: http://clinicaltrials.gov/show/NCT01094496 NLM Identifier Number : NCT01094496.

Cookson M.S., & Sarosday M.F. (1992). Management of stage T1 superficial bladder cancer with intravesical bacillus Calmette-Guerin therapy. *The Journal of Urology,* Vol. 148, No. 3, (September 1992), pp. 797-801

Fuessel, S., Meye, A., Schmitz, M., Zastrow S., Linné C., Richter K., Löbel B., Hakenberg O.W., Hoelig K., Rieber E.P., & Wirth M.P. (2006). Vaccination of hormone-refractory prostate cancer patients with peptide cocktail-loaded dendritic cells: results of a phase I clinical trial. *Prostate,* Vol. 66, No. 8, (June 2006), pp. 811-821.

Feyerabend S., Stevanovic S., Gouttefangeas C., Wernet D., Hennenlotter J., Bedke J., Dietz K., Pascolo S., Kuczyk M., Rammensee H.G., & Stenzl A. (2009). Novel multi-peptide vaccination in HLA-A2+ hormone sensitive patients with biochemical relapse of prostate cancer. *Prostate,* Vol. 69, No. 9, (June 15), pp. 917-927.

Godley, PA., & Taylor M. (2001). Renal cell carcinoma. *Current Opinion in Oncology,* Vol. 13, No. 3 (May 2001), pp. 199-203

Harrop R., & Ryan M. (2005). Active treatment of murine tumors with a highly attenuated vaccinia virus expressing the tumor associated antigen 5T4 (TroVax) is CD4+ T cell dependent and antibody mediated, *Cancer Immunology, Immunotherapy,* Vol. 55. No. 9, (September 2005), pp. 1081–90

Harrop R., Shingler W.H., McDonald M., Treasure P., Amato R.J., Hawkins R.E., Kaufman H.L., de Belin J., Kelleher M., Goonewardena M., & Naylor S. (2006). MVA-5T4-induced immune responses are an early marker of efficacy in renal cancer patients. *Cancer Immunolology, Immunotherapy,* Vol. 60, No. 6, (June 2011), pp.829-37

Hawkins R.E., Macdermott C., Shablak A., Hamer C., Thistlethwaite F., Drury N.L., Chikoti P., Shingler W., Naylor S., & Harrop R. (2009). Vaccination of patients with metastatic renal cancer with modified vaccinia Ankara encoding the tumor antigen 5T4 (TroVax) given alongside interferon-alpha. *Journal of Immunotherapy,* Vol. 32, No. 4, (May 2009), pp.424-429

Higano C.S., Schellhammer P.F., Small E.J., Burch P.A., Nemunaitis J., Yuh L., Provost N., & Frohlich M.W. (2009). Integrated data from 2 randomized, double-blind, placebo-controlled, phase 3 trials of active cellular immunotherapy with sipuleucel-t in advanced prostate cancer. *Cancer,* DOI: 10.1002/cnrc.24429 August 15, 2009

Höltl L., Rieser C., Papesh C., Ramoner R., Herold M., Klocker H., Radmayr C., Stenzl A., Bartsch G., & Thurnher M. (1999). Cellular and humoral immune responses in patients with metastatic renal cell carcinoma after vaccination with antigen pulsed dendritic cells, *Journal of Urology,* Vol. 161, No. 3 (March 1999), pp. 777–82

Iwate Medical University. Phase II Study of Bladder Cancer Using Novel Tumor Antigens for Prevention of the Recurrence for Bladder Cancer After TUR-Bt. In: ClinicalTrials.gov [Internet]. Bethesda (MD): National Library of Medicine (US). 2000- [cited July 2011]. Available from: http://clinicaltrials.gov/ct2/show/NCT00633204 NLM Identifier Number: NCT00633204

Janetzki S., Palla D., Rosenhauer V., Lochs H., Lewis J.J., & Srivastava P.K. (2000). Immunization of cancer patients with autologous cancer-derived heat shock protein GP96 preparations: a pilot study. *International Journal of Cancer*, Vol. 88, No. 2, (October 2000), pp. 232–8

Johnson, L.E., Frye, T.P., Chinnasamy, N., Chinnasamy, D., & McNeel D.G. (2007). Plasmid DNA vaccine encoding prostatic acid phosphatase is effective in eliciting autologous antigen-specific CD8+ T cells. *Cancer Immunolology, Immunotherapy*, Vol. 56, No. 6, (June 2007), pp. 885-895

Jonasch E., Wood C., Tamboli P., Pagliaro L.C., Tu S.M., Kim J., Srivastava P., Perez C., Isakov L., & Tannir N. (2008). Vaccination of metastatic renal cell carcionma patients with autologous tumour-derived vitespen vaccin : clinical findings. *British Journal of Cancer*, Vol. 98, (March 2008), pp. 1336-1341

Kantoff, P.W., Schuetz, T.J., Blumenstein, B.A., Glode M., Bilhartz D.L., Wyand M., Manson K., Panicali D.L. Laus R., Schlom J., Dahut W.L., Arlen P.M., Gulley J.L., Godfrey W.R. (2010). Overall survival analysis of a phase II randomized controlled trial of a poxviral-based PSA-targeted immunotherapy in metastatic castration-resistant prostate cancer. *Journal of Clinical Oncology*, Vol. 28, No. 7, (March 2010), pp. 1099-1105

Kaufman H.L., Taback B., Sherman W., Kim D.W., Shingler W.H., Moroziewicz D., DeRaffele G., Mitcham J., Carroll M.W., Harrop R., Naylor S., & Kim-Schulze S. (2009). Phase II trial of Modified Vaccinia Ankara (MVA) virus expressing 5T4 and high dose Interleukin-2 (IL-2) in patients with metastatic renal cell carcinoma. *Journal of Translational Medicine.*, Vol. 7, No. 7:2, (January 2009).

Kottke, T., Errington, F., Pulido, J., Galivo, F., Thompson, J., Wongthida, P., Diaz, R.M., Chong, H., Ilett, E., Chester, J., Pandha, H., Harrington, K., Selby, P., Melcher, A., & Vile, R. (2011). Broad antigenic coverage induced by vaccination with virus-based cDNA libraries cures established tumors. *Nature Medicine*, (June 2011), DOI: 10.1038/nm.2390

Krege S., Giani G., Meyer R., Otto T., & Rubben H. (1996). A randomized multicenter trial of adjuvant therapy in superficial bladder cancer: transurethral resection plus bacillus Calmette-Guerin. *The Journal of Urology*, Vol. 156, No. 3, (September 1996), pp. 962-6

Kugler A, Stuhler G, Walden P, et al., Regression of human metastatic renal cell carcinoma after vaccination with tumor cell-dendritic cell hybrids, Nat Med, 2000;6:332–6

Lamm DL. (1992). Long-term results of intravesical therapy for superficial bladder cancer. *The Urologic Clinics of North America*, Vol. 19, No. 3., (August 1992), pp. 573–80

McNeel D.G., Dunph ,E.J., Davies J.G., Frye T.P., Johnson L.E., Staab M.J., Horvath D.L., Straus J., Alberti D., Marnocha R., Liu G., Eickhoff J.C., & Wilding G. (2009). Safety and immuniological efficacy of a DNA vaccine encoding prostatic acid phosphatase in patients with stage D0 prostate cancer. *Journal of Clinical Oncology*, Vol. 27, No. 25, (September 2009), pp. 4047-4054

Okazaki I., Mescher M., Curtsinger J., Bostrum N., Fautsch S., & Miller J. (2002). An autologous large multivalent immunogen (LMI) vaccine for the treatment of metastatic melanoma and renal cell carcinoma, *Proceedings of American Society of Clinical Oncology*, 2002;21:20a

Oxford BioMedica & MedSource. A Randomized Phase II Study to Assess the Activity of TroVax® (MVA-5T4) Plus Docetaxel Versus Docetaxel Alone in Subjects With Progressive Hormone Refractory Prostate Cancer. In: ClinicalTrials.gov [Internet]. Bethesda (MD): National Library of Medicine (US). 2000- [cited July 2011]. Available from: http://clinicaltrials.gov/ct2/show/NCT01194960 NLM Identifier Number: NCT01194960

Pardoll, D.M. (2002). Spinning molecular immunology into successful immunotherapy. *Nature Reviews. Immunology*, Vol 2, No. 4, (April 2002), pp. 227-238

Quek M.L., Stein J.P., Nichols P.W., Cai J., Miranda G., Groshen S., Daneshmand S., Skinner E.C., & Skinner D.G. (2005). Prognostic significance of lymphovascular invasion of bladder cancer treated with radical cystectomy. *Journal of Urology*, Vol. 174, No. 1 (July 2005), pp. 103-6

Rieser C., Ramoner R., Holtl L., Rogatsch H., Papesh C., Stenzl A., Bartsch G., & Thurnher M. (1999). Mature dendritic cells induce T-helper type-1-dominant immune responses in patients with metastatic renal cell carcinoma, *Urologia Internationalis*, Vol. 63, No. 3, (1999), pp. 151–9

Tamura Y., Peng P., Liu K., Daou M., & Srivastava, P.K. (1997). Immunotherapy of tumors with autologous tumor-derived heat shock protein preparations, *Science*, Vol., 278, (October 1997), pp.117–20

Thomas-Kaskel, A.K., Zeiser, R., Jochim, R., Robbel, C., Schultze-Seemann, W., Waller, C.F., Veelken, H. (2006). Vaccination of advanced prostate cancer patients with PSCA and PSA peptide-loaded dendritic cells induces DTH responses that correlate with superior overall survival. *International Journal of Cancer*, Vol. 199, No. 10, (November 2006), pp. 2428-2434.

Vaxil Therapeutics Ltd. A Novel Vaccine for the Treatment of MUC1-expressing Tumor Malignancies. In: ClinicalTrials.gov [Internet]. Bethesda (MD): National Library of Medicine (US). 2000- [cited July 2011]. Available from: http://clinicaltrials.gov/show/NCT01232712 NLM Identifier Number: NCT01232712

Vieweg J. & Dannul J. (2005). Technology insight: vaccine therapy for prostate cancer. *Nature*, Vol. 2, No. 1, (January 2005), pp. 44-51.

Waeckerle-Men Y., Allmen E.U., Fopp M., von Moos R., Böhme C., Schmid H.P., Ackermann D., Cerny T., Ludewig B., Groettrup M., & Gillessen S. (2006). Dendritic cell-based multi-epitope immunotherapy of hormone-refractory prostate carcinoma. *Cancer Immunolology, Immunotherapy*, Vol. 55, No. 12, (December 2006), pp. 1524-1533

Wood C.G., Srivastava P., Bukowski R., Lacombe L., Gorelov A.I., Gorelov S., Mulders P., Zielinski H., Hoos A., Teofilovici F., Isakov L., Flanigan R., Gupta R., & Escudier B. (2008). An adjuvant autologous therapeutic vaccine (HSPPC-96;vitespen) versus observation alone for patients at high risk of recurrence after nephrectomy for renal cell carcinoma; a multicentre, open-label, randomized phase III trial, *The Lancet*, Vol. 372, No. 9633, (July 2008), pp. 145-154

Zaharoff D.A., Hoffman B.S., Hooper H.B., Benjamin C.J., Khurana K.K., Hance K.W., Rogers C.J., Pinto P.A., Schlom J., & Greiner J.W. (2009). Intravesical immunotherapy of superficial bladder cancer with chitosan/interleukin-12. *Cancer Research*, Vol. 69, No. (July 2009), pp. 6192–6199

3

Challenges to Prostate Cancer Immunotherapy

Elena N. Klyushnenkova and Richard B. Alexander
*University of Maryland, Department of Surgery,
VA Maryland Health Care System, Baltimore, Maryland,
USA*

1. Introduction

Recent approval of Provenge (Sipuleucel-T, Dendreon Corporation, Seattle, WA) by the United States Food and Drug Administration (FDA) has stimulated a new wave of interest in prostate cancer immunotherapy. Sipuleucel-T is an autologous peripheral blood product (APC8015) comprised of partially purified antigen-presenting cells (including monocytes, dendtritic cells, B cells and T cells) loaded *in vitro* with a recombinant fusion protein PA2024, human prostatic acid phosphatase (hPAP) linked to granulocyte-macrophage colony stimulatory factor (GM-CSF) (Small et al., 2000). The conceptual development of this therapy was derived from the fundamental achievements in several different areas of life science in the past several decades. First, the discovery of dendritic cells (DCs) has led to the exploration of these cells as vaccines for cancer immunotherapy (Steinman & Cohn, 1973). Second, the pioneer studies in melanoma indicated that lineage-specific "self" differentiation antigens can be recognized by the immune system, and could be the targets for the immunotherapy (van der Bruggen et al., 2002). Finally, the technological advances in the blood products manufacturing as well as a satisfactory safety record of other cell-based therapies provided an opportunity for the smooth transition of the basic research ideas into the clinical science (ADIS R&D profile, 2006). However, the road to the approval of the first immunological therapy product was not straightforward. Significant difficulties and controversies surrounded all steps from the initial characterization of the immunogenic properties of hPAP to clinical trials and final regulatory approval of Provenge for the use in patients with asymptomatic metastatic castrate-resistant prostate cancer (mCRPC).

1.1 Provenge: Preclinical studies and clinical trials

The Provenge story has started with an early work by Peshwa et al. that demonstrated the induction of prostate tumor-specific CD8+ cytotoxic T-lymphocytes (CTL) *in vitro* using antigen-presenting cells (APC) pulsed with the synthetic peptide derived from hPAP (Peshwa et al., 1998). These data indicated that PAP-specific CTL precursors exist and could be potentially recruited to elicit an anti-tumor response. Preclinical studies in animal models demonstrated that DCs loaded with recombinant fusion protein PA2024 could induce strong cellular immune responses *in vivo,* cause tumor delay and improve survival (Valone et al., in press, as cited in (Small et al., 2000). Although very limited information about these preclinical studies is available, apparently both DCs as well as GM-CSF portion of the fusion protein were essential for the effective anti-tumor immunity, since injections of the fusion protein alone or injections of soulble PAP protein in Freund's adjuvant failed to induce cellular immune responses (Valone et al., in press, as cited in (Small et al., 2000)).

Sequential phase I/phase II trials were performed to determine the safety and efficacy of Provenge and to assess its capacity to break immune tolerance to the normal tissue antigen hPAP (Small et al., 2000). Twelve men were treated in the phase I portion with increasing doses of Provenge, and six patients received all Provenge that could be prepared from a leukapheresis product. The group was heterogeneous in terms of the disease status and previous treatment. Since PA2024 consisted of hPAP fused to the GM-CSF, T-cell and antibody responses to each of these components were examined. All patients developed immune responses to the recombinant fusion protein used to prepare Provenge, and 38% developed immune responses to hPAP. None of the patients had pre-existing T-cell responses to hPAP. Pre-existing T-cell proliferation responses to GM-CSF were observed in 57% patients, which increased after treatment with Provenge to a total 70% of patients. Overall treatment was well tolerated; most patients had no treatment-related adverse events. Three patients had a more than 50% decline in serum prostate-specific antigen (PSA) level, and another three patients had 25% to 49% decreases in PSA levels. However, no improvements in bone scans or soft tissue disease were observed (Small et al., 2000).

In another phase II study (Burch et al., 2004), 21 patients with histologically documented androgen-independent prostate carcinoma were enrolled. Two patients exhibited a transient 25-50% decrease in serum PSA levels. For one patient, serum PSA level dropped to undetectable level, and remained so for more than 4 years. The patient's retro-peritoneal and pelvic adenopathy also resolved. Most of the patients developed antibody and cellular immune responses to the PA2024 fusion protein. However, the responses to purified hPAP or GM-CSF proteins were not observed. Thus, the antigen-specific immuno-reactivity of Provenge observed in earlier studies was not confirmed in later studies.

The safety and efficacy of sipuleucel-T was evaluated in two identically designed, randomised, double-blind, placebo-controlled phase III trials conducted in men with advanced prostate cancer. In one of the studies, 127 patients with radiological evidence of metastasis, evidence of progressive disease, and an expected survival of at least 3 months were enrolled (Small et al., 2006). Time to progression (TTP) was chosen as the primary end point. Patients were randomly assigned in a 2:1 ratio to receive sipuleucel-T therapy or placebo. In the placebo group, APC were isolated from the leukapheresis product and re-infused without being pulsed with PA2024. This phase III study did not demonstrate an improvement in a primary end point (TTP) in patients treated with sipuleucel-T compared to the placebo group. The median TTP for the sipuleucel-T was 11.7 weeks compared with 10.0 weeks for placebo (p=0.052, log rank test). The study was not powered to detect survival difference between the two treatment arms, however there was a protocol-specified requirement to follow each patient for survival up to 36 months. This analysis demonstrated that patients treated with sipuleucel-T had significant improvement in overall survival. Median survival time was 25.9 months for sipuleucel-T group, and 21.4 months for placebo (p=0.01). The second phase III study revealed no statistically significant benefit in TTP in the overall group (ADIS R&D profile, 2006).

The integrated data from both studies have been recently published (Higano et al., 2009). A total of 225 patients were randomised in both studies to sipuleucel-T (n=147) or placebo (n=78). In the integrated analysis of both studies, patients randomised to sipuleucel-T demonstrated a 33% reduction in the risk of death (hazard ratio, 1.50; 95% confidence interval, 1.10-2.05; P = .011; log-rank test). The treatment effect remained strong after performing adjustments for imbalances in baseline prognostic factors, post-study treatment chemotherapy use, and non-prostate cancer-related deaths. The generally modest toxicity profile, coupled with the survival benefit, suggested a favourable risk-benefit ratio for sipuleucel-T in patients with advanced prostate cancer.

1.2 Provenge: Problems and controversy during regulatory approval

Based on the results of the phase III studies (Small et al., 2006; Higano et al., 2009), Dendreon Corporation submitted the Biologics License Application to the FDA. This decision had raised significant concerns and objections in the scientific community, mostly because the primary endpoint, TTP (for which the study was powered), has not been met, and the claim of the treatment effectiveness (overall survival) was based on the post-hoc analysis. In the opinion of one of the statisticians involved in the initial evaluation of the data, "the trials presented by the company don't provide substantial evidence of efficacy, as required by the FDA regulations. At its best, these trials provided plausibility of efficacy that would justify the conduct of a confirmatory survival trial, and the agent's benefit-to-risk profile remains unknown. The current data are inadequate to make a reliable assessment" (letter from Dr. Flemming, as cited in (Goldberg, 2007a)).

As a part of evaluation process, the application was reviewed by the Cellular, Tissue and Gene Therapies (CTGT) Advisory Committee. However, the process of the approval at the advisory meeting has been conflicting, and required clarification of the approval standards. As the initial discussion at the committee indicated that the data "failed to establish the efficacy" of Provenge, the wording of the question was altered in mid-vote asking whether the sponsor had provided "substantial evidence" of efficacy. This resulted in the vote swing for several members of the advisory panel, and the Committee voted 13 to 4 to recommend Provenge's approval (Goldberg, 2007b). The regulatory terminology for "substantial evidence" and "established efficacy" had led to the vote change by some members, although their position remained the same. For the "established efficacy", the doctor should be able to tell the patient with full confidence that this is established to be an efficacious therapy for the disease. At that time, there were no sufficient grounds for such confidence. However, there was "substantial evidence" that the treatment may work, so the efforts should be continued to evaluate it. Several members of the committee agreed that while the data did not establish efficacy of Provenge, there was substantial evidence that the drug works. There were no significant concerns about the safety of the treatment. Yet, the issue of cerebrovascular events as a potential safety signal was raised. 4.9% of sipuleucel-T-treated patients experienced a cerebrovascular event compared to 1.7% of "placebo" treated group, although the difference was not statistically significant (letter from Dr. Scher, as cited in (Goldberg, 2007b)). The panel voted Provenge was safe by an overwhelming vote of 17 to 0 (Goldberg, 2007b).

The controversy during approval process and continued objections from some members of the CTGT advisory committee as well as from the FDA Oncologic Drug Advisory

Committee (Goldberg, 2007b, 2007c) has led to the delay in the approval of Provenge by the FDA until an ongoing larger Phase III study was completed. The final approval has been granted in 2010 based on the conclusive results of the most recent double-blind, placebo-controlled, multi-center phase III trial in men with mCRPC (Kantoff et al., 2010a). In this study, 512 patients were randomly assigned in a 2:1 ratio to receive either sipuleucel-T (341 patients) or placebo (171 patients). The primary end point was overall survival, analyzed by means of a stratified Cox regression model adjusted for baseline levels of serum PSA and lactate dehydrogenase. In the sipuleucel-T group, there was a relative reduction of 22% in the risk of death as compared with the placebo group (hazard ratio, 0.78; 95% confidence interval [CI], 0.61 to 0.98; P=0.03). This reduction represented a 4.1-month improvement in median survival (25.8 months in the sipuleucel-T group vs. 21.7 months in the placebo group). The 36-month survival probability was 31.7% in the sipuleucel-T group versus 23.0% in the placebo group. While no effect on the time to disease progression was observed, the use of sipuleucel-T prolonged overall survival among men with mCRPC (Kantoff et al., 2010a).

The high level of publicity during of the process of Provenge's approval and significant efforts by public advocates, including advocate patients groups, is understandable since there are not too many options for patients with advanced mCRPC who have a limited life expectancy. Only one drug, docetaxel, has been shown to lengthen overall survival (by approximately 2–3 months) in men with mCRPC (Tannock et al., 2004). The treatment is accompanied by the toxicities so severe that many patients decline to use it at all. Relatively mild and transient toxicity of Provenge compared to the chemotherapy drugs was one of the major factors that have led to its final approval by the FDA.

While Provenge's approval certainly represents a significant achievement in the field of immunotherapy, the controversy surrounding its approval remains unresolved. Recently, the FDA issued a warning letter to Dendreon Corporation for the overstatement of efficacy and omission and minimization of risk information in some promotional materials (http://www.fda.gov/BiologicsBloodVaccines/GuidanceComplianceRegulatory Information/ComplianceActivities/Enforcement/UntitledLetters/ucm221635.htm).

The scientific discussion is also still ongoing, as several issues in the Dendreon's studies design remain disputable from the scientific point of view (Longo, 2010). In the Provenge study, the placebo group received autologous untreated APC, while the treatment group APC treated with received a fusion protein consisting of the antigen (hPAP) as well as an immunomodulatory molecule (GM-CSF). APC treated with GM-CSF alone would serve as a more appropriate placebo control. The role of an antigen-specific component (an immune response to hPAP) is completely unclear. While most of the patients developed antibody responses to the fusion protein, there was no convincing evidence of the humoral immune responses to hPAP. Moreover, the cellular immune responses were not thoroughly evaluated. The proliferation assay using a soluble fusion protein could serve as an indicator of CD4 T-cell responses, however antigen-specific CD8 T-cell responses have not been evaluated at all. While the initial scientific rationale for Provenge was based on the promising effects of the DC-based therapy, Provenge is not a DC product in a strict sense, but a partially enriched peripheral blood product that is cultured *in vitro* in the presence of recombinant GM-CSF to initiate DC differentiation. The product is released for the administration based on the increase in the proportion of cells expressing a surface marker

CD54, which is not a specific marker for DCs. CD54+ cells represent only about 10-20% of the final product, the contribution of the other cell populations and cytokines on the potential therapeutic or toxic effects is not known. While the treatment clearly had a survival benefit in men with mCRPC, Provenge group lived only an average of 4.1 months longer compared with men in the control group. No effect on PSA or any other parameter suggesting anti-tumor effect was found. The mechanism for extension of survival with this agent is unknown and may have nothing to do with an immune response. We agree with the opinion of Dr. Longo that "...the prolongation of survival without a measurable anti-tumor effect is surprising. It is hard to understand how the natural history of a cancer can be affected without some apparent measurable change in the tumor... This lack of tumor effect raises concern that the results could have been influenced by an unmeasured prognostic variable that was accidentally imbalanced in study-group assignments" (Longo, 2010).

The controversy surrounding Provenge also highlights the challenges that investigators in the field of cancer vaccines are facing in the attempt to develop an effective vaccine against prostate cancer, including the selection of target antigen and adjuvant for the vaccine development and the choice of best strategy for immunological monitoring during clinical trials. In this chapter, we will review data generated in our laboratory over a period of more than ten years, and describe our attempts to characterize CD8 T-cell responses to prostate tumor-associated antigens (TAA) and understand the role of CD4 T-cells and humoral immunity in the regulation of the anti-tumor immune response and cancer progression.

2. Evaluation of the CD8 T-cell responses to human PSA in patients with prostate cancer

Pioneering studies in melanoma clearly demonstrated that many cancer antigens were not mutated or abnormal proteins that would be logically expected to be expressed by cells with aberrant function but were, in fact, derived from normal proteins expressed by mature cells of the same lineage from which the tumor was derived (van der Bruggen et al., 2002). The first example of this phenomenon was a demonstration that the enzyme tyrosinase, which is expressed by melanocytes and is required for synthesizing melanin, is an antigen for T-cells in melanoma (Coulie et al., 1994). The link between a successful cancer immunotherapy and the induction of autoimmunity was demonstrated by the fact that the appearance of autoimmune vitiligo correlated with anti-tumor response in patients undergoing melanoma immunotherapy (Rosenberg & White, 1996). Based on melanoma studies, it was reasonable to hypothesize that a successful immunotherapy for prostate cancer could be based on the prostate-specific differentiation antigens. The idea to induce an autoimmune response against normal prostatic proteins was particularly attractive since destruction of the prostate during immunotherapy is of no apparent consequence in men after their reproductive years, as well as in prostate cancer patients who underwent a radical prostatectomy.

Several prostate differentiation antigens, including PSA, PAP and others, have been explored as targets for the prostate cancer immunotherapy (reviewed in (McNeel, 2007)). However, the first step in identifying prostate tumor antigens by studying T-cells specific for prostate tumor cells has not occurred to the extent that it did with melanoma. The identification of T-cells that specifically recognize prostate cancer cells has been hampered by two major problems. First, prostate cancer cells are difficult to grow *in vitro* especially for long periods and second, T-cells specifically recognizing prostate tumor cells have been possible to produce in culture only in rare circumstances (Haas et al., 1990). The T-cell lines can be produced but it is difficult to preserve their function and specificity for an interval long enough to allow for repeated assessments of peptide and whole antigen reactivity that are convincing. These studies have relied upon the *in vitro* cultures of peripheral blood mononuclear cells (PBMC) derived from non-vaccinated cancer patients or normal individuals of known Human Leukocyte Antigen (HLA) types. The responses in such cultures are usually marginal, and may represent fluctuations in the non-specific background or the responses to the impurities in the antigen preparations. Even when peptides show significant immunogenicity *in vitro*, the evidence that CD8 T-cells specific to these peptides could recognize target cells expressing endogenous antigens in Major Histocompatibility Complex (MHC) class I-restricted manner is rarely convincing.

2.1 PSA3 peptide for immunological monitoring and vaccination in patients with prostate cancer

Several computer-based algorithms, either allele-specific, or HLA-unrestricted have also been used to identify immunogenic epitopes (reviewed in (Hattotuwagama et al., 2007)). The major problem of this approach is the low probability that the peptide is made during natural processing and presentation by antigen-presenting cells. This problem is exacerbated by the lack of autologous target cell lines. The data generated using allogeneic partially HLA-matched targets should be interpreted with caution, as this approach is prone to producing false-positive results. In some cases, the epitopes that were selected by this method and initially believed to be naturally processed were later identified as cryptic once lymphocytes from vaccinated patients became available for the analysis.

One of such examples is an HLA-A2.1-restricted peptide $PSA_{154-163}$ (VISNDVCAQV, also known as PSA3). The peptide sequence was selected based on the computer-generated prediction algorithm, and the ability of this peptide to bind HLA-A2 molecule was initially tested in the T2 cell line-based binding assay (Correale et al., 1997). The T2 cell line [(174 x CEM.T2) is deficient in the polymorphic peptide transporter molecule, and expresses very low levels of HLA class I on the surface. An external loading of HLA class I-restricted peptides stabilizes the HLA/peptide complex on the cell surface, which is detected with HLA-specific antibodies by the shift in the immunofluorescence intensity. In the study by Correale at al., the test was performed using a single dose of the peptide (50 μg/ml) at single time point, and demonstrated a reasonably high level of binding (Correale et al., 1997). However, more detailed analysis performed later (Terasawa et al., 2002) using the same assay in a range of peptide doses clearly demonstrated that the PSA3 is a low affinity peptide, as the binding to T2 target cells dramatically decreased at the concentrations lower than 10 μg/ml. Moreover, the analysis of the stability for PSA3 peptide in the T2-based assay also revealed that the PSA3 peptide is unstable, with a half-life of less than 2 hr (Terasawa et al., 2002). PSA3-specific CD8 T-cell lines were established from non-vaccinated HLA-A2.1+ donors but required six or seven *in vitro* stimulation cycles in order to generate a measurable immune response.

Despite its low affinity and stability, PSA3 peptide is still commonly used in PSA-based vaccine clinical trials as a surrogate marker for PSA-specific CD8 T-cell responses. This choice remains highly disputable, and presents significant challenges in the interpretation of the data produced in the immunological assays. A number of recently conducted clinical trails for prostate cancer-specific vaccines reported the successful achievement of the immunological endpoints (Madan et al., 2009; Lubaroff et al., 2009). However, the detailed examination of the data raises significant concerns. One of the problems in the interpretation of the results is lack of actual "raw" data. For example, when the immune reactivity to PSA peptides is measured by interferon (IFN)-γ Enzyme-linked immunosorbent spot (ELISPOT) assay, the results are usually expressed as precursor frequencies or fold increase in precursor frequencies, which makes the interpretation of these data very difficult. In one of the recently published studies in the series of PSA-based vaccine trials, the best responding patient demonstrated PSA3A-specific precursor frequency of 1/35,294 (Gulley et al., 2010). Although no "raw" ELISPOT data were published in this report, the estimation could be made based on the available data for PBMC plating density (Gulley at al., 2002). Simple calculation shows that precursor frequency of about 1/35,000 for a given plating density of $6x10^5$ cells per well would correspond to about 17 positive spots per well. Since the data for absolute magnitude of the response compared to "no peptide" control were not presented, it is not possible to assess the validity of these measurements. Given a significant variation in the non-specific background responses in human PBMC cultures, this is in general a very low count. In our clinical studies, for example, we use very stringent criteria for the distinguishing "positive" and "negative" responses. The ELISPOT result is considered positive if the number of spots in the wells stimulated with specific peptides is 10% higher than the number of spots in the wells without peptide or irrelevant peptide with a cut-off of 20 spots (regardless of plated cell number) above background provided that the difference was statistically significant by 2-sided Student's t-test (Kouiavskaia et al., 2009b).

So far, a scrutinized analysis of the available published data from most of the clinical trials in prostate cancer does not provide a sufficient evidence that CD8 T-cell responses to the naturally processed tumor antigen were induced by the prostate cancer vaccines. In our opinion, the convincing evidence that the vaccines targeting prostatic differentiation antigens are capable of generating a meaningful T-cell-mediated immunity is currently lacking.

2.2 Vaccination with agonist peptide PSA:154-163 (155L) derived from prostate-specific antigen: A phase 2 study in patients with recurrent prostate cancer

Due to the low affinity and stability of PSA3 peptide, a search for amino acid substitutions has been performed to improve peptide binding to HLA-A2.1. A modified agonist peptide PSA:154-163(155L) (also designated PSA-3A, "A" for agonist), which represents a native PSA3 peptide with substitution of leucine at position 155, has been described (Terasawa et al., 2002). The substitution increased the affinity and stability of binding of PSA3A to HLA-A2.1. In this study, CD8 T-cell lines specific for PSA3A were generated by three cycles of *in vitro* stimulation with the peptide, and were capable of recognizing the native PSA3 peptide and lyse peptide-pulsed HLA-A2.1+ tumor target cells. The immunogenicity of PSA3A peptide was also confirmed using *HLA-A2.1* transgenic (tg) mice (Terasawa et al., 2002). The significantly improved immunogenicity of the agonist peptide in human PBMC cultures and in a "humanized" mouse model generated a sufficient level of enthusiasm for the testing this peptide in a clinical trial in patients with prostate cancer.

We have conducted a clinical trial sponsored by the NCI Cancer Therapy Evaluation Program to evaluate the peptide PSA:154-163(155L) as a vaccination strategy for the treatment of prostate cancer in HLA-A2 patients with detectable and rising serum PSA after radical prostatectomy (Clinicaltrials.gov identifier NCT00109811). The results of this study have been recently published in the *Journal of Immunotherapy* (Kouiavskaia et al., 2009a) and are discussed below. The trial was a single dose-level, Phase II pilot trial of 1 mg of PSA3A emulsified with adjuvant (Montanide ISA-51). The primary endpoint was determination of immunogenicity of the vaccine; secondary outcomes were determination of toxicity and effect on serum PSA. In our study, five patients were enrolled and completed all vaccinations. We were not able to detect PSA-3A peptide-specific responses in primary PBMC in a sensitive IFN-γ ELISPOT assay at any time point during the course of vaccination. However, three of five patients demonstrated strong IFN-γ responses, and one patient demonstrated a marginal response to the PSA3A peptide in advanced CD8 T-cell cultures derived from post-vaccination PBMC (Kouiavskaia et al., 2009a). None of the five cultures derived from the baseline PBMC responded to the peptide. These results can be considered as evidence of a successful vaccination in these patients; however, low frequencies of antigen-specific cells could not be detected by direct ELISPOT assay using unfractioned PBMC.

Functional activity of the PSA3A-specific CD8 T-cell lines was also assessed in IFN-γ and Granzyme B ELISPOT assays using various PSA-expressing HLA-A2+ target cells. While strong IFN-γ responses were detected when the PSA3A peptide was presented by HLA-A*0201-expressing HEK293 cells, none of the peptide-specific T-cell lines could recognize HEK293-A*0201 cells expressing endogenous PSA (Kouiavskaia et al., 2009a). We also failed to detect any response to the PSA-producing HLA-A2.1+ prostate adenocarcinoma cell line LNCaP. This cell line is commonly used as a model cell line in prostate cancer studies. The recognition of LNCaP cells by CD8 T-cells specific to the PSA3 or PSA3A peptides has been previously reported (Correale et al., 1997; Terasawa et al., 2002). However, we could not detect any recognition of the LNCaP cells by the PSA3A-specific CD8 T-cell cultures in a sensitive IFN-γ ELISPOT assay, although the same CD8 T-cell lines strongly responded to the stimulation with the peptide presented by other HLA-A2+ tumor cell lines used in the study. The ability of LNCaP cells to express and up-regulate HLA-A2 is highly disputable in the literature. Some studies describe LNCaP subclones that express low but detectable levels of HLA class I presumably sufficient for antigen presentation (Correale et al., 1997) . On the other hand, several studies indicated that HLA class I is under-expressed on LNCaP, rendering the cells poor at presenting antigens in the context of class I. In addition, the LNCaP cell line is unresponsive to IFN-γ treatment due to the lack of JAK1 gene expression (Dunn et al., 2005; Sanda et al., 1995). In our experiments, HLA-A2 was barely detectable on LNCaP cells by flow cytometric analysis, and could not be up-regulated by IFN-γ treatment.

To test the ability of PSA3A-specific CD8 T-cells to recognize tumor target cells expressing endogenous PSA, we have established a PSA-expressing OVCAR3 tumor cells line, and rigorously tested its ability to up-regulate HLA-A2 and process endogenous antigens. CD8 T-cell lines specific to M1 Influenza peptide demonstrated strong reactivity with influenza A virus-infected OVCAR target cells in the IFN-γ ELISPOT assay. In contrast, CD8 T-cell lines specific to PSA3A peptide demonstrated minimal response to OVCAR cells engineered to express endogenous PSA. The responses were observed only in a minority of cultures, and their magnitude was only about 10-20% of the responses against control OVCAR cells (OVCAR-ev) pulsed with PSA3A peptide (Kouiavskaia et al., 2009a). The responses from the only patient that demonstrated the reactivity (Pr159) are shown in Figure 1.

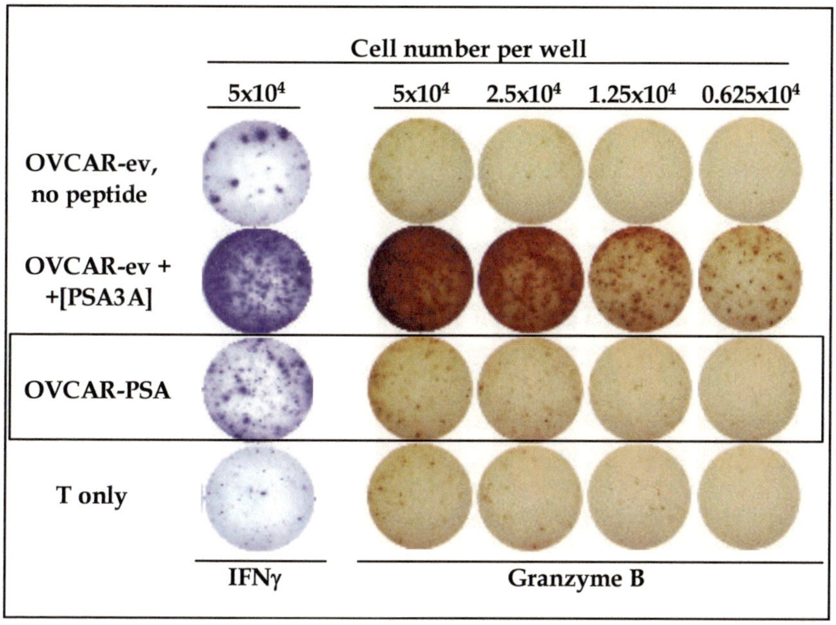

Fig. 1. Recognition of endogenous PSA by PSA3A peptide-specific CD8 T-cells. PSA3A peptide-specific CD8 T-cell line developed from patient's Pr159 PBMC was tested for the reactivity with either specific peptide (presented by OVCAR-ev cells) or PSA-expressing OVCAR tumor cells in IFN-γ (blue dots) or Granzyme B ELISPOT (red dots) assays. Representative wells of triplicates are shown.

Since we detected a weak response to PSA-expressing OVCAR tumor cells in some cultures, we established PSA3A-specific CD8 T-cell clones by limiting dilution from post-vaccination CD8 T-cell cultures of all four responding patients. However, none of the T-cell clones could recognize both the specific peptide and PSA-expressing tumor cells in the same experiment. Interestingly, on a rare occasion we observed clones that reacted with the PSA-expressing tumor cells, but were not reactive with the PSA3A peptide (Figure 2). These data suggest that low levels of reactivity to target cells expressing endogenous PSA that could be detected in some of the cultures were probably due to the non-specific reaction with allogeneic target cells and were not related to the specific anti-PSA immune response. These findings provided evidence that the native peptide, PSA3, is not effectively processed and presented by PSA-expressing tumor cells.

Recent studies in *HLA-A2 tg* mice also confirmed that the PSA3 peptide is poorly immunogenic and is not naturally processed efficiently (Lundberg et al., 2009). In this study, *HLA-A2 tg* mice were immunized with recombinant vaccinia virus encoding whole human PSA, and the CD8 T-cell reactivity with a panel of HLA-A2 restricted peptides was tested by intracellular cytokine staining for IFN-γ. Only a small proportion of CD8 T-cells were reactive against the PSA3 peptide, and the signal was detected only after extensive course of immunization. These data, as well as the findings in our clinical trial, contradict the findings by Terasawa et al. discussed above (Terasawa et al., 2002). One possible explanation of the discrepancy between two studies in *HLA-A2 tg* mice could be the difference in the mouse strains used in both studies. Lundberg et al. used HHD homozygous mice that express a

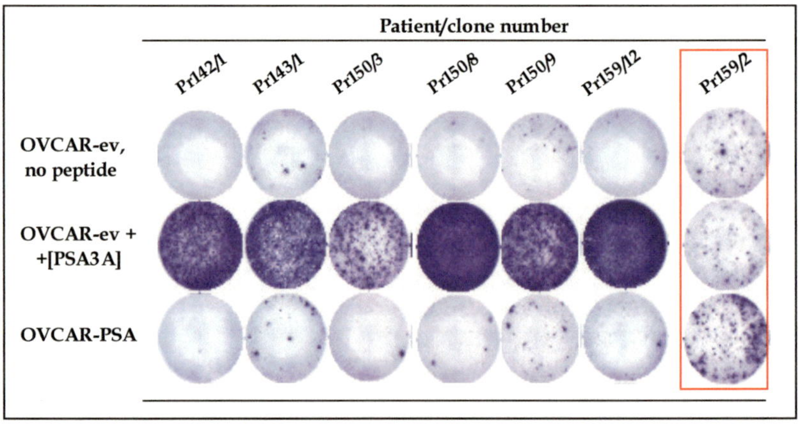

Fig. 2. Lack of recognition of endogenously-expressed PSA by PSA3A peptide-specific CD8 T-cell clones. PSA3A peptide-specific CD8 T-cell clones were developed by limiting dilution (patients Pr142, Pr143, Pr150, Pr159) and tested for reactivity with either specific peptide or PSA-expressing tumor cells in IFN-γ ELISPOT assay. Clone that responded to OVCAR-PSA but lacked peptide-specific reactivity is enclosed into red rectangle (reproduced from Kouiavskaia et al., 2009a).

*HLA-A*0201* chimeric monochain (α1 and α2 domains of *HLA-A*0201* allele and α3 intracellular domain of *H-2D*^{b} allele). The genes for both the *H-2D*^{b} and mouse *β2m* have been disrupted and therefore the HHD mice are deprived of cell surface H-2 molecules (Lundberg et al., 2009). In contrast, Terasawa et al. used different strain of mice that expressed the product of the *HLA-A2.1/K*^{b} chimeric gene as well as native H-2^b molecules (Terasawa et al., 2002). In addition, Lindberg et al. vaccinated mice with a vector encoding whole PSA, hence the responses were detected against naturally processed epitopes. In contrast, Terasawa et al. used a "reversed" approach (immunization with the synthetic peptide in adjuvant), which was appropriate for the evaluation of the peptide immunogenicity but did not address the issues of natural processing. In both studies, mice did not express human PSA as a "self" antigen, hence questions of tolerance could not be addressed in these models. Given a low affinity, low stability, poor natural processing and poor immunogenicity of the PSA3 peptide even in a "foreign" antigen setting, it is not clear why the responses to this peptide are frequently detected in human PBMC cultures.

Significant variations in the methods for the immunological monitoring, and the difficulties in the interpretation of the data generated in different laboratories clearly indicate that there is an overwhelming need for a standardized approach for the data collection and interpretation. Significant attempts have been made recently to unify and integrate immunological monitoring in cancer immunotherapy. The examples of these efforts could be the NCI-supported new initiative, Cancer Immunotherapy Trials Network (http://grants.nih.gov/grants/guide/rfa-files/RFA-CA-10-007.html), or Minimal Information About T-cell Assays ("MIATA") initiative (http://www. miataproject.org). However, these initiatives still do not address all challenges in the interpretation of the immunological data. In many cases, the responses registered in the immunological assays are objectively positive, yet their interpretation could be misleading unless other supportive assays confirm or disprove the original findings. In our clinical trial with the PSA3A peptide, for example, the bulk peptide-specific CD8 T-cell cultures from some patients did display the reactivity against PSA-expressing tumor targets, which could have been interpreted as an indicator that the PSA3 epitope is naturally processed and presented. Only through labour- and time-consuming limiting dilution analysis were we able to demonstrate that the reactivities against the peptide and against the tumor target expressing endogenous protein were clearly separated. Cloning by limiting dilution is one of the examples of the assay that currently cannot be formally standardized. However, utilizing this method in our clinical trial was critical for avoiding a misleading conclusion about potential utility of the PSA3A peptide for the prostate cancer vaccine. Careful selection of target tumor cells tested for the ability to express HLA class I molecules and process endogenous antigens was also critical.

Overall, the immunization with PSA3A peptide in Montanide ISA-51 adjuvant induced a peptide-specific CD8 T-cell response in 4 out of 5 patients. Since the responses can only be detected after CD8 T-cell enrichment and 1–2 rounds of amplification *in vitro*, the vaccine was not very immunogenic, at least in the combination with Montanide ISA-51 adjuvant. We confirmed that CD8 T-cell lines specific to the agonist peptide were capable of recognizing a native PSA3 peptide. However, peptide-specific T-cells failed to recognize HLA-A2 targets expressing endogenous PSA. We concluded that the PSA3 peptide is poorly processed from endogenous PSA and therefore represents a cryptic epitope of PSA in HLA-A2 antigen-presenting cells. There were no significant changes in serum PSA level in any subject. Based on our findings, the trial was terminated.

3. Evaluation of CD4 T-cell-mediated immune responses to prostatic antigens

Given the importance of CD4 T-cells in sustaining effective anti-tumor CTL responses, and their role as effectors mediating autoimmune responses, we studied MHC class II-restricted immune responses to prostatic antigens in patients with prostatic diseases. The identification of the antigens involved in the autoimmune processes in the prostate remains a difficult task since the proliferative responses detected in the peripheral blood of the patients in response to prostatic proteins are weak and difficult to interpret. In our previous work, we were able to establish CD4 and CD8 T-cell clones reactive with human PSA, however we were not able to convincingly establish their epitope specificity using overlapping PSA peptide library (Klyushnenkova et al., 2004). Characterization of immunogenic and naturally processed epitopes derived from human antigens can be significantly facilitated by the use of *HLA tg* mice in which mouse molecules are deleted so that immune-mediated processes are restricted exclusively by human molecules (Taneja & David, 1998).

3.1 Strain-specific differences in the immune response to human PSA in *DR2b tg* mice

The association of multiple sclerosis (MS) with *HLA-DRB1*1501* has led to the development of transgenic mice expressing this allele for the study of experimental allergic encephalomyelitis (EAE) (Madsen et al., 1999). The mice are termed *DR2b tg* in deference to the older designation of *HLA-DRB1*1501* allele. The mice express a hybrid of the $\alpha1$ and $\beta1$ sequences of human alleles *DRA1*0101* and *DRB1*1501* and the $\alpha2$ and $\beta2$ domains of mouse $IE\alpha$ and $IE\beta$, respectively to ensure efficient interaction with mouse CD4. All normal mouse Class II molecules in *DR2b tg* mice have been deleted, hence all CD4 T-cells in these mice are restricted by HLA-DRB1*1501, allowing the CD4 T-cell responses to vaccinated antigens to be studied in detail. Using these mice, we have recently identified two immunogenic epitopes derived from human PSA, $PSA_{171-190}$ and $PSA_{221-240}$. The results of this study have been published in *Clinical Cancer Research* (Klyushnenkova et al., 2005) and are briefly described in Figure 3. In these studies, we immunized *DR2b tg* mice with highly purified human PSA derived from seminal plasma in Complete Freund's Adjuvant (CFA), and screened a library of 20-mer peptides that overlapped by 10 amino acids and spanned the entire protein sequence. Using the "reverse" approach, we also confirmed that immunization with either $PSA_{171-190}$ or $PSA_{221-240}$ induced CD4 T-cell-mediated immunity against whole, naturally processed antigen (Klyushnenkova et al., 2005).

Since *DR2b tg* mice were engineered on C57BL6/J (B6) background, we also compared the immune responses to PSA protein in *DR2b tg* mice and wild type (wt) B6 mice. While *DR2b tg* mice developed a rigorous IFN-γ response to PSA, wt B6 mice developed only marginal response to whole PSA protein, and no significant reactivity was found to any of the 20-mer PSA peptides in the library (Figure 3). These data served as an initial indication that native murine *I-A^b^* allele cannot support a CD4 T-cell-mediated response to human PSA. The MHC class II-dependent strain-specific disparity in the response to PSA had significant consequences for the outcome of tumor growth in our mouse tumor model that will be discussed below in the Section 4.

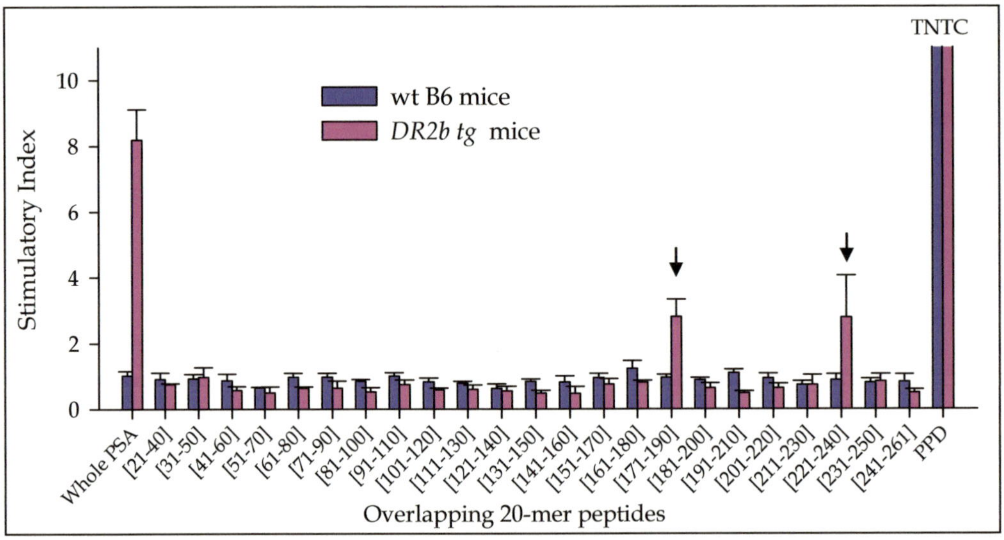

Fig. 3. CD4 T-cell-mediated responses to human PSA in mouse models. *DR2b tg* (pink bars) or wt B6 (blue bars) mice were immunized subcutaneously (s.c.) with human PSA in CFA. Spleens were harvested two weeks later, and lymphocytes were cultured in the presence of PSA protein or a series of overlapping 20-mer peptides derived from the primary amino acid sequence of human PSA. The responses to the purified protein derivate (PPD) of tuberculin served as positive controls. IFN-γ secretion was measured by ELISPOT assay. Stimulatory index was calculated by equation: [Spot number (sample)] / [Spot number (no Ag)]. Data are means ± SD of triplicates. TNTC: "too numerous to count". The 20-mer peptide sequences are published in (Klyushnenkova et al., 2005).

3.2 CD4 T-cell responses to human PAP in mouse models

While our initial efforts were focused on the characterization of the immunogenic properties of PSA, we still do not know whether PSA is an immunodominant antigen or even a particularly strong antigen. Almost exclusive expression of human PAP in normal prostate and prostate tumors makes this protein a promising candidate target for prostate cancer immunotherapy (Fong & Small, 2006). Using *DR2b tg* mice, we studied the immune reactivity to hPAP and identified two immunogenic and naturally processed epitopes within hPAP amino acid sequence. The results of this study have been published in the *Prostate* (Klyushnenkova et al., 2007) and are briefly described in Figure 4.

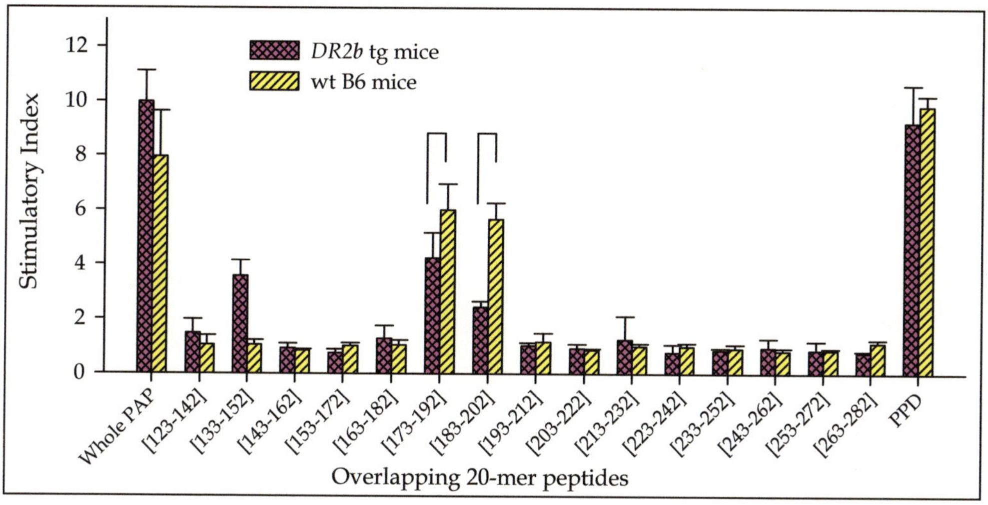

Fig. 4. CD4 T-cell-mediated responses to hPAP in mouse models. *DR2b tg* or wt B6 mice were immunized s.c. with hPAP in CFA. IFN-γ secretion was measured as described in the legend to Figure 3. The peptides from the regions PAP(33-132) and PAP(272-386) showed no significant reactivity and are omitted on the graph. The 20-mer hPAP peptide sequences were published in (Klyushnenkova et al., 2007). Brackets indicate 20-mer peptides common for *DR2b tg* and wt B6 mice.

One of the epitopes was defined by overlapping 20-mer peptides $hPAP_{123-142}$ and $hPAP_{133-152}$, and the other was defined by overlapping peptides $hPAP_{173-192}$ and $hPAP_{183-202}$. These peptides were immunogenic and naturally processed from whole PAP in *DR2b tg* mice and human CD4 T-lymphocyte cultures (Klyushnenkova et al., 2007). Since PSA-specific immunoreactivity demonstrated clear allele-specific differences, we also analyzed hPAP-specific immune responses in wt B6 mice. In contrast to PSA, which showed striking strain-specific differences in CD4 T-cell-mediated reactivity (Figure 3), both *DR2b tg* mice and wt B6 mice developed rigorous immune responses to hPAP protein (Figure 4). Screening of overlapping 20-mer hPAP peptides in wt B6 mice identified an immunodominant *I-A^b^*-restricted epitope defined by overlapping 20-mer peptides $hPAP_{173-192}$ and $hPAP_{183-202}$. This region was identical to the one defined in *DR2b tg* mice (Figure 4) although more detailed analysis would be required to demonstrate whether the anchor residues involved in binding to the I-A^b and DR2b molecule are the same.

3.3 Cross-reactivity between human and mouse PAP: Application to autoimmunity

Given a high level of homology between mouse (mPAP) and human PAP (81% on an amino acid level (Fong et al., 1997)), we examined whether immunization with peptides derived from hPAP could induce cross-reactivity to the corresponding mouse epitope. We chose a 20-mer peptide $hPAP_{173-192}$, which was an immunodominant epitope in both *DR2b tg* and wt B6 mice. As shown in Figure 5, *DR2b tg* mice immunized with $hPAP_{173-192}$ developed strong IFN-γ response to the specific human peptide as well as whole naturally processed hPAP protein, but completely lacked reactivity with a mouse homolog peptide. Similar data were obtained in wt B6 mice (data not shown). Since both $hPAP_{173-192}$ and $hPAP_{183-202}$ overlapping 20-mers showed strong reactivity during peptide library screening in both *DR2b tg* and wt B6 mice (Figure 4), the minimal reactive epitope was most likely located in the region common for these two peptides. As shown in Figure 5, mouse and human PAP differed in 4 amino acids within this overlapping region. These substitutions were sufficient to completely abrogate the response to mPAP in mice immunized with $hPAP_{173-192}$. We also could not detect an antigen-specific inflammation in the prostates of these mice. CD45+ leukocyte infiltrates were present in the prostate stroma, but were attributed to the inflammation induced by the CFA (data not shown).

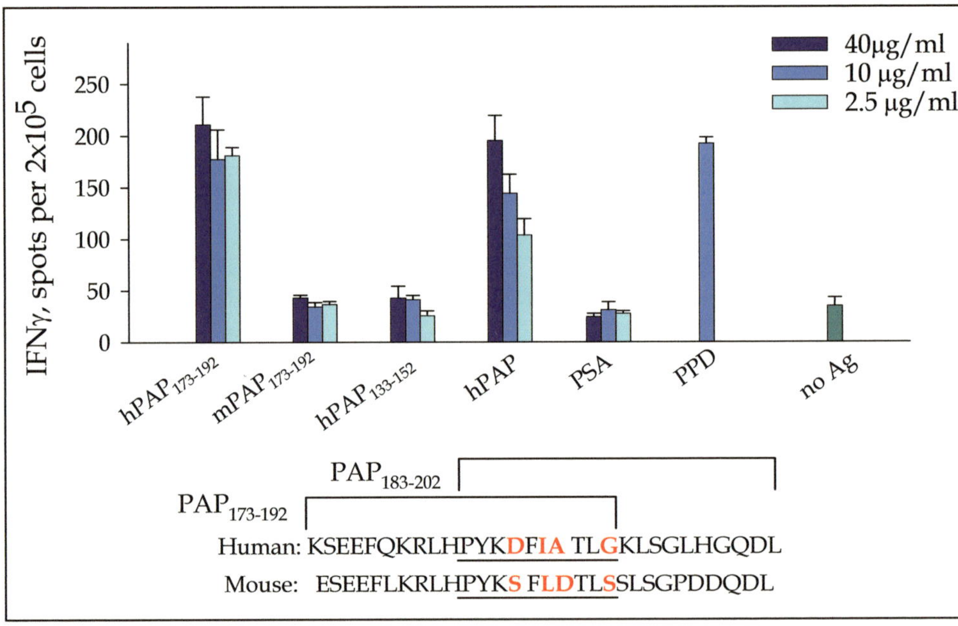

Fig. 5. Lack of cross-reactivity between human and mouse $PAP_{173-192}$ in *DR2b tg* mice. *Top: DR2b tg* mice were immunized s.c. with $hPAP_{173-192}$ peptide in CFA. Spleens were harvested two weeks later and tested for the reactivity with $hPAP_{173-192}$, $mPAP_{173-192}$, or whole soluble hPAP at indicated concentrations. The response to the $hPAP_{133-152}$ and soluble whole PSA served as negative controls; PPD served as a positive control. IFN-γ secretion was measured by ELISPOT assay. Data are means ± SD of triplicates. *Bottom:* amino acid sequences corresponding to human and mouse overlapping peptides $PAP_{171-192}$ and $PAP_{183-202}$ are shown. Overlapping 10-mer regions are underlined. Amino acids that are different between two species are shown in bold red colour.

The cross-reactivity between mouse and human PAP has been previously reported, and served as a rationale for the development of the xenoantigen-based cancer vaccine (Fong et al., 2001; Castelo-Branco et al., 2010). In these studies, wt B6 mice immunized with hPAP developed the immune response to mPAP, which was implied as an underlying mechanism for autoimmune destruction of the prostate gland epithelium in immunized mice. In our experiments, we were not able to establish a molecular basis for the cross-reactivity between human and mouse PAP for the *DR2b* chimeric transgene or the native *I-A^b* allele. Cross-reactivity between human and rodent PAP has been also demonstrated in other models. For example, Copenhagen rats (RT1^{av1} MHC haplotype) immunized with naked DNA vector encoding hPAP developed cross-reactive proliferative and CTL responses to rat PAP that were accompanied by the destructive autoimmune prostatitis (Fong et al., 1997). Similar results were obtained in Lewis rats (RT1^l MHC haplotype) (Johnson et al., 2007). Unfortunately, the molecular mechanism of such cross-reactivity has not been established in these studies. The MHC-restricted epitopes involved into the pathogenic responses in the prostate have not been identified, and the induction of autoimmunity by either immunization with such epitopes or an adoptive transfer of epitope-specific T-cells has not been demonstrated. The pathogenic activity in these models appeared to be associated with CD8 but not CD4 T-cells (Fong et al., 1997; Johnson et al., 2007). These results imply the existence of the H-2^b- and RT allele-restricted epitopes within hPAP amino acid sequence that are identical to or agonistic for the corresponding rodent PAP peptides. Once such epitopes are identified, it would serve as a definitive proof of cross-reactivity between mouse (rat) and human PAP.

3.4 Immune responses to prostatic antigens in patients with chronic prostatitis/chronic pelvic pain syndrome (CP/CPPS)

Several other rodent models of autoimmune prostatitis have been described in the literature (reviewed in (Motrich et al., 2007)), however, it is still unclear how adequate these animal models are for the study of the human disease. Chronic prostatitis/chronic pelvic pain syndrome (CP/CPPS) is a common but poorly understood condition, and is defined only by non-specific symptoms such as pelvic pain, void dysfunction, and lack of bacterial infection (Alexander & Trissel, 1996; Schaeffer et al., 2002). The presence of autoimmune inflammation in CP/CPPS has been suggested based on the cellular and humoral reactivity to the prostatic antigens detected in the peripheral blood (Alexander et al., 1997; Fong et al., 1997; Dunphy et al., 2004; Motrich et al., 2005; Kouiavskaia et al., 2009b), while the histopathological evidence of the autoimmune infiltration in the human prostate is very limited. In contrast, autoimmune prostatitis in animal models is defined based on the presence of inflammatory infiltration accompanied by pathological changes in the prostate epithelium, while the neuro-physiological mechanisms are rarely, if ever, studied.

The assumptions for the autoimmune nature of the CP/CPPS are mostly based on the similarities with other autoimmune diseases and their corresponding animal models (for example, MS and EAE, diabetes etc.) One of the important lessons learned from the rodent models of autoimmunity is the existence of "susceptible" and "resistant" MHC haplotypes. In the"classical" models of autoimmunity, it is a unique combination of an immunogenic epitope and a "susceptible" MHC (usually MHC class II) allele that triggers and governs the process of autoimmune inflammation. In a polymorphic human population, it remains unclear whether T-cells activated by a given prostatic antigen in a context of a given HLA allele are directly involved in the pathogenesis of the disease. We have previously demonstrated that men with a destructive inflammatory process in the prostate gland called granulomatous prostatitis showed the strongest recognition of PSA by the peripheral CD4 and CD8 T-cells, and that CD4 T-cell-mediated recognition occurred in the context of *HLA-DRB1*1501* (Klyushnenkova et al., 2004). In addition, an association of this disease with *HLA-DRB1*1501* in Caucasian men provided the evidence that an autoimmune recognition of a normal self prostatic protein is occurring in a human disease (Alexander et al., 2004). However, we could not establish an association with any common HLA-DR/DQ allele for patients with CP/CPPS (Kouiavskaia et al., 2009b). Some indirect evidence, for example, the presence of autoreactivity with prostatic proteins in the peripheral blood, or the presence of autoantibody response implies the existence of underlying autoimmune process, but the definitive proof is yet to be obtained. In our recent study, we have demonstrated that CD4 T-cells from patients with CP/CPPS have a higher frequency of recognition of the self prostatic proteins PAP and PSA compared to normal male blood donors (Kouiavskaia et al., 2009b). Particularly striking was the difference in the response to $hPAP_{173-192}$ peptide. This peptide has been previously identified in the context of *HLA-DRB1*1501* allele (Klyushnenkova et al., 2007), but showed a significant degree of promiscuity based on the HLA binding assay (Kouiavskaia et al., 2009b). Interestingly, there were no differences between *DR15*+ patients and normal controls in the CD4 T-cell responses to this peptide, while the responses of non-*DR15* patients differed dramatically (Kouiavskaia et al., 2009b). We can speculate that a limited response to $PAP_{173-192}$ in healthy men may be due to the higher threshold of activation for the low affinity/avidity autoreactive T-cells found in the peripheral circulation. Under some conditions, such as inflammatory processes, the lower affinity (or functional avidity) epitopes may become "visible" to the immune cells and facilitate autoimmune reactions. It is possible that the pro-inflammatory environment in CP/CPPS may be contributing to the fact that $PAP_{173-192}$ was the most discriminating peptide between cases and normal male donors. This may also explain broader HLA usage repertoire in response to $PAP_{173-192}$ in CP/CPPS patients compared to the control group. Further experiments using humanized animal models are needed to prove directly that CD4 T-cells specific to $hPAP_{173-192}$ or other antigenic peptides are essential and sufficient to induce a destructive autoimmune response in the prostate.

Since it appears that the induction of an anti-tumor immune response is, in fact, the induction of autoimmunity, many of the principles and models in the study of autoimmunity may be applicable to the field of tumor immunology, and could guide the design of immunotherapy for prostate cancer. Mice co-expressing clinically-relevant or model antigens as "self" antigens in the prostate and HLA class I and/or class II molecules on the genetic background that recapitulate features of prostate carcinogenesis in humans can serve as valuable tools to study the connection between inflammation, autoimmunity, and prostate cancer (see, for example review (Abate-Shen & Shen, 2002)).

4. Autoantibody and regulation of anti-tumor immune responses in prostate cancer

Inflammation is one of the critical factors that may contribute to prostatic carcinogenesis, and there is a considerable evidence for an association between prostate cancer development, inflammation and autoantibody generation against tumor proteins (De Marzo et al., 2007). Various genetic and environmental factors can contribute to the prostate injury, and any of these factors or their combination could lead to a break in immune tolerance and the development of an autoimmune reaction in the prostate. However the exact mechanism that would link autoimmunity and prostate cancer has not been established yet. Since the induction of anti-tumor immunity with prostate differentiation antigens (such as PSA, PAP, PSMA etc), which were logically deduced based on the analogy with melanoma-associated antigens, did not show significant clinical effect, the efforts of the research community have turned to the characterization of naturally occurring anti-tumor immune response in patients with prostate cancer and its role in tumor progression.

The humoral immune responses that occur naturally during the course of tumor development have been extensively characterized during the past decade in an attempt to develop novel, more specific and sensitive assays for early cancer diagnostics, and to identify novel target antigens for the cancer immunotherapy. For example, cancer/testis antigens, a family of molecules with normal expression restricted to male germ cells in the testis but not in adult somatic tissues, are frequently expressed in prostate cancer tumors, and antibodies to these antigens are frequently found in the peripheral circulation in patients with other epithelial cancers (Scanlan et al., 2002; Parmigiani at al., 2006). Other examples include various intracellular antigens over-expressed in prostate cancer (Sreekumar et al., 2004; Bradley et al., 2005; Wang et al., 2005; Arredouani et al., 2009). Because of their very restricted expression pattern in normal tissues and immunogenicity in different types of tumors, these molecules are also considered promising candidates for the prostate cancer immunotherapy.

The tremendous diversity of the target antigens recognized by autoantibodies in different patients represents a significant obstacle for the diagnostics and therapies based on this approach. The development of modern molecular methods including a high throughput methods for identifying personalized tumor-associated antigens would be a significant step in the future development of personalized medicine and can potentially lead to the development of biomarkers for early cancer detection or to distinguish aggressive and indolent forms of prostate cancer. Interpretation of these data in the context of patient's HLA haplotype can provide new insights in the mechanisms that govern the outcome of the anti-tumor immune response.

The list of potential candidate antigens identified by the autoantibody profiling is growing, however the physiological significance of such responses is not completely understood. Many studies in different cancer types, including prostate cancer, have demonstrated that the clinical course of cancer development can be modulated by the naturally occurring anti-tumor immune responses (Taylor et al., 2008). The most intriguing question remains whether or not the autoantibody patterns could serve as a prognostic factor to distinguish aggressive and indolent disease, or to predict the response to the therapy. Our work in *HLA tg* mouse model demonstrated the association between tumor-specific humoral immune responses and tumor progression, and clearly identified a role of "permissive" and "non-permissive" MHC class II alleles in the regulation of anti-tumor immune responses (Klyushnenkova et al., 2009).

In order to understand the role of MHC class II alleles in the development of the anti-tumor immune response we studied the effect of the *HLA-DRB1*1501* expression on the growth of the transgenic adenocarcinoma of the mouse prostate (TRAMP) -C1 tumor line engineered to express human PSA (TRAMP-PSA). The experiments were carried out in the *DR2b* x C57BL/6J (*DR2bxB6*) *F1* mice that accommodate transplantable tumors of B6 origin. In the F1 mice we found that the chimeric *DR2b* transgene was not always expressed in offspring; this allowed us to examine the influence of the MHC class II gene on the growth of the tumor in transgene positive and negative littermates. We observed unexpected and striking differences in the pattern of immunological response and the overall outcome of tumor growth in DR2b+ and DR2b- F1 mice. These results have been recently published in the *Journal Immunology*, Cutting Edge (Klyushnenkova et al., 2009) and are briefly described in Figure 6.

In our *DR2bxB6 F1* model we found that TRAMP-PSA tumors were frequently rejected by DR2b- F1 mice but grew in DR2b+ F1 littermates (Figure 6A). We hypothesized that these differences in tumorigenicity of TRAMP-PSA may be due to the differences in the CTL response to the tumor antigen (PSA). CD8 T-cells-mediated immunity was tested by IFN-γ ELISPOT assay using an immunodominant CD8 T-cell epitope PSA_{65-73}. As shown in Figure 6B, the frequencies of IFN-γ secreting cells in response to PSA_{65-73} peptide or TRAMP-PSA tumor cells were significantly higher in splenocytes from DR2b- F1 mice that rejected TRAMP-PSA cells compared to DR2b+ tumor-bearing F1 littermates. These results were confirmed using an *in vivo* CTL assay based on the fluorescent dye 5-(and 6-) carboxyfluorescein diacetate succinimidyl ester (CFSE) (Figure 6C). This suggested that the expression of the *DR2b* transgene in the mice somehow led to inhibition of the CTL responses to PSA expressed by the tumor cells. In contrast to the CD8 T-cell responses, DR2b+ F1 mice developed strong humoral immune responses to TRAMP-PSA tumors, while PSA-specific antibodies were practically absent in DR2b- F1 mice inoculated with TRAMP-PSA tumors (Figure 6D). The antibody responses in DR2b+ mice were predominantly of IgG1 sub-isotype, which immediately implied the differential CD4 T-cell responses to PSA. Indeed, immunization with soluble PSA protein in CFA, which favors CD4 T-cell-mediated immunity, demonstrated significant strain-specific differences (see Section 3, Figure 3).

Mice expressing chimeric *DR2b* transgene (parental *DR2b tg* and *DR2xB6 F1* mice with DR2b+ phenotype) developed strong immune responses to soluble PSA, and multiple CD4 T-cell epitopes were readily identified by overlapping 20-mer library screening (Figure 3). In contrast, mice lacking *DR2b* transgene (wt B6 and *DR2bxB6 F1* mice with DR2b- phenotype) failed to mount CD4 T-cell responses to PSA, and no epitopes restricted by the native $I\text{-}A^b$ allele were identified during library screening. The simple presence of *DR2b* allele was all that was required in our tumor model for the development of strong humoral immune responses to the tumor antigen (PSA), reciprocal suppression of CD8 T-cell responses and enhanced growth of the tumor.

One of the major mechanisms by which the presence of CD4 T-cell epitopes in PSA can negatively affect anti-tumor immunity may involve a classical pathway of humoral immunity. The mechanisms by which humoral immune response may affect tumor growth have been extensively investigated (reviewed in (Tan & Coussens, 2007)), and may involve antibodies/immune complexes, B cells and Th2 type cytokines. Persistent humoral immune responses can exacerbate recruitment and activation of innate immune cells in neoplastic microenvironments where they regulate tissue remodelling, pro-angiogenic and pro-survival pathways that together potentiate cancer development.

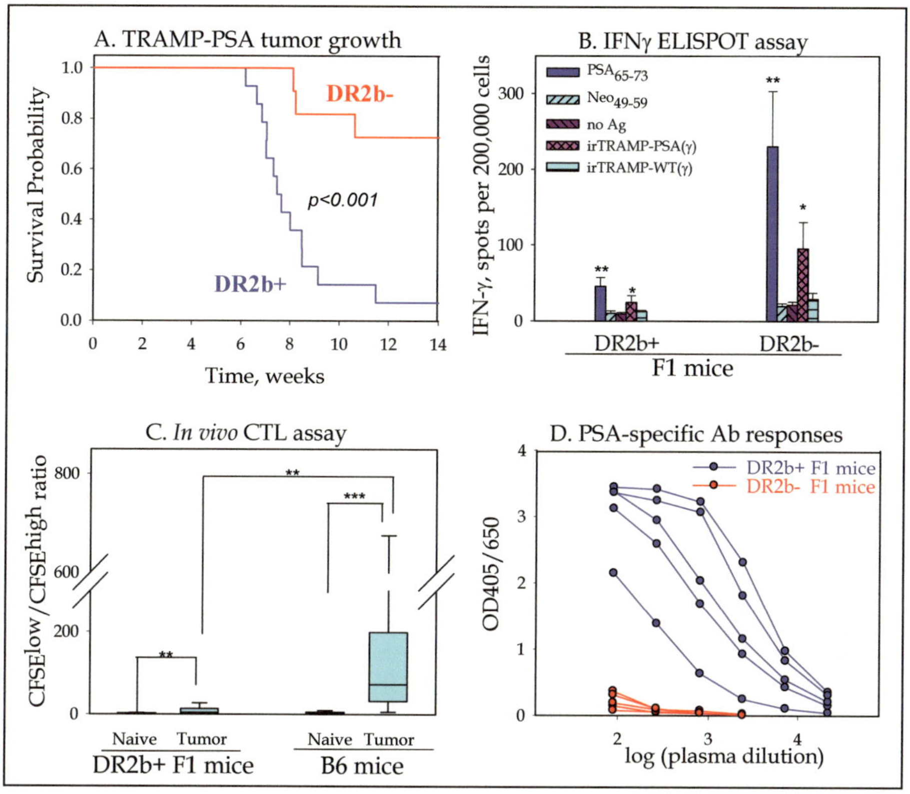

Fig. 6. Strain-specific differences in the pattern of anti-tumor immune responses in the *DR2bxB6 F1* mouse model. *DR2bxB6 F1* male mice (DR2b+ or DR2b- phenotype) were inoculated s.c. with TRAMP-PSA tumor cells. ***A.*** *TRAMP-PSA tumor growth* was monitored for up to 14 weeks. Time-to-event analysis was performed by log rank test using MedCalc software (p value is shown on the graph). Blue line: DR2b+ F1 mice; red line: DR2b- F1 mice. ***B.*** *CD8 T-cell responses to TRAM-PSA tumor cells* were measured by IFN-γ by ELISPOT assay. Splenocytes were cultured with PSA_{65-73} peptide, irrelevant NEO_{49-59} peptide, IFN-γ-treated irradiated TRAMP-PSA or parental TRAMP-C1 tumor cells (irTRAMP(γ)). Spots were counted using ImmunoSpot reader. Mice were tested individually, then means $\pm$ SE were calculated for each group (n=5). Data were analyzed by Mann-Whitney U-test (* $p<0.05$; ** $p<0.01$). ***C.*** *In vivo CTL assay.* Syngeneic splenocytes were used as target cells, and were labeled with two different doses of CFSE. $CFSE^{high}$ cells were pulsed with peptide PSA_{65-73}, and $CFSE^{low}$ cells were left untreated. An equal number of target cells were injected i.v. into either tumor-bearing or naïve mice. B6 mice were used because number of DR2b- F1 mice was not sufficient for the assay. Spleens were analyzed by flow cytometry 16 hr later for the loss of $CFSE^{high}$ population, which served as an indicator of the immunity. $CFSE^{low}/CFSE^{high}$ ratios are presented as box plots, the boundaries of the box show the 5th/95th percentile, a line within the box marks the median. Data were analyzed by Mann-Whitney U-test (** $p<0.01$; *** $p<0.001$). D. *PSA-specific antibody responses to TRAMP-PSA tumor cells* were measured by ELISA two weeks after tumor inoculation. The titration curves are shown for the individual mice (same animals as in Figure 6B). Blue circles: DR2b+ F1 mice; red circles: DR2b- F1 mice. Reproduced from (Klyushnenkova et al., 2009).

The association of the autoantibody responses and cancer outcome may not be straightforward. For example, Fossa et al. demonstrated in a small study that spontaneous serological responses against NY-ESO-1 were correlated with poor survival in mCRPC patients (Fossa et al., 2004). In contrast, several other studies demonstrated that treatment with ipilimumab, a fully human antibody against Cytotoxic T-lymphocyte-Associated protein (CTLA)-4, can induce antibody responses to NY-ESO-1, which was associated with positive clinical effect of the CTLA-4 blockade therapy (Yuan et al., 2008; Fong et al., 2009). Other studies could not find such correlation (Goff et al., 2009). It is clear that not just the presence or absence of autoantibody responses to a particular antigen, but the whole pattern of the response in the context of the cancer type, stage, treatment, as well as patients' HLA and non-HLA genes will dictate the outcome of the anti-tumor immune responses.

The other mechanism by which the presence of a CD4 T-cell epitope(s) in PSA could negatively affect anti-tumor immunity is by induction of TAA (PSA)-specific CD4+CD25+ foxp3+ regulatory T-cells (Treg) that could be selectively activated systemically or at the tumor site in an MHC class II-specific manner in $DR2b^+$ mice. Recent studies are revealing a consistent association of Treg infiltration with tumor formation and progression for many different cancers, including prostate cancer (Sfanos et al., 2008). Regardless of the potential effector mechanisms, the presence of IgG antibody is an excellent indicator of CD4 T-cell specific immune response, which occurs in the context of particular HLA class II alleles. The quality of such response (Th1, Th2, Th17, Treg etc.) depends on many factors including epitope structure of the particular antigen, the HLA haplotype and expression of other genes associated with immune response, the origin of the tumor, and the microenvironment.

Based on our observations in the *DR2b* transgenic mouse model of prostate cancer, we hypothesize that the presence of naturally occurring antibody responses to tumor antigen(s) in advanced prostate cancer is an indicator of an immune response that is ineffective at rejecting the tumor. We hypothesize that, in human malignancies, the diversity of available HLA class II haplotypes in the human population may govern the polarization of anti-tumor immune response. In the polymorphic human population, many tumors may contain antigens that are presented by the patient's HLA class II alleles in this fashion and affect the ability of the host to mount an effective response against the tumor. Our current goal is to identify tumor antigens specific to prostate cancer that can differentially induce CD4 T-cell response in HLA class II allele-specific manner, and to demonstrate the correlation between the expression of "permissive" and "non-permissive" HLA class II alleles, and the magnitude of tumor-specific humoral and cellular immune responses in patients with prostate cancer.

5. Conclusions

An effective immunotherapy against prostate cancer remains a dream. The most successful vaccines against bacterial and viral pathogens are based on the ability to induce strong CTL responses as well as neutralizing antibody responses. For certain categories of diseases, including cancer, this conventional approach does not seem to be effective. The role of humoral responses in anti-tumor immunity is a particularly controversial and highly debated topic. The development of a polarized immune response to the tumor during a natural course of the disease represents a unique challenge for the therapeutic vaccines (such as cancer vaccines) compared to the preventive vaccines against infectious diseases.

The major challenge is not only to induce a strong effector immune response against the tumor, but to simultaneously re-direct already ongoing immune response, which was mounted as a part of the natural course of the disease and already went in the "wrong" direction. Learning to harness the cellular arm of the immune response of proper specificity, diversity, magnitude, function and homing properties is a challenging task that requires significant efforts. Rational antigen design, advanced antigen delivery and adjuvant platforms in combination with the strategies directed toward neutralizing immune suppression hold a new promise for prostate cancer immunotherapy. As new potential target antigens emerge as a result of a next generation screening, their careful validation by "direct" and "reverse" immunology in human lymphocyte cultures and HLA transgenic mice remains an important task. Clinical samples from the patients that underwent treatment with Provenge and other experimental immunotherapies may provide critical clues in the efforts to create an effective treatment for prostate cancer and other epithelial cancers.

6. Acknowledgements

The work described in this chapter has been supported by grants from the National Institutes of Health/ National Institute of Diabetes, Digestive and Kidney Diseases, National Cancer Institute, and the US Department of Veterans Affairs to Richard B. Alexander; and the Institutional Research Grant from the American Cancer Society and intramural research grants from the University of Maryland Greenebaum Cancer Center and Baltimore Research and Education Foundation to Elena N. Klyushnenkova.

7. References

Abate-Shen, C. & Shen, M. M. 2002. Mouse models of prostate carcinogenesis. *Trends in Genetics*, 18(5): S1-S5.

ADIS R&D profile 2006. Sipuleucel-T: APC 8015, APC-8015, prostate cancer vaccine--Dendreon. *Drugs in R&D*, 7(3): 197-201.

Alexander, R. B., Brady, F., & Ponniah, S. 1997. Autoimmune prostatitis: Evidence of T cell reactivity with normal prostatic proteins. *Urology*, 50: 893-899.

Alexander, R. B., Mann, D. L., Borkowski, A. A., Fernandez-Vina, M., Klyushnenkova, E. N., Kodak, J., Propert, K. J., & Kincaid, M. 2004. Granulomatous prostatitis linked to HLA-DRB1*1501. *Journal of Urology*, 171(6 Pt 1): 2326-2329.

Alexander, R. B. & Trissel, D. 1996. Chronic prostatitis: Results of an internet survey. *Urology*, 48: 568-574.

Arredouani, M. S., Lu, B., Bhasin, M., Eljanne, M., Yue, W., Mosquera, J. M., Bubley, G. J., Li, V., Rubin, M. A., Libermann, T. A., & Sanda, M. G. 2009. Identification of the transcription factor single-minded homologue 2 as a potential biomarker and immunotherapy target in prostate cancer. *Clinical Cancer Research*, 15(18): 5794-5802.

Bradley, S. V., Oravecz-Wilson, K. I., Bougeard, G., Mizukami, I., Li, L., Munaco, A. J., Sreekumar, A., Corradetti, M. N., Chinnaiyan, A. M., Sanda, M. G., & Ross, T. S. 2005. Serum antibodies to huntingtin interacting protein-1: a new blood test for prostate cancer. *Cancer Research*, 65(10): 4126-4133.

Burch, P. A., Breen, J. K., Buckner, J. C., Gastineau, D. A., Kaur, J. A., Laus, R. L., Padley, D. J., Peshwa, M. V., Pitot, H. C., Richardson, R. L., Smits, B. J., Sopapan, P., Strang, G.,

Valone, F. H., & Vuk-Pavlovic, S. 2000. Priming Tissue-specific Cellular Immunity in a Phase I Trial of Autologous Dendritic Cells for Prostate Cancer. *Clinical Cancer Research*, 6(6): 2175-2182.

Burch, P. A., Croghan, G. A., Gastineau, D. A., Jones, L. A., Kaur, J. S., Kylstra, J. W., Richardson, R. L., Valone, F. H., & Vuk-Pavlovic, S. 2004. Immunotherapy (APC8015, Provenge) targeting prostatic acid phosphatase can induce durable remission of metastatic androgen-independent prostate cancer: a Phase 2 trial. *Prostate*, 60(3): 197-204.

Castelo-Branco, P., Passer, B. J., Buhrman, J. S., Antoszczyk, S., Marinelli, M., Zaupa, C., Rabkin, S. D., & Martuza, R. L. 2010. Oncolytic herpes simplex virus armed with xenogeneic homologue of prostatic acid phosphatase enhances antitumor efficacy in prostate cancer. . *Gene Therapy*, 17(6): 805-810.

Chen, Y. T., Scanlan, M. J., Sahin, U., Tureci, O., Gure, A. O., Tsang, S., Williamson, B., Stockert, E., Pfreundschuh, M., & Old, L. J. 1997. A testicular antigen aberrantly expressed in human cancers detected by autologous antibody screening. *Proceedings of the National Academy of Sciences of the United States of America*, 94(5): 1914-1918.

Correale, P., Walmsley, K., Nieroda, C., Zaremba, S., Zhu, M. Z., Schlom, J., & Tsang, K. Y. 1997. In vitro generation of human cytotoxic T lymphocytes specific for peptides derived from prostate-specific antigen. *Journal of the National Cancer Institute*, 89(4): 293-300.

Coulie, P. G., Brichard, V., Van Pel, A., Wolfel, T., Schneider, J., Traversari, C., Mattei, S., De Plaen, E., Lurquin, C., Szikora, J. P., Renauld, J. C., & Boon, T. 1994. A new gene coding for a differentiation antigen recognized by autologous cytolytic T lymphocytes on HLA-A2 melanomas. *Journal of Experimental Medicine*, 180(7): 35-42.

De Marzo, A. M., Platz, E. A., Sutcliffe, S., Xu, J., Gronberg, H., Drake, C. G., Nakai, Y., Isaacs, W. B., & Nelson, W. G. 2007. Inflammation in prostate carcinogenesis. *Nature Reviews Cancer*, 7(4): 256-269.

Dunn, G. P., Sheehan, K. C., Old, L. J., & Schreiber, R. D. 2005. IFN unresponsiveness in LNCaP cells due to the lack of JAK1 gene expression. *Cancer Research*, 65(8): 3447-3453.

Dunphy, E. J., Eickhoff, J. C., Muller, C. H., Berger, R. E., & McNeel, D. G. 2004. Identification of antigen-specific IgG in sera from patients with chronic prostatitis. *Journal of Clinical Immunology*, 24(5): 492-502.

Fong, L., Brockstedt, D., Benike, C., Breen, J. K., Strang, G., Ruegg, C. L., & Engleman, E. G. 2001. Dendritic cell-based xenoantigen vaccination for prostate cancer immunotherapy. *Journal of Immunology*, 167(12): 7150-7156.

Fong, L., Kwek, S. S., O'Brien, S., Kavanagh, B., McNeel, D. G., Weinberg, V., Lin, A. M., Rosenberg, J., Ryan, C. J., Rini, B. I., & Small, E. J. 2009. Potentiating endogenous antitumor immunity to prostate cancer through combination immunotherapy with CTLA4 blockade and GM-CSF. *Cancer Research*, 69(2): 609-615.

Fong, L., Ruegg, C. L., Brockstedt, D., Engleman, E. G., & Laus, R. 1997. Induction of tissue-specific autoimmune prostatitis with prostatic acid phosphatase immunization: implications for immunotherapy of prostate cancer. *Journal of Immunology*, 159(7): 3113-3117.

Fong, L. & Small, E. J. 2006. Immunotherapy for prostate cancer. *Current Urology Reports*, 7(3): 239-246.

Fossa, A., Berner, A., Fossa, S. D., Hernes, E., Gaudernack, G., & Smeland, E. B. 2004. NY-ESO-1 protein expression and humoral immune responses in prostate cancer. *Prostate*, 59(4): 440-447.

Goff, S. L., Robbins, P. F., el-Gamil, M., & Rosenberg, S. A. 2009. No correlation between clinical response to CTLA-4 blockade and presence of NY-ESO-1 antibody in patients with metastatic melanoma. *Journal of Immunotherapy*, 32(8): 884-885.

Goldberg, P. Biostatistician Thomas Fleming Warns Against Approval of Provenge. 2007a. *The Cancer Letter*, 33(17): 1-7.

Goldberg, P. Advisors voted for Provenge approval despite fundamental flaws in trials. 2007b. *The Cancer Letter*, 33(14): 1-7.

Goldberg, P. Dear FDA: Provenge provokes letters from opponents, advocates, investors. 2007c. *The Cancer Letter*, 33(16): 1-7.

Gulley, J., Chen, A. P., Dahut, W., Arlen, P. M., Bastian, A., Steinberg, S. M., Tsang, K., Panicali, D., Poole, D., Schlom, J., & Michael, H. J. 2002. Phase I study of a vaccine using recombinant vaccinia virus expressing PSA (rV-PSA) in patients with metastatic androgen-independent prostate cancer. *Prostate*, 53(2): 109-117.

Gulley, J. L., Arlen, P. M., Madan, R. A., Tsang, K. Y., Pazdur, M. P., Skarupa, L., Jones, J. L., Poole, D. J., Higgins, J. P., Hodge, J. W., Cereda, V., Vergati, M., Steinberg, S. M., Halabi, S., Jones, E., Chen, C., Parnes, H., Wright, J. J., Dahut, W. L., & Schlom, J. 2010. Immunologic and prognostic factors associated with overall survival employing a poxviral-based PSA vaccine in metastatic castrate-resistant prostate cancer. *Cancer Immunology, Immunotherapy*, 59(5): 663-674.

Haas, G. P., Solomon, D., & Rosenberg, S. A. 1990. Tumor-infiltrating lymphocytes from nonrenal urological malignancies. *Cancer Immunology, Immunotherapy*, 30(6): 342-350.

Hattotuwagama, C. K., Doytchinova, I. A., & Flower, D. R. 2007. Toward the prediction of class I and II mouse major histocompatibility complex-peptide-binding affinity: in silico bioinformatic step-by-step guide using quantitative structure-activity relationships. *Methods in Molecular Biology*, 409: 227-245.

Higano, C. S., Schellhammer, P. F., Small, E. J., Burch, P. A., Nemunaitis, J., Yuh, L., Provost, N., & Frohlich, M. W. 2009. Integrated data from 2 randomized, double-blind, placebo-controlled, phase 3 trials of active cellular immunotherapy with sipuleucel-T in advanced prostate cancer. *Cancer*, 115(16): 3670-3679.

Johnson, L. E., Frye, T. P., Chinnasamy, N., Chinnasamy, D., & McNeel, D. G. 2007. Plasmid DNA vaccine encoding prostatic acid phosphatase is effective in eliciting autologous antigen-specific CD8+ T cells. *Cancer Immunology, Immunotherapy*, 56(6): 885-895.

Kantoff, P. W., Higano, C. S., Shore, N. D., Berger, E. R., Small, E. J., Penson, D. F., Redfern, C. H., Ferrari, A. C., Dreicer, R., Sims, R. B., Xu, Y., Frohlich, M. W., & Schellhammer, P. F. 2010a. Sipuleucel-T immunotherapy for castration-resistant prostate cancer. *New England Journal of Medicine*, 363(5): 411-422.

Kantoff, P. W., Schuetz, T. J., Blumenstein, B. A., Glode, L. M., Bilhartz, D. L., Wyand, M., Manson, K., Panicali, D. L., Laus, R., Schlom, J., Dahut, W. L., Arlen, P. M., Gulley, J. L., & Godfrey, W. R. 2010b. Overall survival analysis of a phase II randomized controlled trial of a Poxviral-based PSA-targeted immunotherapy in metastatic castration-resistant prostate cancer. *Journal of Clinical Oncology*, 28(7): 1099-1105.

Klyushnenkova, E. N., Kouiavskaia, D. V., Berard, C. A., & Alexander, R. B. 2009. Cutting edge: Permissive MHC class II allele changes the pattern of antitumor immune response resulting in failure of tumor rejection. *Journal of Immunology*, 182(3): 1242-1246.

Klyushnenkova, E. N., Kouiavskaia, D. V., Kodak, J. A., Vandenbark, A. A., & Alexander, R. B. 2007. Identification of HLA-DRB1*1501-restricted T-cell epitopes from human prostatic acid phosphatase. *Prostate*, 67(10): 1019-1028.

Klyushnenkova, E. N., Link, J., Oberle, W. T., Kodak, J., Rich, C., Vandenbark, A. A., & Alexander, R. B. 2005. Identification of HLA-DRB1*1501-restricted T-cell epitopes from prostate-specific antigen. *Clinical Cancer Research*, 11(8): 2853-2861.

Klyushnenkova, E. N., Ponniah, S., Rodriguez, A., Kodak, J., Mann, D. L., Langerman, A., Nishimura, M. I., & Alexander, R. B. 2004. CD4 and CD8 T-lymphocyte recognition of prostate specific antigen in granulomatous prostatitis. *Journal of Immunotherapy*, 27(2): 136-146.

Kouiavskaia, D. V., Berard, C. A., Datena, E., Hussain, A., Dawson, N., Klyushnenkova, E. N., & Alexander, R. B. 2009a. Vaccination With Agonist Peptide PSA: 154-163 (155L) Derived From Prostate Specific Antigen Induced CD8 T-Cell Response to the Native Peptide PSA: 154-163 But Failed to Induce the Reactivity Against Tumor Targets Expressing PSA: A Phase 2 Study in Patients With Recurrent Prostate Cancer. *Journal of Immunotherapy*, 32(6): 655-666.

Kouiavskaia, D. V., Southwood, S., Berard, C. A., Klyushnenkova, E. N., & Alexander, R. B. 2009b. T-cell recognition of prostatic peptides in men with chronic prostatitis/chronic pelvic pain syndrome. *Journal of Urology*, 182(5): 2483-2489.

Longo, D. L. 2010. New therapies for castration-resistant prostate cancer. *New England Journal of Medicine*, 363(5): 479-481.

Lubaroff, D. M., Konety, B. R., Link, B., Gerstbrein, J., Madsen, T., Shannon, M., Howard, J., Paisley, J., Boeglin, D., Ratliff, T. L., & Williams, R. D. 2009. Phase I clinical trial of an adenovirus/prostate-specific antigen vaccine for prostate cancer: safety and immunologic results. *Clinical Cancer Research*, 15(23): 7375-7380.

Lundberg, K., Roos, A. K., Pavlenko, M., Leder, C., Wehrum, D., Guevara-Patino, J., Andersen, R. S., & Pisa, P. 2009. A modified epitope identified for generation and monitoring of PSA-specific T cells in patients on early phases of PSA-based immunotherapeutic protocols. *Vaccine*, 27(10): 1557-1565.

Madan, R. A., Arlen, P. M., Mohebtash, M., Hodge, J. W., & Gulley, J. L. 2009. Prostvac-VF: a vector-based vaccine targeting PSA in prostate cancer. *Expert Opinion on Investigational Drugs*, 18(7): 1001-1011.

Madsen, L. S., Andersson, E. C., Jansson, L., krogsgaard, M., Andersen, C. B., Engberg, J., Strominger, J. L., Svejgaard, A., Hjorth, J. P., Holmdahl, R., Wucherpfennig, K. W., & Fugger, L. 1999b. A humanized model for multiple sclerosis using HLA-DR2 and a human T-cell receptor. *Nature Genetics*, 23(3): 343-347.

McNeel, D. G. 2007. Prostate cancer immunotherapy. *Current Opinion in Urology*, 17(3): 175-181.

Motrich, R. D., Maccioni, M., Molina, R., Tissera, A., Olmedo, J., Riera, C. M., & Rivero, V. E. 2005. Presence of INFgamma-secreting lymphocytes specific to prostate antigens in a group of chronic prostatitis patients. *Clinical Immunology*, 116(2): 149-157.

Motrich, R. D., Maccioni, M., Riera, C. M., & Rivero, V. E. 2007. Autoimmune prostatitis: state of the art. *Scandinavian Journal of Immunology*, 66(2-3): 217-227.

Parmigiani, R. B., Bettoni, F., Vibranovski, M. D., Lopes, M. H., Martins, W. K., Cunha, I. W., Soares, F. A., Simpson, A. J., de Souza, S. J., & Camargo, A. A. 2006. Characterization of a cancer/testis (CT) antigen gene family capable of eliciting humoral response in cancer patients. *Proceedings of the National Academy of Sciences of the United States of America*, 103(48): 18066-18071.

Peshwa, M. V., Shi, J. D., Ruegg, C., Laus, R., & van Schooten, W. C. 1998. Induction of prostate tumor-specific CD8+ cytotoxic T-lymphocytes in vitro using antigen-presenting cells pulsed with prostatic acid phosphatase peptide. *Prostate*, 36(2): 129-138.

Rosenberg, S. A. & White, D. E. 1996. Vitiligo in patients with melanoma: normal tissue antigens can be targets for cancer immunotherapy. *Journal of Immunotherapy*, 19(1): 81-84.

Sanda, M. G., Restifo, N. P., Walsh, J. C., Kawakami, Y., Nelson, W. G., Pardoll, D. M., & Simons, J. W. 1995. Molecular characterization of defective antigen processing in human prostate cancer. *Journal of the National Cancer Institute*, 87(4): 280-285.

Scanlan, M. J., Gure, A. O., Jungbluth, A. A., Old, L. J., & Chen, Y. T. 2002. Cancer/testis antigens: an expanding family of targets for cancer immunotherapy. *Immunological Reviews*, 188: 22-32.

Schaeffer, A. J., Landis, J. R., Knauss, J. S., Propert, K. J., Alexander, R. B., Litwin, M. S., Nickel, J. C., O'Leary, M. P., Nadler, R. B., Pontari, M. A., Shoskes, D. A., Zeitlin, S. I., Fowler, J. E., Jr., Mazurick, C. A., Kishel, L., Kusek, J. W., & Nyberg, L. M. 2002. Demographic and clinical characteristics of men with chronic prostatitis: the national institutes of health chronic prostatitis cohort study. *Journal of Urology*, 168(2): 593-598.

Sfanos, K. S., Bruno, T. C., Maris, C. H., Xu, L., Thoburn, C. J., DeMarzo, A. M., Meeker, A. K., Isaacs, W. B., & Drake, C. G. 2008. Phenotypic analysis of prostate-infiltrating lymphocytes reveals TH17 and Treg skewing. *Clinical Cancer Research*, 14(11): 3254-3261.

Small, E. J., Fratesi, P., Reese, D. M., Strang, G., Laus, R., Peshwa, M. V., & Valone, F. H. 2000. Immunotherapy of Hormone-Refractory Prostate Cancer With Antigen-Loaded Dendritic Cells. *Journal of Clinical Oncology*, 18(23): 3894-3903.

Small, E. J., Schellhammer, P. F., Higano, C. S., Redfern, C. H., Nemunaitis, J. J., Valone, F. H., Verjee, S. S., Jones, L. A., & Hershberg, R. M. 2006. Placebo-controlled phase III trial of immunologic therapy with sipuleucel-T (APC8015) in patients with metastatic, asymptomatic hormone refractory prostate cancer. *Journal of Clinical Oncology*, 24(19): 3089-3094.

Sreekumar, A., Laxman, B., Rhodes, D. R., Bhagavathula, S., Harwood, J., Giacherio, D., Ghosh, D., Sanda, M. G., Rubin, M. A., & Chinnaiyan, A. M. 2004. Humoral immune response to alpha-methylacyl-CoA racemase and prostate cancer. *Journal of the National Cancer Institute*, 96(11): 834-843.

Steinman, R. M. & Cohn, Z. A. 1973. Identification of a novel cell type in peripheral lymphoid organs of mice. I. Morphology, quantitation, tissue distribution. *Journal of Experimental Medicine,* 137(5): 1142-1162.

Tan, T. T. & Coussens, L. M. 2007. Humoral immunity, inflammation and cancer. *Current Opinion in Immunology,* 19(2): 209-216.

Taneja, V. & David, C. S. 1998. HLA transgenic mice as humanized mouse models of disease and immunity. *Journal of Clinical Investigation,* 101(5): 921-926.

Tannock, I. F., de, W. R., Berry, W. R., Horti, J., Pluzanska, A., Chi, K. N., Oudard, S., Theodore, C., James, N. D., Turesson, I., Rosenthal, M. A., & Eisenberger, M. A. 2004. Docetaxel plus prednisone or mitoxantrone plus prednisone for advanced prostate cancer. *New England Journal of Medicine,* 351(15): 1502-1512.

Taylor, B. S., Pal, M., Yu, J., Laxman, B., Kalyana-Sundaram, S., Zhao, R., Menon, A., Wei, J. T., Nesvizhskii, A. I., Ghosh, D., Omenn, G. S., Lubman, D. M., Chinnaiyan, A. M., & Sreekumar, A. 2008. Humoral response profiling reveals pathways to prostate cancer progression. *Molecular & Cellular Proteomics,* 7(3): 600-611.

Terasawa, H., Tsang, K. Y., Gulley, J., Arlen, P. M., & Schlom, J. 2002. Identification and characterization of a human agonist cytotoxic T- lymphocyte epitope of human prostate-specific antigen. *Clinical Cancer Research,* 8(1): 41-53.

van der Bruggen, P., Zhang, Y., Chaux, P., Stroobant, V., Panichelli, C., Schultz, E. S., Chapiro, J., Van Den Eynde, B. J., Brasseur, F., & Boon, T. 2002. Tumor-specific shared antigenic peptides recognized by human T cells. *Immunological Reviews,* 188: 51-64.

Wang, X., Yu, J., Sreekumar, A., Varambally, S., Shen, R., Giacherio, D., Mehra, R., Montie, J. E., Pienta, K. J., Sanda, M. G., Kantoff, P. W., Rubin, M. A., Wei, J. T., Ghosh, D., & Chinnaiyan, A. M. 2005. Autoantibody signatures in prostate cancer. *New England Journal of Medicine,* 353(12): 1224-1235.

Yuan, J., Gnjatic, S., Li, H., Powel, S., Gallardo, H. F., Ritter, E., Ku, G. Y., Jungbluth, A. A., Segal, N. H., Rasalan, T. S., Manukian, G., Xu, Y., Roman, R. A., Terzulli, S. L., Heywood, M., Pogoriler, E., Ritter, G., Old, L. J., Allison, J. P., & Wolchok, J. D. 2008. CTLA-4 blockade enhances polyfunctional NY-ESO-1 specific T cell responses in metastatic melanoma patients with clinical benefit. *Proceedings of the National Academy of Sciences of the United States of America,* 105(51): 20410-20415.

4

Prostate Cancer Immunotherapy – Strategy with a Synthetic GnRH Based Vaccine Candidate

J.A. Junco[1] et al.*
[1]*Department of Cancer,*
Center for Genetic Engineering and Biotechnology of Camaguey,
Ave. Finlay y Circunvalación Norte, Camaguey,
Cuba

1. Introduction

Recent clinical trials have shown therapeutic vaccines to be promising treatment modalities for prostate cancer. Additional strategies are being investigated that combine vaccines and standard therapeutics as anti-hormone treatment to optimize the vaccines' effects.

Previous studies with Gonadotropin Releasing Hormone (GnRH/LHRH) vaccines have demonstrated the usefulness of immunization against this hormone in prostate cancer. To this purpose, we generated the completely synthetic GnRHm1-TT peptide which has been validated in a proof of concept formulated together with Montanide ISA 51 adjuvant. Such vaccine preparation induced a significant anti-GnRH immune response and correspondingly reduced testosterone to castration levels and thus produce a biological response in hormone-dependent tumors. As a novel strategy the GnRHm1-TT peptide has been also emulsified with the adjuvant combination Montanide ISA 51 and VSSP. The use of this candidate in healthy animal models showed a significant increase in the anti GnRH immune response in comparison with the previous candidates, including their advantages regarding prostate and its testicle atrophy. Moreover, the use of the GnRHm1-TT/Montanide ISA 51/VSSP vaccine candidate produced a significant inhibition of tumor growth in mice transplanted with hormone-sensitive murine tumor Shionogi SC-115. The development of a Phase I clinical trial in patients with advanced prostate cancer using GnRHm1-TT/Montanide/VSSP vaccine, demonstrated the safety of using this candidate in humans as well as the therapeutic elements which must be demonstrated more widely in future clinical trials.

---

*F. Fuentes[1], R. Basulto[1], E. Bover[1], M.D. Castro[1], E. Pimentel[1], O. Reyes [2], R. Bringas[2], L.Calzada[1], Y. López[1], N. Arteaga[1], A. Rodríguez[3], H. Garay[2], R. Rodríguez[4], L. González-Quiza[4], L. Fong[4] and G.E. Guillén[2]
[1]*Department of Cancer, Center for Genetic Engineering and Biotechnology of Camaguey, Ave. Finlay y Circunvalación Norte, Camaguey, Cuba*
[2]*Center for Genetic Engineering and Biotechnology, Havana, Cuba*
[3]*University of Medical Sciences of Camaguey, Carretera Central SN, Camaguey, Cuba*
[4]*Marie Curie Oncologic Hospital of Camaguey, Carretera Central SN, Camaguey, Cuba*

2. Epidemiology of prostate cancer

Prostate cancer is the most commonly diagnosed malignancy in men in the Western Hemisphere, with 33% incidence rate and the second leading cause of cancer death in men, exceeded only by lung cancer despite the efforts to achieve early diagnosis of disease through the use of the serological marker "prostate specific antigen" (PSA). Worldwide, there are about 650 000 reported new cases of prostate cancer each year and a mortality of about 200 000 cases. Autopsy studies in men show that 70% of men develop prostate cancer sometime in their lives, although many of them are clinically irrelevant (Russel et al, 1994; Cancer Statistics, 2008).

Prostate cancer is diagnosed in a clinically relevant stage in one out of six men around the world and is usually diagnosed by elevated levels of prostate specific antigen (PSA) or the presence of an abnormal digital rectal examination.

The Prostate Specific Antigen (PSA), is a protein produced by normal and pathological prostate cells. This protein is found in relatively small levels in the bloodstream of men with normal prostate, however, is considerably increased in most individuals suffering from a malignant disease of the prostate, but also tends to increase in benign diseases of the gland such as prostatitis and benign prostatic hyperplasia (BPH).

While assessing the levels of PSA takes into account the individual's age, it is generally considered that these values may reach up to 4 ng/mL (Sonpavde et al, 2010). Unfortunately, however, the PSA does not distinguish between the stages of the disease.

3. Prostatic tumurogenesis

Prostate cancer seems to develop over a period ranging from 20 to 30 years (Kabalin et al, 1989; Sacker et al, 1996). In most cases, the tumurogenesis begins as a prostatic inflammatory atrophy which progresses to prostatic intraepithelial neoplasia (PIN), which in some cases leads to carcinoma (De Marzo et al 2003, Nelson et al, 2007). In addition to genetic changes occurred, androgens act as promoters of proliferation and prostate growth. Thus, testosterone passes into the prostate cell where the action of the enzyme 5 alpha reductase is converted to its metabolically active form, dihydrotestosterone (DHT). Once DHT binds to the receptor in the cytoplasm, this favors the formation of dimers crossing the nuclear membrane where the complex binds to genes with androgen-responsive elements, a process modulated by co-activators and co-repressors (You and Tindall, 2004).

Thus, if normal prostatic epithelial cells are deprived of testosterone, this progresses to death by apoptosis. Similarly, the majority of prostatic adenocarcinomas are androgen-dependent, which means they are responders to testosterone hormone ablation. This behavior of prostate cells has influenced therapeutic concepts in prostate cancer for decades (Culig et al, 2005). Thus even in cases of metastatic disease, the first therapeutic step is represented by androgen suppression, which causes death by apoptosis in most prostate cells and leads to remission in about 85% to 90% of individuals.

4. Current therapies in prostate cancer

Prostate cancer patients at initial stages of the disease are treated successfully with radical prostatectomy or radiation therapy, however, approximately 30–40% of them will ultimately develop recurrent diseases (Roehl et al, 2004).

Once prostate cancer reach the prostatic capsule and seminal glands, the androgenic ablation represents the most useful therapeutic procedure since the decade of the 40´s of the last century (Culig et al, 2005; Pienta et al, 2006). The normal intervention of the prostate cancer includes: the surgical castration, the use of estrogens, anti-androgenic therapy to inhibit the testosterone actions and, the use of GnRH analogues which prevent the production of androgens in the testicles.

The anti-hormones therapies, although very much in use, have various inconveniences. Thus, the surgical castration is not ethically accepted by most patients. The estrogens, such as the diethyl-stilbestrol (DES) are highly toxic to the cardiovascular system and the anti-androgens frequently produce severe gastro-intestinal toxicity (Finstad et al, 2004) while pituitary adenomas and hot flush during the first weeks of treatment are reported for GnRH analogs treatment. However, the most important drawback of anti-hormonal therapy in prostate cancer consists in that the benefit of this therapy last for an average of between 18 and 36 months (Casper et al, 1991). At that stage those clones of cells that escaped to the requirements of the absence of testosterone or lower levels, begin to grow or proliferate as castration resistant prostate cancer (CRPC) and emerge as the predominant cell phenotype. When CRPC appears, chemotherapy and steroids represent the alternative palliative treatment left for patients who no longer respond to hormone therapy. The half-life for these patients ranges between 18 and 24 months (Tannock et al, 2004). Of the many treatment approaches for recurrent prostate cancer that no longer responds to hormonal agents, immunotherapy is particularly promising, due to several unique characteristics of both the disease and the treatment.

5. Prostate cancer immunotherapy

Prostate cancer is a relatively indolent disease, allowing time for the immune system to generate an immunologic response. Furthermore, since the prostate is a nonessential organ, targeting prostate cancer-associated antigens are unlikely to have significant negative side effects. Finally, therapeutic cancer vaccines have been shown to be much less toxic than chemotherapy, hormonal therapy or targeted therapies, thus significantly improving a patient's quality of life.

Studies in animals and humans developed over decades using non-specific immune therapies, suggest the usefulness of these therapies in prostate cancer. However, these therapies have been used mainly in advanced stages of cancer. Immunotherapies are classified as passive and active. The former include the treatment with immunomodulatory substances, the infusion of cytokines and immune effector agents such as antibodies or lymphocytes.

In medical practice the most widely used cytokine-stimulating factor has been the Granulocyte-Macrophage Colony-Stimulating Factor (GM-CSF). This cytokine is known to act at different levels of the immune response which includes the stimulation to arachidonic acid release in neutrophils and active cellular response mediated by antibodies (Weisbart et al, 1985).

An active immunotherapy vaccine includes strategies in which the goal is to produce an immune response against the tumor/host factors that aid the maintenance and growth of metastatic tumor (Rini et al, 2004).

Ideally, therapeutic prostate cancer vaccines should induce a focused antitumor immune response by targeting defined tumor-associated antigens (TAAs) through TH1 cell stimulation. The ideal TAA should be specific to, or overexpressed on the surface of prostate cancer cells. Several prostate-associated TAAs have been identified and that include: the prostate specific antigen (PSA), a 34-kD kallikrein-like serine protease expressed almost exclusively by prostate epithelial cells and is the most widely used serum marker for diagnosis and monitoring of prostate cancer (Freedland et al, 2008; Madan et al, 2009). The prostate specific membrane antigen or PSMA which is a 100-kD transmembrane glycoprotein commonly found on the surface of late stages, undifferentiated metastatic prostate cancer and is an imaging biomarker for staging and monitoring of therapy. It also represents an attractive antigen for antibody-based diagnostic and therapeutic intervention in prostate cancer, since it is highly restricted to the prostate and overexpressed in all tumor stages (Fishman et al, 2009). The prostatic acid phosphatase or PAP is a secreted glycoprotein (50 kDa) that serve as a well-known tumor marker of differentiated prostate epithelial cells (Becker et al, 2010) whose primary biologic function is still unclear. Another potential target, TARP, is a protein expressed in patients with prostate and breast cancer and is present in both normal and malignant prostate cancer tissue. It is found in about 95% of prostate cancer specimens, making TARP a promising target antigen for cancer vaccines (Maeda et al 2004; Epel et al, 2008). Recently, a prostate-specific gene encoding a protein named NGEP has been discovered. The full length protein (NGEP-L) is expressed in normal, hyperplastic and cancer prostate tissue (Cereda et al, 2010).

Despite the long list of tumor markers, PSA has been the most useful TAA as a diagnostic tool and for immunotherapy. In this sense, PSA has been used as part of the PSA-TRICOM vaccine design, which showed a beneficial impact on metastatic CRPC patients and is currently in Phase III clinical trial (Bavarian Nordic, 2011).

As part of the immune response modulation, Cytotoxic Lymphocite Antigen 4 (CTLA-4), represents an important immune checkpoint molecule expressed after activation by an APC. CTLA-4 blocking could disrupt the transmission of the regulatory signal and may increase the immune response of CTLs against tumor cells (Fong et al, 2008). In this sense, Ipilimumab is a fully humanized monoclonal antibody against CTLA-4 that demonstrated PSA decline in a Phase I clinical trial (Small et al, 2007) and is currently in Phase III trial. (http://www.clinicaltrials.gov).

The most successful prostate cancer immunotherapy intervention is represented however, by the ex vivo vaccine called "Provenge" or "Sipuleucel T", which is generated from each patient's own Peripheral Mononuclear Blood Cells (PMBCs), that are later "charged" with the fusion protein PAP/GM-CSF and the GM-CSF. (Burch et al, 2000). These immunotherapy demonstrated a significant improvement in the overall survival for Sipuleucel-T (25.8 months) vs. placebo (21.7 months) (Kantoff et al, 2010) and has been registered by the FDA in the United States and is the only therapeutic vaccine of its kind in the world for this condition.

Combining therapeutic cancer vaccines with hormonal therapies is a potential approach for hormone-sensitive tumors, such as breast and prostate cancer. Preclinical data indicate that testosterone suppression affects not only prostate tumors, but also the immune system (Aragon et al, 2007). Increasingly data suggest that androgen deprivation therapy (ADT) in prostate cancer can augment the immune response by increasing T-cell infiltration into the prostate (Mercader et al, 2001). Furthermore, ADT has been shown to decrease immune tolerance of TAAs, increase the size of the thymus (where CTLs are produced), and enhance the T-cell repertoire (Drake et al, 2005; Sutherland et al, 2005; Aragon et al, 2007; Goldeberg et al, 2007). It may also stimulate CTLs by reducing the number of regulatory Tcells (Tregs), improving immune-mediated tumor-specific response (Wang et al, 2009).

6. Vaccines design with autologous molecules

Immunization against endogenous molecules requires a sufficient level of neutralizing antibodies during the treatment period to obtain the desired effect. To produce an immune response against these molecules, several of which are not immunogenic thenselves, many strategies, such as the coupling to a carrier protein and the use of powerful adjuvants are required (McKee et al, 2010).

6.1 Prostate cancer immunotherapy based on GnRH. State of the art

GnRH-based vaccines represent a promising anti-hormonal treatment alternative in prostate cancer, because these can reduce serum testosterone to castration levels, avoid the "hot flushes" produced by GnRH analogues and can be administered in acute and complicated forms of prostate cancer. In turn, the ability to generate a memory immune response in vaccinated patients allows them to do without medications for relatively long periods of time which also results in lower medication costs and marketing. This aspect gives vaccines high added-value and very competitiveness in the market.

6.1.1 Carriers molecules to GnRH vaccine delivery

The most often used approach to make a peptide immunogenic, is to couple it to a protein molecule. Commonly used carrier proteins are KLH, TT, DT, OVA, BSA and HSA. The origin of the carrier protein could be of importance for the level of immunogenicity of the conjugate. The use of "foreign" proteins is expected to result in conjugates with a stronger immune response. In general, most exogenous proteins can be used as carriers, although non-mammalian proteins are expected to be more immunogenic. Additionally, the site of conjugation may determine the efficacy of the immunization. Conjugation via glutamine at position 1 induced a higher GnRH specific antibody response and reduced testosterone levels in rabbits more effectively than conjugation via positions 6 or 10. Similarly, no difference in GnRH antibody response has been observed in male sheep when GnRH was conjugated to KLH via a substituted cysteine either at position 1, 6 or 10 (Goubau et al, 1989). These results have been confirmed in mice. At the same time, specificity of the antisera depend on the site of conjugation. So, experiment carried out by conjugation via cysteine on position 1 resulted in C-terminal directed antibodies, conjugation via cysteine on position 10 generated N-terminal directed antibodies, while conjugation via cysteine at position 6 generated both N- and C-terminal antibodies (Silversides et al, 1988). In contrast, Ferro et al. (1998) showed that the N-terminal conjugation via a cysteine substitution at position 1 resulted in effective immunization of rats, while conjugation via cysteine substitution at position 10 was not effective. Other groups used native GnRH extended with glycine and cysteine, conjugated to a carrier protein (Ferro et al., 1996; Miller et al., 2000) or longer spacer peptides (Simms et al., 2000; Parkinson et al., 2004). Thus, it seems that immunization with GnRH peptides, conjugated to a carrier protein via the N-terminus results in more effective antibody titers than conjugation via the C-terminus. However, this was not confirmed in all studies and may depend on the chemical approach used and substitution of amino acids required for coupling.

One of the most promising vaccine candidate based on GnRH have been developed by United Biomedical (UBI, Hauppauge, USA), which is a complete synthetic vaccine comprising the GnRH decapeptide, several promiscuous T-cell epitopes and a domain from Yersinia invasin protein to improve the immunogenicity of the GnRH-T cell epitope constructs (Finstad et al., 2004). Although the single constructs were not completely effective in rats, mixtures of constructs caused serum testosterone to drop to very low levels, whereas testes weights were less than 25% of the controls. The antigens in a water-in-oil formulation and oil-in-water formulation were effective in baboons and dogs, respectively. Phase I clinical trials have been planned recently using this vaccine candidate, however, no results have been published so far.

In the hope of developing a better anti GnRH vaccine apart from the mentioned carrier molecules, some alternatives have been used like the *Mycobacterium tuberculosis* hsp 70, linked to GnRH-6-DLys by elves and Roitt's group employing either Ribi adjuvant or incomplete Freund's adjuvant. With either adjuvant, all mice produced sufficient antibodies to cause atrophy of the uro-genital complex. LHRH-6-DLys was also employed after conjugation to albumin and mixed with Specol as adjuvant. These vaccine candidate have been used in pigs as an alternative to castration (Zeng *et al,* 2002).

Previous studies of the Population Council group (Ladd *et al,*1990) found that the conjugation of TT at the N-terminal was better than at the C-terminal. Desirability of keeping the LHRH C-terminal free has also been advocated by Ferro *et al.* (2002). Linkage of TT at the N-terminal in Des 1-GnRH, where glutamic acid at position 1 is replaced by cysteine, gives better conjugate that induces antibodies specific to the classical GnRH-1. Dimerization enhances antibody titers but the monomer conjugate was found to be more effective (Ferro *et al.*, 2002).

6.1.2 Recombinant vaccines against LHRH/GnRH

Enough data have accumulated to conclude that the vaccines against GnRH-I can be employed in humans and in animals without side-effects. These vaccines are beneficial in the treatment of prostate carcinoma patients to reduce fertility of wild animals and sex steroid hormone production thus regulating estrus and libido of animals raised for meat production.

Recombinant vaccines would be substantially cheaper to produce at industrial scale than synthetic vaccines conjugating multiple copies of GnRH with receptor-binding domain of *Pseudomonas* exotoxin (Hsu *et al,* 2000). This recombinant protein containing 12 repeats of LHRH along with this carrier generated high antibody titres in rabbit and is recommended for the treatment of hormone-sensitive cancer. At the same time, genes for three repeats of GnRH linked through an eight amino acid hinge fragment of human IgG1 to a helper T-cells peptide of measles virus have been constructed in order to increase immunogenicity. The DNA coding for a dimer of this complex assembly was fused to the C-terminal (199–326)-encoding sequence of asparaginase (Jinshu *et al.*(2006). This protein was expressed in *E. coli* and generated an anti LHRH response .

Talwar *et al.* (2004) reported the ability of a multimer recombinant anti-LHRH vaccine to cause decline of testosterone to castration level and atrophy of rats prostate. In the design of this vaccine, DT/TT used as carriers in the previous semisynthetic vaccines were replaced by four or five T non-B-cell peptides interspersed in four or five LHRH units. This was done to avoid carrier-induced epitope suppression brought by DT/TT carrier conjugates (Sad *et al.*, 1991), and also to communicate through an array of these T-cell determinants with MHC across the spectrum in a polygenetic population. The genes were assembled, cloned and expressed at high level (15% of total cellular protein) in *E. coli* (Gupta *et al.*, 2004). Employing a buffer at pH 3, it was possible to extract the protein from inclusion bodies employing low concentrations of chaotropic reagents (2 mol/l urea instead of 8 mol/L). The protein was purified and refolded to native immunoconformation (Raina *et al.*, 2004).

The company Biostar, (Saskatoon, Canada), developed a GnRH vaccine comprising a recombinant fusion protein produced in *E. Coli* bacteria. Several copies of a GnRH-tandem molecule were fused to the terminal ends of leukotoxin. This vaccine has shown full efficacy in young pigs and cats (Manns and Robbins, 1997; Robbins et al., 2004), while antibody responses were variable in heifers (Cook et al., 2001). For application in prostate cancer patients, the vaccine called Norelin™, was out-licensed to York Medical BioSciences (Mississauga, Canada). In 2001 clinical studies indicated that the vaccine with an aluminium salt-based adjuvant was safe to be used in humans, however it was not immunogenic enough to raise a sufficiently strong immune response. In 2003, a second clinical trial was initiated. This vaccine was well tolerated with ´no major adverse events (www.ymbiosciences.com). In a recent press release it has been announced a trial in prostate cancer patients in China (www.unitedbiomedical.com). On the other hand Proterics developed a GnRH vaccine containing the GnRH decapeptide with an additional glycine and cysteine ´Prolog´, which was out-licensed to ML Laboratories. They completed phase II clinical studies in 2000, but at present no results have been published (www.mllabs.co.uk). Most recently, the chimeric peptide called GnRH3-hinge-MVP which contains three linear repeats of GnRH (GnRH3), a fragment of the human IgG1 hinge region, and a T-cell epitope of measles virus protein (MVP). The expression plasmid contained the GnRH3-hinge-MVP construct ligated to its fusion partner (AnsB-C) via a unique acid labile Asp-Pro linker. The recombinant fusion protein was expressed in an inclusion body in *Escherichia coli* under IPTG or lactose induction and the target peptide was easily purified using washing with urea and ethanol precipitation. The target chimeric peptide was isolated from the fusion partner following acid hydrolysis and purifed using DEAE-Sephacel chromatography. Further, immunization of female mice with the recombinant chimeric peptide resulted in generation of high-titer antibodies specifc for GnRH. The results showed that GnRH3-hinge-MVP could be considered as a candidate anti-GnRH vaccine, however the reports just include their use as immunocastration vaccine (Jinshu X, 2006). In 2008, the group of Li Yu and colleagues at Department of Biochemistry, Medical College, Jinan University in China developed GnRH-PE40, one of the recombinant single-chain fusion proteins consisting of GnRH fused to a binding defective form of *pseudomonas aeruginosa* exotoxin A (PE40), which has been developed as a preparation with potential functions of immune castration in male reproductive system (Li et al, 2008).

6.1.3 Adjuvants and other strategies employed for enhancement of immune response

The adjuvants most commonly used in human and veterinary vaccines are oil-based adjuvants and aluminum hydroxide (Alum). Responses to Alum are often low and of short duration. Oil-based adjuvants are effective in generating a high immune response, but may cause inflammatory reactions. Complete Freunds adjuvant (CFA) is a mineral oil, which forms a water-in-oil emulsion, and contains killed and dried bacteria to stimulate the immune response. This combination induces high antibody responses; because of these characteristics and CFA being one of the oldest adjuvants used, it is ´the gold standard´ among adjuvants. However, due to the inflammatory side effects, which may occur at the site of injection, its use is limited to experimentation in laboratory animals.

Instead of whole bacteria, bacterial compounds such as muramyl dipeptide (MDP), lipopolysaccharide (LPS) or monophosphoryl lipid A (MPL) can be used to stimulate the immune system. Alternative immune stimulating compounds are saponins, i.e. Quil A and the purified QS21 fraction, bacterial DNA, microparticles, Iscoms, liposomes, virus-like particles, block polymers and dimethyldioctadecylammonium bromide(DDA).

Among the new adjuvant in development we count Titermax, which contains non-mineral oil and a block polymer that forms a water-in-oil emulsion, and RIBI adjuvant, which contains non-mineral oil with microbial components that forms an oil-in-water emulsion (Bennett et al., 1992; Kiyma et al, 2000). The comparison of CFA to Montanide ISA 51, which forms a water-in-mineral oil emulsion, showed that CFA was superior to ISA 51 with respect to antibody titers and subsequent effects on testosterone levels when tested in sheep. In contrast, others found effective GnRH antibody responses using ISA 51 combined with DDA in baboons (Finstad et al., 2004). In conclusion, effective antibody titers can be generated with adjuvants other than CFA, however, responses may differ among studies due to differences in target species, number of immunizations, antigen type and dose.

A novel retro-inverso GnRH composed of D-amino acids assembled in reverse order (C to N terminus) was found to induce high titers of antibodies reactive with native GnRH without conjugation to a carrier or use as an adjuvant (Fromme *et al.*, 2003). On the other hand non-ionic surfactant vesicles, aluminium hydroxide, Quil A, polylactide co glycolide acid (PLGA) and Quil A/PLGA combination, with their cysteine-modified LHRH linked to TT have been the best adjuvant used by Ferro *et al.* (2004) and interestingly, there exist reports from 1998 that the encapsulation of GnRH-6-DLys-TT in PLGA microspheres induces a bio-effective antibody response within 15 days after a single administration, obliterating the necessity of repeated injections (Diwan *et al*, 1998)

7. Clinical trials in prostate carcinoma patients

Several GnRH vaccines have been developed for the treatment of prostate cancer. Clinical trials in patients with advanced prostate cancer revealed that in contrast to rodents and monkeys, high antibody titers were obtained in some, but not all treated patients. A reduction in prostatic size was observed in 3 out of 6 patients treated with 400 µg conjugate in Alum and in 1 out of 6 patients treated with 200 µg conjugate (Talwar et al., 1995). The same group used a vaccine comprising a modified GnRH decapeptide with a D-Lysine at position 6 linked to DT in the development of a Phase I/ II clinical trials in 28 patients of advanced stage carcinoma of prostate (12 patients at the All India Institute of Medical Sciences, New Delhi, India, 12 at the Post Graduate Institute of Medical Education and Research, Chandigarh, India, and 4 at the Urologizche Klinikum, Salzburg, Austria). The vaccine employed alhydrogel, an adjuvant permissible for human use. It was used at 200 µg and 400 μg dose, and three injections were given at monthly intervals. The vaccine was well tolerated by all patients with no side-effects attributable to immunization. A 400 μg dose produced antibody titres >200 pg dose. Patients generating >200 pg of antibodies/ml benefited clinically and testosterone declined to castration levels. The prostate-specific antigen (PSA) and acid phosphatase declined to low levels. Ultrasonography and serial nephrostograms showed the regression of prostatic mass (Talwar *et al.*, 1998). A preclinical study was previously developed by Fuerst in rats bearing androgen-dependent prostatic tumors R3327-PAP. As a result of this study carried out in Copenhagen rats implanted SC with the tumor fragments, after three immunizations tumor growth was suppressed compared to untreated controls. Surprisingly, tumor growth was also suppressed in rats implanted with androgen-independent Dunning tumor cells R3327-AT2.1. This Phenomenon is suggested to be related with the presence of a local GnRH-loop in the prostate, which is affected by GnRH neutralizing antibodies and produce a tumor growth reduction even in testosterone-independent tumors.

A very promising approach using the GnRH antigen was developed by the Aphton company in USA. That comprises the GnRH molecule extended with a linker peptide of 6 amino acids conjugated to DT. Two clinical trials with a GnRH-DT vaccine have been carried out at Nottingham, UK by Bishop's group. In the first study (Simms *et al.*, 2000), the vaccine was used at two doses 30 μg and 100 μg, administered three times over 6 weeks in 12 patients with advanced prostate cancer. It was well tolerated and in five patients a significant reduction in serum testosterone and PSA levels was seen. Testosterone declined to castration level in four patients for 9 months. Since the modest results obtained in this trial, 3 and 15 μg doses were evaluated in order to determine how the doses reduction can work (Parkinson et al, 2004). As result of this approach, suppression of testosterone to castrate levels was detected in 2 out of 6 patients treated with 15 μg antigen, whereas none of the patients treated with 3 μg responded. The above-mentioned clinical studies in India, Austria and UK confirmed the safety of LHRH or GnRH linked to DT vaccine in prostate carcinoma patients. These studies further showed that in patients generating adequate antibodies, testosterone declined to castration levels with concomitant decline of PSA, and there was clinical benefit to the patients.

8. GnRHm1-TT, a new strategy to prostate cancer immunotherapy

The development of the vaccine candidate GnRHm1-TT has as its main invention the substitution of L-glycine in position 6 of the GnRH molecule by the amino acid L-proline and the addition of a T helper epitope of TT (Bringas et al, 2000). With this modification we expected to guarantee a "change" in the "U" native conformation of the natural GnRH peptide structure, which is known to play a pivotal role in binding to the receptor (Millar et al, 1977; Millar et al, 2008) and on the other hand, to generate a more rigid molecule that makes it more available to the immune system in the hope to break the B cells tolerance (Goodnow et al, 1991; Bizzini and Achour,,1995) while the incorporation of the TT 830-844 promiscuous epitope give an additional "immunologic target" to recognize this molecule. (Hoskinson et al, 1990, Ferro and Stimson, 1998, Finstad et al, 2004).

The high production of natural antibodies against GnRH, induced by the GnRHm1-TT peptide in AF and in the two types of Montanide, demonstrated the immunogenicity of the peptide used and its potential to "fool" the physiological mechanisms of immunologic tolerance together with the fact that the Montanide ISA 51 showed some superiority over the FA in terms of antibody titers.

An important fact in the development of a GnRH based vaccine has been the decision about the peptide doses to employ. In this sense, experiments carried out with doses ranging from 125 to 750 µg in rats addressed the usefulness of the 750 µg doses in comparison with lower doses according to the time to develop the anti immune response and the anti GnRH titres. That demonstrate the desirability of using high peptide doses of GnRHm1-TT to achieve the breaking of B cell tolerance and at the same time the utility of using fortnightly and monthly immunization schedules. That is in correspondence with previous works using similar candidates (Talwar et al, 1997, Finstad et al, 2004)

In the hope to demonstrate the feasibility of generating an effective immune response with the vaccine candidate GnRHm1-TT/ Montanide ISA 51 in other species of mammals, given that although GnRH is a hormone that is 100% homologous in all of them (Talwar et al, 1997, Millar et al, 2008), HLA system among species produces a different behavior of the immune response (Friederike et al, 2008), experiments were carried out in two animal models that share different genetic homology; the New Zealand rabbits and Macacus monkeys.

The development of an immunization schedule in both species showed that 100% of the animals generated anti-GnRH antibody titres, regardless of the dose used (750 µg or 1mg). However, the increase in dose up to 1mg, produced a significant rise in antibody titres generated, although this increase did not result in different levels of testosterone.

In this sense, the results suggest that, once antibodies against GnRH hormone reach "critical" levels, they achieve the formation of nearly 100% of circulating immune complexes with GnRH and they will result in the fall of testosterone levels. That observation is in accordance with some reports that suggest that rather than their isotype or antibody affinity, the biological effect of anti-GnRH antibodies depends on the speed of its appearance and its maintenance in sufficient concentrations (Talwar et al 2004, Miller et al, 2006). The use of doses over 1 mg did not improve significantly the characteristics of the immune response produced, neither seemed to generate a phenomenon of immunological tolerance.

These results have great relevance for making decisions regarding the selection of the peptide dose in the following of experiments in other animal models and in humans. In turn, the increased robustness of the *Macacus irus* model, allowed to explore how the immune response would behave when using the intramuscular route (IM). The results found with GnRHm1-TT formulated in Montanide ISA 51, corresponded to those obtained by other authors that report similar immunogenicity between IM and SC routes (Talwar et al, 1997). These similar behavior can be related to the ability of the adjuvant Montanide ISA 51, similar to the AF, to produce a reservoir of antigen and its slow release to the immune system, which allows a better efficiency of antigen presentation by macrophages and Dendritic cells (DC) to T cells (Guerrero et al, 1982; Forsbucher et al, 1996). That approach demonstrates the feasibility of using IM route in human trials where both, the Montanide ISA 51 and Montanide ISA 51 VG, produce a marked local toxic effect when administered subcutaneously (manufacturer's data SEPPIC, France).

In a step forward, the vaccine candidate GnRHm1-TT/Montanide ISA 51 was evaluated in the Dunning R3327-H tumor model, which shares similar characteristics to cancer in humans (Isaacs et al, 1994). The results of the high anti-GnRH seroconversion (88%) in the model demonstrated the feasibility of the vaccine in generating a consistent humoral immune response, despite the presence of established tumor. So, despite the variability in the anti-GnRH titres it droped testosterone levels until castration in all the animals that seroconverted and in consequence a significant tumor growth inhibition was observed (Table 1).

Animal number	Time to seroconversion (in days)	Anti GnRH titres (day 90)	Testosterone (nmol/L) (day 90)	Survival (in days)
32-	60	1/ 200[e]	1,70±0,04[a]	150[b]
36-	45	1/ 400[c]	0,07±0,02[a]	150[b]
43	45	1/400[c]	0,01±0,00[a]	265[a]
46-	45	1/800[b]	0,07±0,02[a]	195[b]
49-	45	1/ 800[b]	0,00±0,00[a]	265[a]
51-	45	1/ 1600[a]	0,00±0,00[a]	95[c]
55-	45	1/200[d]	0,84±0,28[a]	60[c]
56-	60	1/100[d]	0,18±0,01[a]	265[a]
60-	-	0/00	1,9 0±0,3[b]	85[c]

Table 1. Effects of the immunization with vaccine candidate GnRHm1-TT/Montanide in Copenhagen rats implanted with the Dunning R3327-H tumor.

Different letters denote significant differences calculated according to the U Mann Whitney test. The differences in the anti-GnRH antibody titres and Testosterone were calculated using a simple ANOVA and for the survival a Log Rank test was carried out.

As an important fact it was noted that despite the uncontrolled tumor growth observed in cases beyond the hormone-dependence, Dunning R3327-H tumor does not generate distant metastases (Isaacs et al, 1978, 1986; Canena-Adams, 2007, Cho et al, 2009; Peschke et al, 2011).

In order to determine the direct role of the anti GnRH antibodies in the described immunocastration effects in healthy and tumor implanted animals, purified serum obtained from rabbits immunized with the GnRHm1-TT/Montanide ISA 51 vaccine candidate was used and tested in the mammalian COS-7 cells model (Millar et al, 2003). As a result, a gradual decrease in the Inositol Phosphate (IP) concentration was detected once the anti GnRH antibodies concentration was increased from 0,65 µg to 12.5 mg, showing the neutralizing capacity of the anti GnRH antibodies generated with the vaccine candidate.

Despite the satisfactory results obtained with the use of the vaccine candidate GnRHm1-TT/Montanide ISA 51 in the different tested models, the slow appearance of anti-GnRH antibodies (after 3 immunizations) and hence; the consequently slow fall in testosterone levels and the heterogeneity in the atrophy effects in prostate and testes in the vaccinated individuals, led us to a new strategy to include the use of a combination of adjuvants in order to enhance the immune-response attributes induced and the biological effects.

The use of combinations of potent adjuvants to promote the inflammatory cells to escape from the regulatory circuit, is an attractive idea, well addressed by the scientific literature that has been recently practiced in the development of preventive vaccines (Ambrosino et al, 1992; Udono et al, 1993; Nestle et al, 1998). This strategy, however, has not been used so far in the development of therapeutic vaccines based on poorly immunogenic self-molecules as GnRH. In the current vaccine design, a Montanide ISA 51/VSSP adjuvant combination was explored.

The VSSP belongs to the range of pathogen-derived adjuvants which have the ability to stimulate dendritic cells (DC) through receptors similar to those described in Drosophila Tolls (TLR). This adjuvant has within its active molecules, those classified as "dangerous", according to the so-called danger theory (Andersen et al, 1989, Lowell et al, 1990; Zollinger, 1990, 1994, Jeannin et al, 2000; 2003; Matzinger et al, 2001).

As a result of the immunization of rats with the GnRHm1-TT peptide emulsified with the adjuvant combination Montanide ISA 51/VSSP, a strong humoral response manifested as three-fold increase in anti-GnRH antibody titres and a significant improvement in the speed of the anti-GnRH was produced (Fig.1).

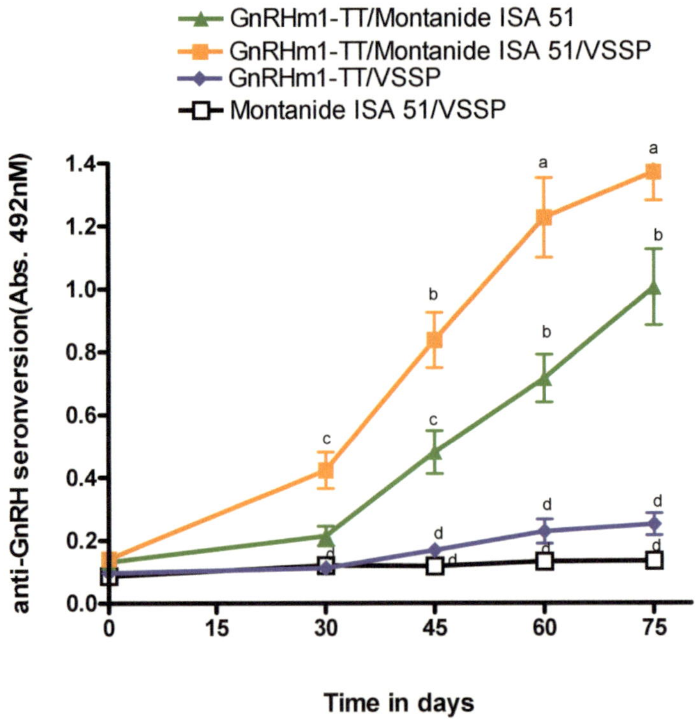

Fig. 1. Graphic representation of anti GnRH seroconversion generated in male rats immunized with the vaccine composition GnRHm1-TT, with or without the presence of VSSP. Serums from different experimental groups were obtained at days 0, 30, 45, 60, and 75. These were diluted in a blocking buffer 1:50. The T bars for each point convey the absorbance mean ± DE. Different letters denote statistical differences between the points according to the non-parametrical Kruskal Wallis analysis.

It also highlights the fact that this formulation, is the first to allow to obtain mean levels of castration at day 60 after the beginning of the immunization. In addition the adjuvant combination generated a reduction of over 60% of the size of the prostate and testes which was significantly higher than that achieved with the traditional vaccine candidate GnRHm1-TT/Montanide and represents an unprecedented result in the development of such vaccines.

The VSSP classifies as a type 2 adjuvant, acting by stimulating antigen presenting cells through TLR 2 and 6 by a mechanism independent of LPS, producing increased maturation of the humoral immune response in a Th1 pattern (personal communication) and together with the adjuvant Montanide ISA 51, favors the direct stimulation of the innate immune response (Aguiar et al, 2009). To evaluate the antitumoral potentiality of the GnRHm1-TT/Montanide ISA 51 VG /VSSP vaccine candidate, the hormone-sensitive Shionogi SC-115 murine prostate tumor model was used.

Similar to the pattern described in healthy rats, immunization of DD/S mice bearing the Shionogi tumor generated a fast seroconversion and high antibody titers against GnRH after 2 administrations. These results, although expected, are further evidence of the immunogenicity of the GnRHm1-TT peptide in a new species of rodents. In accordance with those anti GnRH antibodies, testosterone ablation was observed in all the immunized mice and a controlled tumor growth was seen in most cases (Fig. 2).

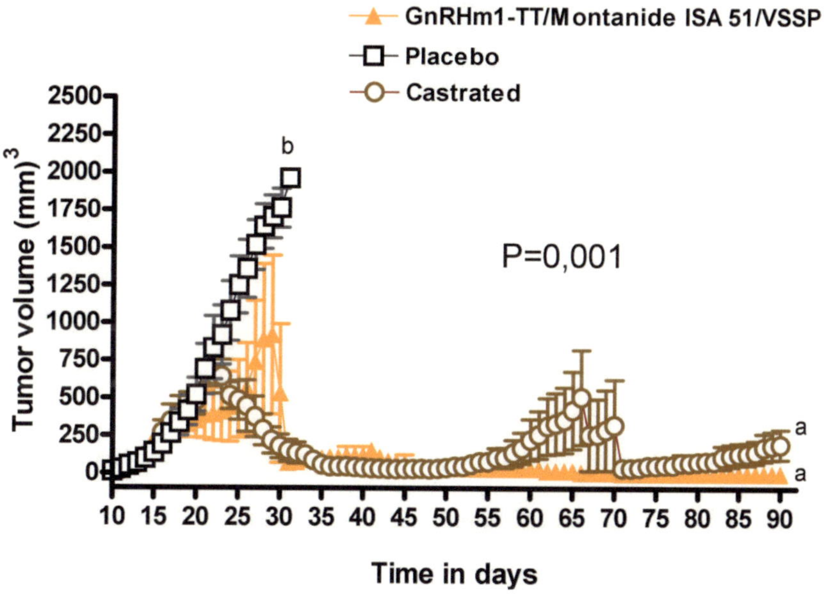

Fig. 2. Tumor growth behaviour of the Shionogi tumor in DD/S mice immunized with the vaccine candidate GnRHm1-TT/Montanide/VSSP. The mice were immunized with the vaccine candidate GnRHm1-TT/Montanide/VSSP at days 0, 15, 30, 45, and 60. (n=5). The castrated group was orchiectomized at day 15 after the tumor cells were inoculated. The placebo group was immunized with the same frequency as the immunized one. The former group received a mixture of Montanide ISA 51 VG/VSSP. The curve comparison was made using the Kruskal Wallis test. Different letters denote significant differences ($p<0,05$).

Although routine prostate cancer immunotherapy refer to those interventions related to the use of specific TAA or cell based vaccines, and GnRH vaccines are considered just as hormonal ablation therapy; the introduction of powerful adjuvant as part of the GnRH vaccines open the possibility to works at the same time as enhancers of antigen spreading and DC stimulation and suppression of T regs cell population. Additionally there are published results (Nesslinger et al, 2007), that argue that castration alone is capable of inducing antibodies against tumor in both, animal models and in humans as a result of efficient presentation of tumor antigens obtained from apoptotic bodies.

In the case of the vaccine candidate under study, which has the powerful components, Montanide ISA 51 and VSSP, we hypothesized that the apoptotic bodies resulting from testosterone ablation of prostate cancer cells in the presence of the "danger" signals produced by VSSP through TLR 2 and 6 in a context of the inflammatory enviroment, produce an immunological spreading of specific CTL that recognizes the most representative TAA. Similarly, a specific humoral response against tumor antigens can be reached contributing to a better antitumoral effect (Nesslinger et al, 2007). These aspects must be studied in depth in new preclinical and clinical studies to characterize a more efficient vaccine candidate GnRHm1-TT/Montanide ISA 51/VSSP as an advantageous alternative for the treatment of prostate cancer. In Clinical setting an important milestone of the trial was to demonstrate the safety of this candidate. As evidence of vaccine efficacy, recently the GnRHm1-TT/Montanide ISA 51/VSSP candidate (Heberprovac), have been employed in a Phase I clinical trial in advanced prostate cancer patients. The vaccine was well tolerated and no important side effects were detected. As results of immunization, all the 6 patients that concluded the treatment developed anti GnRH antibodies and had depleted the testosterone until castration levels and, in concordance normalized their PSA values. After 4 year of clinical and haematological follow up of the clinical trial, 5/6 patients are alive and keep a favourable clinical picture and normal PSA behaviour.

9. Concluding remarks

Therapeutic cancer vaccines have been in use for several years now. At the beginning, with disappointing results, but after many attempts our understanding growth in the sense of figuring out how the immune system works. This knowledge permitted the successful development of more potent vaccines and other immunotherapeutic agents that are currently in advanced clinical trial or registered as Sipuleucel-T.

GnRH-based vaccines represent a promising anti-hormonal treatment alternative in prostate cancer, because these can reduce serum testosterone to castrate levels, avoid the "hot flushes" produced by GnRH analogues and can be administered in acute and complicated forms of prostate cancer.

Although regularly prostate cancer immunotherapy refer to those interventions related with the use of specific TAA or cell based vaccines, the introduction of powerful adjuvants as part of the GnRH vaccines enables them to work similarly as enhancers of antigen spreading and DC stimulation and immune response modulation.

The development of the vaccine candidate GnRHm1-TT have as main invention the substitution of L-glycine in position 6 of the GnRH molecule by the amino acid L-proline and the addition of a T helper epitope of TT (Bringas et al, 2000) and the use of the

Montanide ISA 51/VSSP adjuvant combination in order to improve the immunogenicity and antitumoral effects of such vaccine. Additionally, it is supposed that the vaccine candidate GnRHm1-TT/Montanide/VSSP take advantage of the tumor apoptosis produced by the testosterone ablation and the special conditions available with the use of the VSSP adjuvant to stimulate a successful antigen presentation to DC and a prominent immunological spreading of effector T cell directed to prostate TAA. Additionally as Nesslinger states, castration alone is capable of inducing antibodies against tumor in both, animal models and in humans as a result of efficient presentation of tumor antigens obtained from apoptotic bodies. (Nesslinger et al, 2010).

In this context, we consider GnRH vaccine like GnRHm1-TT/Montanide/VSSP to represent a powerful weapon that could be employed by uro-oncologist to control the course of prostate cancer toward the CRPC.

10. Acknowledgments

The authors acknowledge Dr. Peter Peschke, at DKFZ, Heidelberg, Germany, Dr. Brad Nelson at DRC BCCRC at Vancouver island, Canada and Dr. Robert Millar MRC Human Reproductive Sciences Unit, Edinburgh, UK for their support of this study.

We specially thanks the Union for International Cancer Control (UICC) and Deutscher Akademischer Austausch Dienst (DAAD), Germany, for the fellowships and support to carry out this work. We also are thankful to Lic. Orestes Padrón Yordi for the manuscript revision.

11. References

[1] Ambrosino DM, Bolon D, Collard H, Van Etten R, Kanchana MV, Finberg RW. Effect of Haemophilus influenzae polysaccharide outer membrane protein complex conjugate vaccine on macrophages. J Immunol 1992; 149:3978-83.

[2] Andersen BM. Endotoxin releases from Neisseria Meningitides. Relationship between key bacterial characteristics and meningococal disease. Scand J Infect Dis Suppl 1989; 64:1-43.

[3] Aragon-Ching JB, Williams KM, Gulley JL. Impact of androgen-deprivation therapy on the immune system: implications for combination therapy of prostate cancer. Front Biosci 2007;12:4957-71.

[4] Bavarian Nordic Receives Special Protocol Assessment Agreement from the FDA for Phase 3 Trial of PROSTVAC®. Accessed: April 2011; Available from: http://www.bavariannordic. com/investor/announcements/2010-40.aspx

[5] Becker JT, Olson BM, Johnson LE, Davies JG, Dunphy EJ, McNeel DG. DNA vaccine encoding prostatic acid phosphatase (PAP) elicits long-term T-cell responses in patients with recurrent prostate cancer. J Immunother 2010;33(6):639-47.

[6] Bennett, B., Check, I.J., Olsen, M.R., Hunter, R.L., 1992. A comparison of commercially available adjuvants for use in research. J. Immunol. Methods, 153: 31-40.

[7] Bizzini B y Achour A. "Kinoids": the basis for anticytokine immunization and their use in HIV infection. Cell. Mol. Biol 1995; 41: 351–356.

[8] Bringas R, Basulto R, Reyes O. De la Fuente J. Vaccine preparation for reversible mammals immunocastration 2000. PCT patent N0. A61K37/38, C07K 7/00.

[9] Burch PA, Breen JK, Buckner JC, Gastineau DA, Kaur JA, Laus RL, Padley DJ, Peshwa MV, Pilot HC, Richardson RL, Smits BJ, Sopapapan P, Strang G, Valone FH, Vuk-Pavlovic S. Priming tissue specific cellualr immunity in a phase I trial of autologous dendritic cells for prostate cancer. Clin Cancer Res 2000; 6:2175-82.
[10] Cancer statistics. CA Cancer J Clin 2008; 58: 71-96.
[11] Canene-Adams K, Lindshield BL, Wang S, Jeffery EH, Clinton SK, Erdman JW. Combinations of tomato and broccoli enhance antitumor activity in dunning r3327-h prostate adenocarcinomas.. Jr. Cancer Res. 2007; 7(2):836-43.
[12] Casper RF. Clinical uses of gonadotropin-releasing hormone analogues. Can Med Assoc J 1991; 144:53–158.
[13] Cereda V, Poole DJ, Palena C, Das S, Bera TK, Remondo C, et al. New gene expressed in prostate: a potential target for T cell-mediated prostate cancer immunotherapy. Cancer Immunol Immunother 2010;59(1):63-71.
[14] Cho H, Ackerstaff E, Carlin S, Lupu ME, Wang Y, Rizwan A, O'Donoghue J, Ling CC, Humm JL, Zanzonico PB, Koutcher JA. Neoplasia 2009; 11(3):247-59.
[15] Cook T, Sheridan WP. Development of GnRH antagonists for prostate cancer: New approaches to treatment. Oncologist 2001; 5:162–168.
[16] Culig Z, Steiner H, Bartsch G and Hobisch A. Mechanisms of endocrine therapy-responsive and-unresponsive prostate tumors. Endocrine-Related Cancer 2005; 12:229-244.
[17] De Marzo A.M, Nelson W.G, Isaacs W.B, and Eptein J.I. Pathologic and molecular aspects of prostate cancer. Lancet 2003; 361:955-964.
[18] Diwan M, Dawar H and Talwar GP (1998) Induction of early and bioeffective antibody response in rodents with the anti LHRH vaccine given as a single dose in biodegradable microspheres along with alum. Prostate 35,279–284.
[19] Drake CG, Doody AD, Mihalyo MA, Huang CT, Kelleher E, Ravi S, et al. Androgen ablation mitigates tolerance to a prostate/prostate cancer-restricted antigen. Cancer Cell 2005;7(3):239-49.
[20] Epel M, Carmi I, Soueid-Baumgarten S, Oh SK, Bera T, Pastan I, et al. Targeting TARP, a novel breast and prostate tumor-associated antigen, with T cell receptor-like human recombinant antibodies. Eur J Immunol 2008;38(6):1706-20.
[21] Ferro VA, Costa R, Carter KC, Harvey MJ, Waterston MM, Mullen AB, Matschke C, Mann JF, Colston A and Stimson WH (2004) Immune responses to a GnRH-based anti-fertility immunogen, induced by different adjuvants and subsequent effect on vaccine efficacy. Vaccine 22,1024–1031.
[22] Ferro, V.A, O'Grady, J.E., Notman, J, Stimson, W.H. An investigation into the immunogenicity of a GnRH analogue in male rats: a comparison of the toxicity of various adjuvants used in conjuction with GnRH glycys. Vaccine 1996; 14: 451-457.
[23] Ferro, V.A., Stimson,.W.H,. Investigation into suitable carrier molecules for use in an anti-gonadotrophin releasing hormone vaccine. Vaccine 1998; 16: 1095-1102.
[24] Finstad C.L, Wang C.Y, Kowalsky J, Zhang M, Li M, Li X, Xia W, Bosland M, Murthy k.k, Walfield A, Koff W.C, Zamb T.J. Synthetic luteinizing hormone releasing hormone (LHRH) vaccine for effective androgen deprivation and its application to prostate cancer immunotherapy. Vaccine 2004; 22:1300-1313.

[25] Fishman M. A changing world for DCvax: a PSMA loaded autologous dendritic cell estrogen by anastrozole enhances the severity of experimental polyarthritis. Exp Gerontol 2009;44(6-7):398-405

[26] Fong L, Small EJ. Anti-cytotoxic T-lymphocyte antigen-4 antibody: the first in an Matzinger P. Essay 1: the danger model in its historical context. Scand J Immunol 2001; 54:4–9.

[27] Forsthuber T, Yip HC, Lehmann PV. Induction of TH1 and TH2 immunity in neonatal mice. Science 1996; 271:1728-30.

[28] Freedland SJ, Hotaling JM, Fitzsimons NJ, Presti JC, Jr., Kane CJ, Terris MK, et al. PSA in the new millennium: a powerful predictor of prostate cancer prognosis and radical prostatectomy outcomes--results from the SEARCH database. Eur Urol 2008;53(4):758-64;discussion 65-6.

[29] Friederike F, Heinen T, Wunderlich FT, Yogev N, Buch T, Roers A, Betelli E, Muller W, Anderton S, Waisman A. Tolerance without clonal expansion: A self -antigen-expressing B cell program self reactive T cells for future deletion. The journal of immunology 2008; 181:5748-5769.

[30] Goodnow C. C., Brink R., Adams E. Breakdown of self tolerance in anergic B Lymphocytes. Nature 1991, 532-536.

[31] Goubau S, Silversides D.W, Gonzalez A, Laarveld B, Mapletoft, R.J, Murphy B.D. Immunisation of sheep against modified peptides of gonadotropin releasing hormone conjugated to carriers. Domest. Anim. Endocrinol 1989; 6: 339-347.

[32] Gupta JC, Raina K, Talwar GP, Verma R and Khanna N (2004) Engineering,cloning and expression of genes encoding the ultimeric luteinising- hormone-releasing-hormone linked to T-cell determinants in *Escherichia coli*.Protein Express Purif 37,1-7.

[33] HoskinsonR.M, Rigby R.D, Mattner P.E, Huynh V.L, D'Occhio M, Neish A, Trigg T.E, Moss B.A, Lindsey M.J, Coleman G.D, Schwartzkoff C.L. Vaxtrate®: an anti-reproductive vaccine for cattle. Aust. J. Biotechnol 1990; 4: 166-170.

[34] Hsu CT, Ting CY, Ting CJ, Chen TY, Lin CP, Whang-Peng J and Hwang J (2000) Vaccination against gonadotropin-releasing hormone (GnRH) using toxin receptor-binding domain-conjugated GnRH repeats. Cancer Res 60,3701–3705.

[35] Isaacs J .T, Lundmo P.I, Berges R, Martikainen P, Kyprianou N, English H .F. Androgen regulation of programmed death of normal and malignant prostatic cells. 1992. Journal of andrology 1992; 13(6):457-64.

[36] Isaacs J.T, Isaacs W.B, Feitz W.F, Scheres J. Establishment and characterization of seven Dunning rat prostatic cancer cell lines and their use in developing methods for predicting metastatic abilities of prostatic cancer. Prostate 1986; 9:261-81.

[37] Isaacs JT, Heston WD, Weisman RM, Coffey DS. Animal models of the hormone-sensitive prostatic adenocarcinomas, Dunning R-3327-H, R-3327-HI, and R-3327-AT. Cancer Res 1978; 38:4353-4359.

[38] Jeannin P, Renno T, Goetsch L, Miconnet I, Aubry J.P, Deineste Y. et al. OmpA targets dendritic cells, induces their maturation and deliver antigen into the MHC class I presentation pathway. Nat Immunol 2000; 6:502-9.

[39] Jinshu Xu, Zheng Zhu, Peng Duan, Wenjia Li, Yin Zhang,Jie Wu, Zhuoyi Hu, Rouel, Roque , Jingjing L. Cloning, expression, and puriWcation of a highly immunogenic

recombinant gonadotropin-releasing hormone (GnRH) chimeric peptide. Protein Expression and PuriWcation 50 (2006) 163–170.
[40] Kabalin, J.M., et al.. Unsuspected adenocarcinoma of the prostate in patients undergoing cystoprostatectomy for other causes: Incidence, histology and morphometric observations. J. Urol 1989; 141:1091-1094.
[41] Kantoff PW, Higano CS, Shore ND, Berger ER, Small EJ, Penson DF, et al. Sipuleucel-T immunotherapy for castration-resistant prostate cancer. N Engl J Med 2010;363(5):411-22.
[42] Kiyma, Z., Adams, T.E., Hess, B.W., Riley, M.L., Murdoch, W.J., Moss, G.E, 2000. Gonadal function, sexual behavior, feedlot performance, and carcass traits of ram lambs actively immunized against GnRH. Journal of Animal Science 78: 2237-2243.
[43] Ladd A, Tsong YY, Lok J and Thau RB (1990) Active immunization against LHRH: Effects of conjugation site and dose. Am J eprod Immunol Microbiol 22,56–63.
[44] Li Yu, Zhong-Fang Zhang, Chun-Xia Jing, Feng-Lin Wu. Intraperitoneal administration of gonadotropin-releasing hormone-PE40 induces castration in male rats. *World J Gastroenterol* 2008; 14(13): 2106-2109.
[45] Madan RA, Arlen PM, Mohebtash M, Hodge JW, Gulley JL. Prostvac-VF: a vectorbased vaccine targeting PSA in prostate cancer. Expert Opin Investig Drugs 2009;18(7):1001-11.
[46] Maeda H, Nagata S, Wolfgang CD, Bratthauer GL, Bera TK, Pastan I. The T cell Receptor gamma chain alternate reading frame protein (TARP), a prostate-specific protein localized in mitochondria. J Biol Chem 2004;279(23):24561-8.
[47] Manns J.G, Robbins S.R. Prevention of boar taint with a recombinant based GnRH vaccine. In: Bonneau, M., Lundström, K. and Malmfors, B. (Eds.) Boar taint in entire male pigs. Wageningen Pers, Wageningen 1997; 92:137-140.
[48] McKee AS, MackLeod KL, Kappler JW, Marrack P. Immune mechanism of protection: Can adjuvants rise to the chalenge? BMC Biology 2010; 8:37, 1-10.
[49] Mercader M, Bodner BK, Moser MT, Kwon PS, Park ES, Manecke RG, et al. T cell infiltration of the prostate induced by androgen withdrawal in patients with prostate cancer. Proc Natl Acad Sci U S A 2001;98(25):14565-70.
[50] Millar R.P, Pawson A.J, Morgan K, Emilie F, Rissman E.F. Zi-Liang Lu. Diversity of actions of GnRHs mediated by ligand-induced selective signaling. Frontiers in Neuroendocrinology 2008; 29:17–35.
[51] Miller, L.A., Johns, B.E., Killian, G.J., 2000. Immunocontraception of white-tailed deer with GnRH vaccine. Am. J. Reprod. Immunol. 44: 266-274.
[52] Nesslinger N.J, Sahota R.A, Stone B, Johnson K, Chima N, King C, Rasmusen D, Bishop D, Rennie P.S, Gleave M, Blood P, Pai H, et al. Standard treatments induce antigen specific immune responses in prostate cancer. Clin Cancer Res 2007; 13: 1493-502.
[53] Nesslinger NJ, Ng A, Tsang KY, Ferrara T, Schlom J, Gulley JL, et al. A viral vaccine encoding prostate-specific antigen induces antigen spreading to a common set of self-proteins in prostate cancer patients. Clin Cancer Res 2010;16(15):4046-56.
[54] Nestle FO, Alijagic S, Gilliet M, Sun Y, Grabbe S, Dummer R, Burg G, Schadendorf D. Vaccination of melanoma patients with peptide- or tumor lysate-pulsed dendritic cells. Nat Med 1998; 4:328-32.

[55] Parkinson R.J, Simms M.S, Broome P, Humphreys J.E, Bishop M.C. A vaccination strategy for the long-term suppression of androgens in advanced prostate cancer. Eur. Urol 2004; 45: 171-175.
[56] Patients: long-term results. J Urol 2004;172(3):910-4. 2008;26(32):5275-83.
[57] Peschke P, Karger CP, Scholz M, Debus J, Huber PE. Relative biological effectiveness of carbon ions for local tumor control of a radioresistant prostate carcinoma in the rat.. Int J Radiat Oncol Biol Phys 2011; 79(1):239-46.
[58] Phase 3 Study of Immunotherapy to Treat Advanced Prostate Cancer. Accessed: April 2011; Available from: http://www.clinicaltrials.gov/ct2/show/NCT01057810?term=NCT01057810&rank=1.
[59] Pienta K.J, and Brandley D. Mechanisms underlaying the androgen-independent prostate cancer. Clin. Can. Res 2006; 12:1665-1671.
[60] Raina K, Panda AK, Ali MM and Talwar GP (2004) Purification, refolding,and characterization of recombinant LHRH-T multimer. Protein Express Purif 37,8–17.
[61] Rini B. Recent clinical development of dendritic cell-based immunotherapy for prostate cancer. Expert Opin Biol Ther 2004; (11):1729-1734.
[62] Robbins S.C, Jelinski M.D, Stotish R.L. Assessment of the immunological and biological efficacy of two different doses of a recombinant GnRH vaccine in domestic male and female cats (Felis catus). J. Reprod. Immunol 2004; 64: 107-119.
[63] Roehl KA, Han M, Ramos CG, Antenor JA, Catalona WJ. Cancer progression and
[64] Russel DW, Wilson J.D. 5 alpha reductase: Two genes/to enzimes. Annu Rev Biochem 1994; 63:25-61.
[65] Sacker W.A, et al. Age and racial distribution of prostatic intraepithelial neoplasia. Eur. Urol 1996; 30:138-144.
[66] Sad S, Gupta H.M, Talwar G.P, Raghupathy R. Carrier induced suppression of the antibody response to self hapten. Immunlogy 1991; 74:223-7.
[67] Silversides D.W, Allen A.F, Misra V, Qualtiere L, Mapletoft R.J, Murphy B.D. A synthetic luteinizing hormone releasing hormone vaccine I. Conjugation and specificity trials in BALB/c mice. J. Reprod. Immunol 1988; 13: 249-261.
[68] Simms M.S, Scholfield D.P, Jacobs E, Michaeli D, Broome P, Humphreys J.E, Bishop M.C. Anti-GnRH antibodies can induce castrate levels of testosterone in patients with advanced prostate cancer. Br. J. Cancer 2000; 83: 443-446.
[69] Small EJ, Tchekmedyian NS, Rini BI, Fong L, Lowy I, Allison JP. A pilot trial of CTLA-4 blockade with human anti-CTLA-4 in patients with hormone-refractory prostate cancer. ClinCancer Res 2007;13(6):1810-5.
[70] Sutherland JS, Goldberg GL, Hammett MV, Uldrich AP, Berzins SP, Heng TS, et al. Activation of thymic regeneration in mice and humans following androgen blockade. J Immunol 2005;175(4):2741-53.
[71] Talwar G.P, Diwan M, Dawar H, Frick J, Sharma S.K, Wadhwa S.N.. Counter GnRH vaccine. In: M. Rajalakshmi and P.D. Griffin (Editors). Proceedings of the Symposium on 'Male Contraception: present and future. New Delhi 1995: 309-318.
[72] Talwar G.P, Raina K, Gupta J.C, Ray R, Wadhwa S, Ali M.M. A recombinant luteinising-hormone-releasing hormone immunogen bioeffective in causing prostatic atrophy. Vaccine 2004; 22:3713-3721.
[73] Talwar G.P. Vaccines for control of fertility and hormone-dependent cancers. Immunology and Cell Biology 1997; 75:184–189.

[74] Tannock I.F, et al. Docetaxel plus prednisone or mitoxantrone plus prednisone for advanced prostate cancer. N. Engl. J. Med 2004; 351:1502-1512.
[75] Udono H, Srivastava P.K. Heat shock protein 70-associated peptides elicit specific cancer immunity. J Exp Med 1993; 178:1391-6.
[76] Vaccine for prostate cancer. Expert Opin Biol Ther 2009;9(12):1565-75.
[77] W.G. Prostate cancer prevention. Curr. Opin. Urol 2007; 17:157-167.
[78] Wang J, Zhang Q, Jin S, Feng M, Kang X, Zhao S, et al. Immoderate inhibition of
[79] Weisbart R.H, Golde D.W, Clarck S.C, Wong G.G, Gasson J.C. Human GMCSG is a neutrofil activator. Nature 1985; 314:361-3.
[80] Yu L, Wang L, Wang H and JW Xuan. Application of Gleason analogous grading system and flow cytometry DNA analysis in a novel knock-in mouse prostate cancer model. Postgrad. Med. J 2006; 82: 40-45.
[81] Zeng W, Ghosh S, Lau YF, Brown LE and Jackson DC (2002) Highly immunogenicand totally synthetic lipopeptides as self-adjuvanting immunocontraceptive vaccines. J Immunol 169,4905–4912.
[82] Zollinger W.D. New and improved vaccines against meningococal disease. In: Woodrow GC, Levine MM, editors. New generation vaccines. Marcel Dekker: NY 1990; 325-48.

5

Immune-Therapy in Cutaneous Melanoma – Efficacy Immune Markers

Monica Neagu and Carolina Constantin
"Victor Babes" National Institute of Pathology, Splaiul Independentei, Bucharest, Romania

1. Introduction

The chapter presents updated results of immune-therapy in cutaneous melanoma in the light of the well-known resistance of this disease and the unrelenting efforts in overcoming it. The types of immune-therapy are correlated intrinsically with the efficacy immune-markers utilized for thorough monitoring of treated patients.

This life threatening disease has a recently reported increased incidence; in the United States, this continues to rise from 4% to 6% annually, despite steps towards primary prevention. Similar increases are being noted worldwide. It has been estimated that the current lifetime risk for developing invasive melanoma is 1 in 58 and it has been reported that over 8,000 Americans died of melanoma in 2009 (Rigel, 2010). These statistics highlight the need to find both new efficient therapies and improved markers for predicting disease evolution and therapy monitoring.

Immune markers related to therapy monitoring are an important field for at least two reasons: the lack of good clinical responses in immune-therapy and the need for accumulating knowledge regarding the molecular processes that governate tumour progression (Riker et al., 2006). The intent of this chapter is to describe the immune-therapies approaches in the intimate link with the immune markers as therapy efficacy monitoring. Immune monitoring is valuable not only for efficacy purposes but also for immune-tailored individualized therapy.

2. Immune therapy – The ultimate solution in cutaneous melanoma?

Up to date immunotherapy approaches that are in the stage of clinical development include: cytokines (IL-2, IFN, TNF, IL-7, IL-12, IL-21), cytokine-antibody fusion proteins or immunocytokines, whole tumour cell vaccines, genetically modified tumour cells, heat shock protein vaccines, peptide vaccines, dendritic cells pulsed with tumour antigens, tumour antigen-naked DNA vectors, recombinant viral vectors, adoptive transfer of cloned tumour antigen-specific T cells, Toll-like receptor ligands, antagonistic antibodies to

Cytotoxic T Lymphocyte-Associated Antigen 4 (CTLA-4), activating antibodies that target CD40 and CD137.

All the therapeutical approaches seek to induce cytotoxic T-cell responses to tumours ranging from mono-specific immunotherapy, targeting only one specific tumour antigen, to polyvalent immunotherapy, which attempts to induce immune responses to multiple antigenic components, to gene-based therapy, which manipulates the immunogenicity of the tumour. Each of these therapies' goal is to induce proliferation and differentiation of anti-tumoral antigen-specific memory T-cells.

The FDA approved immune therapies for cutaneous melanoma comprise: IL-2, IFN and the most recent anti-CTL-4.

2.1 Immune therapy and Immune markers

There are still no validated immune markers to be used in monitoring immune-therapy in cutaneous melanoma, although it is the domain that would benefit the most from immune monitoring biomarkers and that surrogate immunologic markers of efficacy have not been reported thus far.

One of the most used immune-marker in cutaneous melanoma is the "immune cell". As an established disease with a high immune-suppressive background, peripheral immune cells were quantified both in relation to the monitoring of the patients immune status, and in therapy efficacy monitoring. We have previously published that peripheral blood CD4+/CD8+ ratio can monitor a good therapeutic response and that monitoring the dynamics of this subpopulations ratio can detect a good therapeutical response (Neagu et al., 2010). In the first reported study of high-risk melanoma patients immunized with gp100 and tyrosinase peptides (Cassarino et al., 2006) no difference in nevi tissue was found regarding CD3, CD4, CD8, MHC-I, MHC-II, CD1a, HMB-45, MART-1, tyrosinase, but an increase in p53 and bcl-2 staining, in the nevi post-treatment has been found. Authors explain that activating melanoma-specific T cells for preventing melanoma recurrence a response mediated by p53 and bcl-2 is triggered in benign melanocytes (Cassarino et al., 2006). Another group showed that following transcutaneous delivery, gp100 vaccination activates Langerhans cell and antibody production, markers of definitely immune activation (Frankenburg et al., 2007).

In a phase I/II trial for melanoma vaccine comprising six melanoma-associated peptides (MAGE proteins, MART-1/MelanA, gp100, and tyrosinase), patients' follow-up was performed using the *in vitro* proliferation of CD4+ lymphocytes. After vaccination, the monitoring of a good response was marked by an increased proliferation of T cells to relevant peptides in over 80% of patients correlated with good clinical response as well (Slingluff et al., 2008). Another study enrolling stage III/IV melanoma patients showed the data regarding patients vaccinated with Melan-A/Mart-1 peptide and Klebsiella outer membrane protein p40 as an adjuvant. In this trial the therapy was monitored by *ex vivo* analysis of Melan-A/Mart-1 specific CD8 T cells. Increased percentages of T cells, memory/effector T cell differentiation, positive IFN-gamma and antibody responses to p40 were observed in all patients and positive clinical response in half of the treated patients (Lienard et al., 2009).

3. Immune-therapy – *Ups and downs*

Each of the immunosuppressive mechanisms that underlie cutaneous melanoma development can be a target for clinical manipulation and it is obvious that immune-related parameters are useful in immunotherapy monitoring of the melanoma.

3.1 Immunomodulatory antibodies

Therapeutic antibodies induce cellular/complement-dependent cytotoxicity against tumour cells, or can modify immune responses by blocking the inhibitory signal pathways or stimulating the excitatory signal pathways.

The surface molecules involved in this type of therapy are CD28, CTLA-4 (CD152), Toll-like receptor and many more. Both clinical and preclinical data indicate that CTLA-4 blockade using anti-CTL-4 antibodies results in direct activation of CD4+ and CD8+ effector cells in melanoma. Immune cells as parameters for immune-therapy efficacy should be evaluated in terms of progression-free survival and overall survival.

In a very comprehensive recent paper (Joel et al., 2010) it was demonstrated that the receptors for the Fc region of the antibodies FcγR (FcγRIIB) expresed by the tumour act as „decoy receptors", binding the IgGs that have an anti-melanoma action. Through this mechanism, the Fc recognition by the effector cells is hindered and the tumour escapes the immune effectors and can evolve toward metastasis. This group demonstrated that FcγRIIB inhibits *in vitro* antibody dependent cell cytotoxicity. It seems that FcγR suffer a selection process during the metastasis and that if the cutaneous melanoma evolves, their expression increase in the liver or in the lymph nodes. The FcR action is described in its dual mode as follows: FcγRIIB1 are not detected in melanocytes and have a low expression in primary tumours, while FcγRIIB1 is highly expressed in metastatic tumours in spleen and lymph nodes (Cassard et al., 2008). Knowing the potential of these receptors to modulate the immune response, therapeutic antibodies with an optimized Fc region can trigger an increased Antibody-Dependent Cell-Mediated Cytotoxicity (ADCC), Antibody Dependent Cell Phagocytosis (ADCP) and Complement Dependant Cytotoxicity (CDC). The authors propose (Joel et al., 2010) to lower the Fc binding capacity to the FcγRIIB and to increase Fc binding to FcγRIIIA and FcγRI. It is of high probability that these improvements could trigger an enhanced efficiency of therapeutical anti-melanoma antibodies.

3.1.1 Targeting cytotoxic T-lymphocyte antigen-4

Cytotoxic T lymphocyte-associated antigen 4 (CTLA-4) is expressed by activated T cells and a subset of regulatory T cells being a co-inhibitory molecule. Its physiological role is to maintain an immune homeostasis by limiting T cell responses and inducing tolerance to self (Yuan et al., 2008). CTLA-4 has binding affinity for the B7 surface molecules of antigen-presenting cell (APC), its affinity exceeding that of CD28. The binding induces T-cell anergy and inhibits secretion of mainly IL-2. When CD28 is bound, costimulatory pathways are triggered and T-cell proliferation and IL-2 production are enhanced (Weber, 2008). Therefore, this type of cell has a crucial negative role in the development of cutaneous melanoma.

Antibodies targeting CTLA-4, in their therapeutical form of ipilimumab and tremelimumab, have proven good clinical results. From early-phase clinical trials anti-CTLA-4 antibodies showed good results in melanoma and manageable toxicities. Then in phase II overall and long-term survival were increased in combined or in individual therapies (Tarhini et al., 2010). Recently published results from a phase III clinical trial (ClinicalTrials.gov number, NCT00324155) (Robert et al, 2011) performed in several centres and institutes showed that in untreated metastatic melanoma overall survival of patients receiving ipilimumab plus dacarbazine was significantly longer compared to the other arms of the clinical trial. Side effects did not occur in the ipilimumab-dacarbazine group. This year, FDA approved ipilimumab and it was considered the „major breakthrough" in cancer immunotherapy.

Side effects in anti-CTLA-4 therapy are named "immune-related adverse events" (irAEs). IrAEs mainly include digestive related negative effects, dermatitis, hepatitis and endocrinopathies, among other occasionally reported ones. It is clear that irAEs are the direct consequence of CTLA-4 blockade but can be managed by the physician (Phan et al., 2008; Di Giacomo et al., 2010).

The markers involved in this type of immunotherapy are several and compile both soluble/circulatory and tissue related groups. Therefore, anti-CTLA-4 treatment was monitored through Treg evaluation (Menard et al., 2008). After this therapy, the effector and memory CD4+ and CD8+ T-cell pool and TCR-dependent T-cell proliferation were restored. In this case, free survival and overall survival were directly correlated with the resistance of peripheral lymphocytes to Treg-inhibitory effects (Menard et al., 2008). The authors state that the biological activity marker of memory T-cell resistance to Treg resulting from anti-CTLA-4 treatment is a good efficacy marker (Langer et al., 2007). At the tissue level, after anti-CTL4 treatment diffuse intra-tumoral infiltrates of CD8+ T cells correlated with good clinical outcome of the patients. Moreover patients with regressing tumours had an increased frequency of CD8+ cells with/without a concomitant increase in CD4+ cells (Neagu et al., 2010).

Immunomodulatory therapy in melanoma needs thorough efficacy monitoring in both circulatory and tissue immune markers.

3.2 Dendritic cell therapy

Skin's immune system has several cellular components, mainly regulatory T cells, natural killer T cells (NKT), and distinct subsets of immature and mature dendritic cells (DCs). All these cellular components comprise the immunosuppressive network (Rabinovitch et al., 2007). DCs are more therapy tools than actual immune-markers. The reason is that DC release large quantities of dexosomes, their function being the transfer of antigen-loaded MHC class I / II and other associated molecules, to naive DC potentially leading to the amplification of the cellular immune response (Delcayre et al, 2005). Few years ago, using these DC "products" - dexosomes, two phases I clinical studies were published. In these studies, the monitoring was performed using T and NK cells as markers for cellular immune responses (Escudier et al., 2005; Hao et al., 2006). Dexosomes (Dex) are stable and carry defined proteins and lipids that can be standardized. The authors report that they could generate 10 vaccines of NK cell-stimulating Dexosomes. Using these dexosomes, melanoma patients can be boosted for DC-mediated T- and NK-cell responses (Viaud et al., 2010).

One of the first pilot trials using DC pulsed with autologous tumour lysate has shown that among all the advanced cancer patients entering the study one melanoma patient with extended metastases had a partial response lasting 8 months, while seven patients were stable for more than 3 months, and 7 had progression of the disease. Dendritic cells immune-therapy can induce a cell-mediated antitumour immune response in patients giving good clinical outcome (Mayordomo et al., 2007). In another study, isolated DCs were activated with CD40L, loaded with antigenic melanoma peptides and then injected into patients with resected melanoma. The patients were monitored for antigen-specific immune responses, namely skin reactions to peptides alone or peptide-pulsed DCs and circulating T-cells responses (Davis et al., 2006).

When vaccinated with DC, clinical investigators monitor the efficacy by the presence of vaccine-related tumour antigen-specific T cells in delayed type hypersensitivity (DTH) skin biopsies, in correlation to the clinical outcome. Punch biopsies taken from positive DTH sites proved clusters of CD2+ and CD3+ infiltrating cells, out of which over 50% were CD4+, the rest being CD8+ T cells (Aarntzen et al, 2008).

It seems that there is an effervescent period of publication on dendritic cell therapy in cutaneous melanoma, but all the papers underlie some crucial points in using DC therapies. When using *ex vivo* generated DC, the effective migration of DCs to the T-cell areas in the lymph node is necessary; therefore, adding inflammatory cytokines would be beneficial (Aarntzen et al, 2008). Moreover, the addition of synergistic immunomodulatory agents to enhance immunogenicity (Erdmann & Schuler-Thurner, 2008) can enhance the clinical response.

Monitoring the DC therapy comprises several steps to be taken. The inoculated DCs have to be monitored for their migratory potential to the tumour site. It is commonly agreed on the efficacy monitoring of the vaccine by detecting T-cell responses in vaccinated patients using biopsies derived from DTH sites in good correlation with the clinical outcome in melanoma patients (Aarntzen et al, 2008).

3.3 Vaccines with melanoma antigens

The processes that induce effective antitumour immunity by cancer vaccines implie several events: antigen delivery to antigen-presenting cells, migration of dendritic cells that carry the processed antigen to draining lymph nodes, antigen presentation to circulating T cells that enter the lymph nodes through the high endothelial venules, expansion of antigen reactive T-cells in the lymph nodes, dissemination of specific T-cells to tumour site, and tumour destruction by activated tumour-reactive T-cells (Slingluff Jr et al., 2008).

The vaccines that were built until now against melanoma are based on strategies for activating the protective immunity by Tregs depletion and blockade of T-cell inhibitory molecules such as CTLA-4. All these approaches have developed multiple new proteomic/genomic tools to monitor immune responses in vaccinated patients. Several published clinical trials emphasized that melanoma antigen vaccination should be monitored using peripheral immune cells as the principal parameter. Some types of vaccination with melanoma-associated antigens will be highlighted in this section.

Developing cancer vaccines implies complex monitoring of the immune responses. Firstly, the efficacy of the vaccine in inducing/augmenting a specific T-cell response has to be tested. Secondly, the spontaneous tumour-directed immune responses, the functional characteristics of T-cell responses and, last but not least, the relationship between immune monitoring assay results and clinical end points have to be evaluated (Neagu et al, 2010).

Giving a three decades view on cutaneous melanoma vaccination, important points have been highlighted (Sondak et al., 2006). Some of the vaccines, in late stages of clinical trials were discontinued due to regulatory and commercialization technicalities. Vaccines from autologous samples are reduced to patient groups still having accessible, surgically removable and sufficient tumour tissue for a complete treatment. Vaccines of allogeneic source can have common antigens, but they can lack the actual individual molecular particularities of an autologous tumour (Sondak et al., 2006).

In a review of the National Cancer Institute's experience with 440 patients (mostly melanoma patients) receiving 541 different vaccines, only 4 complete and 9 partial responses were seen, for an overall response rate of 3% (Rosenberg et al., 2004). A randomized comparison of a peptide-pulsed dendritic cell vaccine to the cytostatic agent dacarbazine (DTIC) in patients with advanced melanoma showed similarly low levels of objective response for the vaccine; the median time to progression and a median survival was relatively the same when DTIC alone was used (Rosenberg et al., 2004).

One of the largest randomized clinical trials involving vaccines for the adjuvant therapy of melanoma was published several years ago. The trial compared a GM2 ganglioside vaccine (GMK vaccine, Progenics, Tarrytown, NY) to high-dose IFN in the adjuvant therapy of patients with resected melanoma at high risk of recurrence. In this trial, antibody responses to the vaccinated ganglioside were achieved by many patients. Unfortunately, the overall results were far more better for IFN treatment in both relapse-free and overall survival (Kirkwood et al., 2001, 2004) and the clinical trial was stopped. Then two randomized trials of a polyvalent whole cell melanoma vaccine (Canvaxin, CancerVax, Carlsbad, CA) were performed on patients with resected stage III and IV melanoma (an even higher-risk population than in the aforementioned ganglioside study); they were also stopped early because of a poor vaccine efficacy (Cancer Vax Corporation, 2005).

A different polyvalent melanoma vaccine phase III trial (Melacine, Corixa, Seattle, WA) was conducted in patients with resected stage II melanoma. Analyzing the data, an effect of the vaccine on relapse-free survival (Sosman et al., 2002) and overall survival (Sondak et al., 2004) for vaccine-treated patients expressing HLA antigens (HLA-A2 or HLA-C3) was obtained. This subset of patients (over half of the enrolled patients) was intended to be followed in order to verify the results, probably a follow-up of several years. In the end, the manufacturer of this vaccine simply decided not to support the development of Melacine.

3.3.1 Autologous tumour vaccines

Autologous vaccines derived from the patient's own tumour have the main advantage of containing unique or rare tumour antigens that develop during mutational events. Autologous tumour vaccines are designed as appropriately HLA-matched for optimum antigen presentation to T lymphocytes host. Until recently, no autologous melanoma vaccine had ever been successfully tested in a phase III clinical trial. A phase III clinical trial using heat shock proteins (HSP) extracted from autologous tumour (Oncophage, Antigenics, New York, NY) was developed. In the cell, these proteins act as "chaperones" for peptide antigens and have the potential to present tumour antigens to the immune system (Rivoltini et al., 2003; Lewis, 2004). Even though the preliminary results indicated no statistically significant effect for the heat shock vaccine compared with the physician's choice of therapy, an intriguing observation of this trial is that the group of patients with M1 stage of disease treated with the vaccine, lived longer than those receiving other therapy, although not significant (Antigenics press release, 2005).

3.3.2 Allogeneic vaccines

A different type of vaccine developed in parallel with the previously presented one, are the allogeneic vaccines. These are composed of intact or modified melanoma cells from other patients selected for the presence of shared antigens found on a large percentage of melanomas. Compared with autologous tumour vaccines, the allogeneic ones have significant advantages in terms of availability for patients in all stages of the disease, and providing the capability to administer multiple vaccinations over an extended period. They may also be more naturally recognizable by the patient's immune system than an autologous cell preparation. However, they may lack unique or rare antigens that could be important antigenic targets in any given patient's melanoma.

Canvaxin is a polyvalent irradiated melanoma auto/allo vaccine, originally developed by Dr. Donald Morton and commercially developed by CancerVax in partnership with Serono (Geneva, Switzerland) (Hsueh & Morton, 2003; Motl, 2004). This vaccine has been studied in two multi-centre randomized phase III trials in patients with resected stage III and IV melanoma. Recently, the Data Safety Monitoring Board overseeing these two studies determined that the trials were unlikely to provide efficacious results and the protocols were discontinued. The authors' state that there are multiple reasons for a vaccine to prove its usefulness in earlier stage patients compared with the ones diagnosed in later stage disease (Salazar & Disis, 2005). Firstly, increasing evidence suggests that tumour progression leads to increased immunosuppression mechanisms directly mediated by tumour cells and/or by their microenvironment. The immune suppression is also induced by the presence of increasing numbers of Tregs (Viguier et al., 2004). Moreover, increasing numbers of tumour cells are increasingly likely to express antigenic heterogeneity that would limit the ability of an induced immune response to completely eradicate the tumour (Riker et al., 1999). Finally, in a patient with a relatively high residual tumour burden (patients stage IV melanoma), tumour progression could readily occur during the period required for induction of an immune response post-vaccination. In that case, the vaccination "failure" conclusion is not true as it did not have the chance to even naturally develop. To overcome this, it has been proposed that measuring the T-cell response from lymph nodes draining the cutaneous sites of vaccination could be a sensitive assessment of immunogenicity developed by a melanoma vaccine administration (Slingluff Jr et al., 2008).

Surprisingly, in some studies, induction of T-cell responses is not reliably associated with clinical tumour regression. As an example, vaccination with a modified gp100 peptide led to detectable CTL responses in the peripheral blood in over 90% of patients, but no clinical tumour regressions were observed. In another section of the same study, in which patients were received in addition high-dose of IL-2, there was a noticeable clinical tumour regressions in 41% of patients, but T-cell responses were registered in only a small minority of patients (Rosenberg et al., 1998). Nevertheless, optimization of cancer vaccines will benefit from complex immune monitoring in multiple lymphoid compartments. Critical compartments for immune monitoring are comprising the lymph node as the site of T-cell response induction, the circulating peripheral blood lymphocytes (PBL) and the sites of primary and metastatic tumour as well (Slingluff Jr et al., 2008). Cancer vaccine clinical trials meant to induce T cell - mediated immunity are evaluated routinely by measuring the immune response in the PBL but not in the other two compartments. Some murine and human studies suggest that, even after a single immunization, epidermal Langerhans cells migrate and mature to draining nodes within hours, with a peak of T-cell accumulation in the draining lymph nodes at day 5–10 (Macatonia et al., 1987; Rosato et al., 1996; Yoshizawa et al., 1991). Thus, it has been hypothesized that evaluation of T-cell responses in the draining lymph node would permit a more sensitive measure of immunogenicity than evaluation of T-cell responses in the peripheral blood alone (Slingluff Jr et al., 2008). From patients enrolled in clinical trials of experimental melanoma peptide vaccines, sentinel immunized nodes (SIN) were harvested a week after the third vaccine round, in order to identify the peak time of T-cell accumulation. T-cell responses to defined peptides were detected 25% more often in the SIN compared with PBL. Combining the evaluation of PBL and SIN leads to increased sensitivity in detecting immunogenicity to nearly 75%. Moreover, the T-cell responses in a SIN were detected at a high level, when they were either absent or at low level in both blood and the involved lymph node prior to vaccination (Yamshchikov et al., 2001). This finding supports the continued evaluation of the SIN for monitoring T-cell responses to melanoma peptide vaccination.

The challenges in melanoma vaccination are extensive, but they can be surmounted by a thorough understanding of immune mechanisms and proper guided clinical trials (Sondak et al., 2006). We can add to these relevant conclusions that careful monitoring of anti-tumour T-cell responses, directed toward tumour peptides/proteins/antigens, developing complex monitoring of the patient's immune responses and establishing an intricate relation with clinical end points would definitely add important value to vaccination treatment in melanoma.

3.4 Immune-therapy with cytokines

Using combinations of chemotherapy with cytokines, clinical parameters of patients were improved. All the promising new therapeutic agents have to be related to identification of predictors of response leading towards personalized therapy. IL-2, IFN, IL-12 and other therapeutical combinations were used and monitoring their efficacy was performed using immune markers.

Melanoma is resistant to standard chemotherapy, having a response rate for any single agent or combination of agents of 15% - 25%. Using combinations of chemotherapy, IFN and IL-2 the response rate was improved, but with no clear effect on overall survival (Chapman, 2007).

3.4.1 IL-2

Particularly IL-2 was involved in cutaneous melanoma immune-therapy in the last 20 years. Several years ago, it has been published that over the course of IL-2 based immunotherapy, difficulties associated with the monitoring of anti-tumour immune responses arise (Andersen et al., 2003). A couple of years ago, despite promising phase II data, phase III studies have failed to show meaningful clinical benefit for the combination of cytokines with cytotoxic chemotherapy (Andersen et al., 2003) and now the effort is focused on identifying predictors of therapeutic response, therefore an increased efficacy in term of patients benefit (Atkins, 2006). Following high-dose IL-2 administration, the number and frequency of regulatory T cells (Tregs) were monitored in patients with progressive disease and the values returned to normal in patients with objective clinical responses (Cesana et al., 2006) or the monitoring was performed analyzing pSTAT5 in patient's PBMC (Varker et al., 2006). Investigating patients with intralesional IL-2 treatment authors pointed out an increase in the CD4+/CD8+ ratio and a rise in the percentage of CD25+ cells in the CD4+ population, the majority of this population being activated T cells. The local IL-2 is able to induce a systemic beneficial immunological effect (Green et al, 2008).

There are several studies that combine IL-2 with vaccines or growth factors. Thus when combining IL-2 with Melan-A-specific CTL, an anti-tumour response was elicited and monitored by an elevated frequency of circulating Melan-A + T cells, an increase in eosinophils and a selective loss of Melan-A expression in lymph node metastases without major adverse effects (Makensen et al., 2006). Another phase II clinical trial using a combination of IL-2 with GM-CSF (Elias et al., 2005), showed the DC activation, and an increased IL-2 receptor expression on T cells. The treatment was intended to high-risk melanoma patients and no significant side-effects were registered. Continuing their work (Elias et al., 2008) the same group reported the clinical benefit of using GM-CSF and IL-2 with or without autologous vaccine in patients with resected melanoma. Just recently published, a phase III clinical trial (Schwartzentruber et al., 2011) with melanoma patients diagnosed in stage III and IV (ClinicalTrials.gov number, NCT00019682) receiving IL-2 and gp100 peptide vaccine showed that the response rate was improved and progression-free survival increased when combining these two immune therapeutical agents in comparison to IL-2 administered individually.

3.4.2 IFN

IFN-alpha is one of the most used immune-therapy agent and IFN treatment was demonstrated to significantly prolong relapse-free survival of patients diagnosed in stage IIB-III melanoma. When these patients were subjected to IFN-alpha2b therapy, a significant decrease of serum levels of immunosuppressive / tumour angiogenic/growth stimulatory factors (Vascular Endothelial Cell Growth Factor - VEGF, Epidermal Growth Factor - EGF and hepatocyte growth factor- HGF), increased levels of anti-angiogenic IFN-gamma inducible protein 10 (IP-10) and IFN-alpha along with their good clinical outcome (Yurkovetski et al., 2007) have been noted. As therapeutic monitoring tools, gene microarray analysis of the transcriptional profile of peripheral T cells, NK, and monocytes as a response to IFN-alpha therapy was demonstrated. Authors point out that the transcriptional profiles of PBMCs from IFN-alpha treated patients may be a useful predictor of the *in vivo* response of immune cells to IFN-alpha immunotherapy (Zimmerer et al., 2008).

In a prospective neoadjuvant trial for IFNalpha2b, in which tissue samples were obtained before and after therapy, double immunohistochemistry for pSTAT1 and pSTAT3 was done. The pSTAT1/pSTAT3 ratios were augmented by IFNalpha2b both in melanoma cells and in lymphocytes. Antigen peptide transporter 2, involved in the transport of various molecules across extra- and intra-cellular membranes (TAP2), was augmented by IFNalpha2b (but not TAP1 and MHC class I/II). The authors prove that IFNalpha2b significantly modulates the balance of STAT1/STAT3 in tumour cells and host lymphocytes, mechanisms that lead to the up-regulation of TAP2 and an augmented host antitumour response. The baseline of pSTAT1/pSTAT3 ratio in tumour cells may serve as a useful predictor of the therapeutic effect of IFN (Wang et al., 2007).

3.4.3 IL-12

IL-12 as therapy agent has both immunoregulatory function and anti-tumour activity mediated by stimulation of T and NK effector cells. Authors propose IL-12 as a therapeutical agent using a protocol to pre-screen melanoma patients for IL-12Rbeta2 expression to stratify the potential responders, administrate non-toxic doses and target IL-12R+ tumour cells, by local administration or injection of IL-12 fused to an antibody specific to tumour cells (Cocco et al., 2009). This interleukin is recently highly involved in cutaneous melanoma genetic therapy (see section).

Cytokines are the molecular messengers that control almost any physiological function of immune cells and are involved in the neoplastic transformation of normal cells. Cytokines are involved in immune recognition, proliferation and effector functions of immune cells. From the beginning of the research in the biomarkers discovery field, cytokines and their receptors were searched in association to diagnostic, prognostic and/or therapy. Some of the cytokines became therapeutic agents, such as IL-2 and all the recent papers on the clinical efficacy of cytokines state that this type of immune-therapy gets its best place in therapeutical combinations.

3.5 Targeting innate-immunity

Toll-like receptors (TLR) are involved in the regulation and activation of both innate and adaptive immunity (Takeda et al., 2003), activating therefore the anti-tumoural activity of lymphocytes. In a recently published experimental model, synthetic agonists for TLR 3 and 9 activated T cells improving their anti- melanoma activity (Amos et al., 2011) action that was supposed to take place *via* IFN-γ production. Moreover, TLR agonists can be good adjuvants in immune therapy.

In a phase I clinical study with synthetic agonists of TLR 9 in advanced stages melanoma, a complete regression was obtained in one of the 5 tested patients. The immune monitoring was performed testing the serum concentrations of IL-6, IP-10, IL-12p40, TNF-alpha. The immune treatment proved good clinical response metastatic melanoma (Hofmann et al., 2008). In a case study with a long period of treatment with TLR 9 agonist, it was reported that this compound induced strong tumour-specific immune response (Stoeter et al., 2008).

A phase II clinical study using TLR 7 agonist administered in patients with metastatic melanoma published its results several years ago and showed a prolonged stabilization of the disease. Monitoring was performed measuring IFN and IP-10 and peripheral blood immune cells. Out of 13 patients, 4 had disease stabilization and one patient had a partial remission. CD86 expression on monocytes, IFN and IP-10 increased in most patients upon therapy (Dummer et al., 2008).

Combining DTIC with the topical application of a TLR agonist in an experimental model decreased the rate of tumour evolution and enhanced animal survival. In this study authors stated that the topical application of TLR agonist is more efficient than intratumoural inoculation. Immune monitoring showed that the antitumour effect is both CD4+ and CD8+ dependent, the B220+CD8+ subset of dendritic cells and NK1.1+ CD11c+ cells within the tumours were enhanced, thus a more effective immune response against melanoma (Najar & Dutz, 2008). When using another combination, namely topical application of TLR agonist and intra-tumoural inoculation of DCs a good immune response was obtained in an experimental model. This therapeutical combination resulted in a significant tumour regression and a therapeutical approach to be considered (Lee et al., 2007).

In patients topically treated with TLR-7 agonists, the tumour infiltrate showed an increased population of CD3+, CD4+ and CD8+ T cells, cytotoxic T cells (TIA-1+, granzyme B+) and DC CD 123+ (Wolf et al., 2007).

Overall, agonists that address Toll-like receptors act through enhancing anti-tumoural cellular activity and systemically by an increased production of cytokines and chemokines.

3.6 Gene therapy

In cutaneous melanoma the genetic patterns can be the starting point for developing new molecular targets for therapeutic intervention and diagnostic biomarkers for melanoma (Su et al., 2009). In melanoma several altered tumour suppressor genes (p53, CDKN2A, Ras) are frequently found in primary and metastatic melanomas and are incriminated for the invasive and metastatic potential (Lalou et al., 2010). Gene therapy has been a rapidly expanding field in cancer in the last years and evermore in cutaneous melanoma. In this disease, the gene therapy tendency is the manipulation of interleukin genes. Thus, this year, in mouse experimental models, the results of an interesting attempt of gene therapy have been published. DCs genetically altered to express IL-12 can induce cytotoxic CD8+ T cell antitumoural response. The immune-intervention has good therapeutical potential as peptides from tumour-associated stromal antigens can be recognized by peripheral blood CD8+ T cells from melanoma patients after *in vitro* stimulation (Zhao et al., 2011). In addition, this year, in IL-10-knockout mouse model it was demonstrated that these mice are more resistant to melanoma development, IL-12 and IFN-γ being secreted in increased quantities (Marchi et al., 2011). The authors have constructed a plasmid containing the murine IL-10 receptor. When treating the animals with this plasmid, their survival time extended post-inoculation with melanoma cell lines. Associating this gene therapy with IL-12 gene therapy a beneficial therapeutical response could be obtained.

Several years ago, the first report on the clinical safety of *in vivo* particle-mediated epidermal delivery (PMED) as a cancer gene therapy was published (Ryan et al., 2007). PMED is transferring to specific location genes without viral carrier, the procedure has no viral potential risks, presents multipotency in cell transfections and multi gene transfer. For this therapy, authors have chosen the genes for gp100 and GM-CSF. Using PMED, they delivered these genes to patients with melanoma. The immune monitoring of treated patients was multifaceted: a complex array of auto-antibodies, rheumatoid factor, peripheral blood lymphocytes CD69+ expression, CD1a+ dendritic cells in biopsies and so on. The first reported clinical trial transferring cDNAs for gp100 and GM-CSF to patients concluded that the procedure is safe and that it can induce transgene expression in the treated skin.

Gene therapy's future and clinical benefit rely on the genotypic pattern of the patients. Therefore, several years ago it was reported on a large number of patients that the presence of chemokine receptor 5 gene (CCR5Delta32) polymorphism in patients diagnosed in advanced stages subjected to immunotherapy can indicate a decreased survival and, moreover, this gene pattern can be useful in selecting patients that have the best clinical outcome when subjected to immune therapy (Ugurel et al., 2007).

Gene therapy has still to overcome clinical compliances and prove its lack of deleterious side-effects in order to conquer the immune therapy field in melanoma.

3.7 Epigenetic therapy

The investigations regarding cancer alterations have gained, in the recently years, a new thrilling way for defining novel clinical settings and therapies, namely the epigenetic research (Selcuklu & Spillane, 2008). In contrast with genetic events involving irreversible changes in the genome (e.g. deletions), epigenetic changes imply alterations in gene expression without modifications of the primary DNA sequence. In addition, an epigenetic profile should be concurrently self-perpetuating, heritable and reversible (Bonasio et al., 2010; Howell et al., 2009). It is now accepted that malignant transformation of melanocytes occurring in cutaneous melanoma, is greatly accompanied by epigenetic modifications (Sigalotti et al., 2010). Such "epimutations" could be turned on in defining new therapies considering the high incidence, poor prognosis and resistance of metastatic melanoma to conventional therapies (Howell et al., 2009).

The epigenetic modifications of mammalian DNA involve at a glance cytosines methylation from CpG dinucleotide islands, deacetylation of DNA-binding histones and noncoding RNA profiles (miRNA) (Esteller, 2007). However, it is still under debate if post-translational modifications of histones and miRNAs signature are considered epigenetic events; in addition, some authors sustain that methylation of cytosines C-5 is the only clearly identified epigenetic modification of DNA in mammalian cells (Howell et al., 2009; Bird, 2002).

The ***DNA methylation*** process is under the balance of complex equipment consisting of DNA methyltransferases (DNMTs) responsible for genome-wide DNA methylation patterns, and methyl-CpG-binding proteins dedicated to deciphering the methylation profile. A normal cellular development is characterized by a properly specified DNA methylation outline but any deviation from this established pattern is one of the important characteristics for the majority of human cancers. As a general characteristic, neoplastic transformation is accompanied by complex disturbances of the genomic DNA methylation homeostasis. There is a variable and still relatively unknown extent of methylation range, (Howell et al., 2009) with both gene-specific hypermethylation and genome-wide hypomethylation as a consequence (Sigalotti et al., 2010; Jones & Baylin, 2007).

Histones are DNA-binding proteins mostly responsible for packaging of DNA into chromatin (Bird, 2002) and DNA segregation from the transcriptional machinery (Jones & Baylin, 2007). The acetylated histones at lysine residues are associated with transcriptionally active DNA whereas ***histone deacetylation*** means transcriptionally inactive DNA.

Histone deacetylases (HDACs) are involved in the development of various tumours through the alteration of normal gene expression and inhibition of DNA repair machinery (Hadnagy et al., 2008) thus representing one of the main epigenetic targets in cancer therapy (Howell et al., 2009). Despite the substantial information regarding the DNA methylation pattern in cutaneous melanoma, the existing data for abnormal post-translational modifications of histones are limited and someway indirect; these resulting from subsequent observations post-therapy with pharmacologic inhibitors of histone-modifying enzymes (i.e., HDACi) (Sigalotti et al., 2010).

Although relatively new entry and still not fully accepted as steady players in the epigenetic research of cancer, ***microRNAs*** gained a special attention in melanoma studies. MicroRNAs (miRNAs) are endogenous small noncoding RNAs (≈22-nt) with a regulatory nature upon gene expression by inhibiting mRNA translation (Bartel, 2004) or by causing mRNA degradation (Sood et al., 2006). Nowadays there are hundreds of confirmed miRNAs in humans (Molnár et al., 2008) and current evidence is emerging to the important role of particular miRNAs in human cancer epigenetic pathogenesis (Howell et al., 2009). Thus, data regarding miRNA deregulation in melanoma is rather limited, the majority of studies about miRNA involvement in tumourigenesis are completed especially on melanoma cell lines. However, the altered pattern of miRNA in melanoma seems to be related with apoptosis (miR-15b), cell cycle (miR-193b) and invasion/metastasis (miR-182) (Satzger et al., 2009; Chen et al., 2010; Segura et al., 2009).

Taking into account the epigenetic deregulation imprinting described so far in cutaneous melanoma, the intervention therapy from this point of view is focused on the DNMT and/or HDAC inhibitors. DNMT inhibitors (Lyko & Brown, 2005) are consisting of cytosine analogues and thus mimic the substrate for DNMT. 5-azacytidine (Vidaza), 5-AZA-CdR (Dacogen), S110 and zebularine (Yoo et al., 2007) are among the most accepted cytosine analogues exploited in melanoma *epitherapeutics*. Such analogues are incorporated in genomic DNA during the S-phase of the cell cycle and upon methylation a covalent bond between modified DNA and enzyme are formed, resulting the inactivation of DNMT, cellular depletion of enzyme and, therefore, the demethylation of DNA (Schermelleh et al., 2005). Along with DNMT inhibitors, histone deacetylase inhibitors (HDACi) have been hailed as a powerful new class of anticancer drugs. One of these inhibitors, trichostatin A (TSA), is thought to promote immune responses against tumours by an epigenetic control of cell cycle progression in G1 and G2-M phase, leading the growth arrest, differentiation or apoptosis (Setiadi et al., 2008). TSA treatment enhance the expression of some components of the antigen processing equipment and of MHC class I molecules on the carcinoma cell surface, leading to an enhanced vulnerability to killing by antigen-specific CTLs. Thus, immunotherapeutic anti-tumour approaches for eliminate cell cancers could be perceived differently by these novel insights defined by epigenomics (Setiadi et al., 2008).

4. Summary

Immune-therapy in cutaneous melanoma has to evaluate antitumour efficacy, autoimmunity, and reconstitution of a functioning immune system. Clinical studies and experimental research have gathered significant results to conclude that complex vaccines, combination of different therapeutical approaches, dendritic cell-based therapies in conjunction with co-stimulatory molecules, are superior to conventional immunization protocols in the induction of tumour-specific immune responses.

Target Agent	**Immune markers therapy monitoring**	**Comments**	**Stage**	**Ref.**
		Immunomodulatory antibodies		
CTL-4	peripheral CD4+ CD8+ T, CD8+; tumour infiltrates	Progression-free and overall survival	FDA appr.	Robert et al., 2011
		Anti-TLR synthetic agonists		
TLR 7	IFN, IP-10, peripheral blood immune cells, intratumoral infiltrates	Stabilization of the disease	Phase II	Dummer et al., 2008 Wolf et al., 2007
TLR 3 TLR 9	anti-tumoral T cells, IFNγ	Good clinical response metastatic melanoma	Phase I	Amos et al., 2011 Hofmann et al., 2008 Stoeter et al., 2008
		Dendritic cell		
Dex	T and NK cells	Activation of T-cells and NK cells	Phase I	Escudier et al., 2005 Hao et al., 2006 Viaud et al., 2010
DC	Cell mediated anti-tumoral immune response DTH reaction	Good clinical outcome	Pilot Phase I Phase II	David et al., 2006 Mayordomo et al., 2007
		Vaccines with melanoma antigens		
HSP	T cell stimulation	Longer survival	Phase III	Rivoltini et al., 2003, Lewis, 2004
gp100 peptide	T cytotoxic activation	Tumour regression	Phase III	Schwartzentruber et al., 2011
		Cytokines		
IL-2	Number and frequency of Tregs	Good clinical responses	FDA appr.	Cesana et al., 2006
IL-2 and Melan-A-specific CTL	Circulating % of Melan-A + T cells, eosinophils	Good clinical responses	Phase II	Makensen et al., 2006
IL-2 and gp100 vaccine	CD4, CD8, Tregs	Response rate and progression-free survival increased	Phase III	Schwartzentruber et al., 2011

IFN-alpha2b	IP-10, VEGF, EGF, HGF, peripheral NK, T and monocytes Tissue pSTAT1/pSTAT3	Prolong relapse-free survival Adjuvant therapy Predictor of the therapeutic effect	FDA appr.	Yurkovetski et al., 2007 Wang et al., 2007
IL-12	Stimulation of T and NK	Marker for stratifying the potential responders	Phase I/II	Cocco et al., 2009
		Gene therapy		
DC express IL-12	CD8 anti-tumoral response	Extended survival time	Animal models	Zhao et al., 2011
Plasmid - IL-10R gene	IL-12 and IFN secretion	Extended survival time	Animal models	Marchi et al., 2011
		Epigenetic immune-therapy		
TSA	CTL antigen-specific	Decreased invasion and cell cycle arrest	Cellular models	Setiadi et al., 2008

Table 1. Immune-therapies and immune efficacy markers in cutaneous melanoma (FDA appr. = FDA approval; Dex.= Dexosomes)

The immune parameters that efficiently monitor the evolution of the patients subjected to immune therapy comprise circulatory and tissue immune-related components. Hundreds of opened/approved clinical trials testing immune-therapy efficacy in cutaneous melanoma are using the immune monitoring of enrolled patients. All the authors agree that when using immuno-therapeutic agents in cutaneous melanoma, the systemic immune response is to be monitored (for a "at a glance" perspective see Table 1).

5. Conclusions and future perspectives

All the recent studies and research regarding melanoma immunotherapy have demonstrated that complex vaccines and the combination of different approaches, such as the use of dendritic cell vaccines in conjunction with co-stimulatory molecules, are superior to conventional immunization protocols in the induction of tumour-specific immune responses. Evaluation of clinical parameters and patient's-specific real-time immunological parameters may identify the most effective immunotherapy in melanoma. There are at least hundreds of approved clinical trials in immune-therapy related to cutaneous melanoma and the majority is foreseeing the utility, if not actively using, immune monitoring of enrolled patients.

Besides the approved cytokines in the immune-therapy of cutaneous melanoma, antibodies targeting CTLA-4 have demonstrated their feasibility, safety, and clinical activity and were approved as therapeutic agent in melanoma.

The failure of immune-therapies underlined in various sections probably reside in the immunological profile of the patient, thus the need of finding predictive markers is mandatory in order to detect treatment outcome in melanoma. Molecules that arise in the processes of neoplastic transformation, invasion and metastasis, are interrelated with the components of the immune responses. Future molecular patterns of cutaneous melanoma will compulsory comprise immune-related molecules. Nowadays forces are gathered to search for immune markers that specifically indicate the disease stage and eventually develop new targets for personalized efficient therapy.

We expect melanoma vaccination to become clinical routine therapy in the very near future. In this respect, a thorough monitoring is foreseen and in the future-to-be biomarkers panel, immune markers will have their foremost role. As the pathophysiology of melanoma is complex it is more convincing that only a combination of markers from genomics, transcriptomics, metabolomics and proteomics can cover the array of processes comprising the development of cutaneous melanoma. In this future set of markers, MHC allele expression in the individual patient's tumour and T-cell mediated immune responses specific for autologous melanoma will be evaluated.

As the incidence of melanoma is steadily increasing, an individualized immunological profile of the patient can reorient/personalize immune-therapy and monitor the efficacy of the treatment approach and the molecular diagnostic of cutaneous melanoma will have important immune components. Although far from being exhaustive, this chapter was intended to overview the main immune therapy possibilities used in the management of cutaneous melanoma patient. In all the stages of cutaneous melanoma development, immune elements are involved; they are associated with tumour initiation, tumour evasion, suppressed immune response and probably many more unknown mechanisms.

6. Acknowledgement

Authors contributed equally to this chapter funded by NATO SPF project 982838/2007, PN 09.33 - 01.01/2008. Authors would like to thank student Irina Radu for technical assistance.

7. References

Aarntzen, E.H.; Figdor, C.G.; Adema, G.J.; Punt, C.J. & de Vries I.J. (2008). Dendritic cell vaccination and immune monitoring. *Cancer Immunol. Immunother*, Vol.57, No.10, (Oct 2008), pp. 1559-1568, ISSN: 1432-0851

Amos, S.M.; Pegram, H.J.; Westwood, J.A.; John, L.B.; Devaud, C.; Clarke, C.J.; Restifo, N.P.; Smyth, M.J.; Darcy, P.K. & Kershaw, M.H. (2011). Adoptive immunotherapy combined with intratumoral TLR agonist delivery eradicates established melanoma in mice. *Cancer Immunol Immunother.*, Vol.60, No.5, (May 2011), pp. 671-683, ISSN: 1432-0851

Andersen, M.H.; Gehl, J.; Reker, S.; Pedersen, L.Ø.; Becker, J.C.; Geertsen, P. & Straten, P. (2003). Dynamic changes of specific T cell responses to melanoma correlate with IL-2 administration. *Semin. Cancer Biol*, Vol.13, No.6, (Dec 2003), pp. 449-459, ISSN: 1044-579X

Antigenics press release, October 10, 2005. Accessed October 31, 2005, Available from: http://www.antigenics.com/news/2005/1010.phtml.

Atkins, M.B. (2006). Cytokine-based therapy and biochemotherapy for advanced melanoma. *Clin. Cancer Res.*, Vol.12, No.(7 Pt 2), (April 2006), pp. 2353s-2358s, ISSN: 1557-3265

Bartel, D.P. (2004). MicroRNAs: genomics, biogenesis, mechanism, and function. *Cell*, Vol.116, No.2, (Jan 2004), pp. 281-297

Bird, A. (2002). DNA methylation patterns and epigenetic memory. *Gene Dev*, Vol.16, No.1, (Jan 2002), pp. 6-21, ISSN: 1549-5477

Bonasio, R.; Tu, S. & Reinberg, D. (2010). Molecular signals of epigenetic states. *Science*, Vol.330, No.6004, (Oct 2010), pp. 612-616, ISSN: 1095-9203

Cancer Vax Corporation media release, October 3, 2005. Accessed October 31, 2005, Available from: http://news.cancervax.com/phoenix.zhtml?c=147045&p=irol-newsArticle&t=Regular&id=763722&.

Cassaday, R.D.; Sondel, P.M.; King, D.M.; Macklin, M.D.; Gan, J.; Warner, T.F.; Zuleger, C.L.; Bridges, A.J.; Schalch, H.G.; Kim, K.M.; Hank, J.A.; Mahvi, D.M. & Albertini, M.R. (2007). A Phase I Study of Immunization Using Particle-Mediated Epidermal Delivery of Genes for gp100 and GM-CSF into Uninvolved Skin of Melanoma Patients, *Clin Cancer Res*, Vol.13, (Jan 2007), pp. 540-549, ISSN: 1557-3265

Cassard, L.; Cohen-Solal, J.F.G.; Fournier, E.M.; Camilleri-Broët, S.; Spatz, A.; Chouaïb, S.; Badoual, C.; Varin, A.; Fisson, S.; Duvillard, P.; Boix, C.; Loncar, S.M.; Sastre-Garau, X.; Houghton, A.N.; Avril, M.-F.; Gresser, I.; Fridman, W.H. & Sautès-Fridman, C. (2008). Selective expression of inhibitory Fcγ receptor by metastatic melanoma impairs tumor susceptibility to IgG-dependent cellular response. *International Journal of Cancer*, Vol.123, No.12, (Sep 2008), pp. 2832–2839, ISSN: 1097-0215.

Cassarino, D.S.; Miller, W.J.; Auerbach, A.; Yang, A.; Sherry, R. & Duray, P.H. (2006) The effects of gp100 and tyrosinase peptide vaccinations on nevi in melanoma patients. *J Cutan Pathol*, Vol.33, No.5 (May 2006), pp. 335-342, ISSN: 1600-0560

Cesana, G.C., DeRaffele, G., Cohen, S., Moroziewicz, D., Mitcham, J., Stoutenburg, J.; Cheung, K.; Hesdorffer, C.; Kim-Schulze, S. & Kaufman, H. L. (2006). Characterization of CD4+CD25+ regulatory T cells in patients treated with high-dose interleukin-2 for metastatic melanoma or renal cell carcinoma. *J. Clin. Oncol.*, Vol.24, No.7, (March 2006), pp. 1169-1177, ISSN: 1527-7755

Chapman, P.B. (2007). Melanoma vaccines. *Semin. Oncol.*, Vol.34, No.6, (Dec 2007), pp. 516-523

Chen, J.; Feilotter, H.E.; Pare, G.C.; Zhang, X.; Pemberton, J.G.; Garady, C.; Lai, D.; Yang, X. & Tron, V.A. (2010). MicroRNA-193b represses cell proliferation and regulates cyclin D1 in melanoma. *Am J Pathol*, No.176, (May 2010), pp. 2520-2529, ISSN: 1525-2191

Cocco, C.; Pistoia, V. & Airoldi, I. (2009). New perspectives for melanoma immunotherapy: role of IL-12. *Curr. Mol. Med.*, Vol.9, No.4, (May 2009), pp. 459-469, ISSN: 1566-5240.

Cohen-Solal, J.F.G.; Cassard, L.; Fournier, E.M.; Loncar, S.M.; Fridman, W.H. & Saut`es-Fridman, C. (2010). Metastatic Melanomas Express Inhibitory Low Affinity Fc Gamma Receptor and Escape Humoral Immunity. Dermatology Research and Practice Vol.2010, (Aug. 2010) , 11 pages, ISSN: 1687-6113

Davis, I.D.; Chen, Q.; Morris, L.; Quirk, J.; Stanley, M.; Tavarnesi, M.L.; Parente, P.; Cavicchiolo, T.; Hopkins, W.; Jackson, H.; Dimopoulos, N.; Tai, T.Y.; MacGregor, D.; Browning, J.; Svobodova, S.; Caron, D.; Maraskovsky, E.; Old, L.J.; Chen, W. & Cebon, J. (2006). Blood dendritic cells generated with Flt3 ligand and CD40 ligand prime CD8+ T cells efficiently in cancer patients. J. Immunother, Vol.29, No.5, (Sep/Oct 2006), pp. 499-511, ISSN: 1537-4513

Delcayre, A.; Shu, H. & Le Pecq, J.B. (2005). Dendritic cell-derived exosomes in cancer immunotherapy: exploiting nature's antigen delivery pathway. *Expert Rev. Anticancer Ther,* Vol.5, No.3, (June 2005), pp. 537-547, ISSN: 1473-7140

Di Giacomo, A.M.; Biagioli, M. & Maio, M. (2010). The emerging toxicity profiles of anti-CTLA-4 antibodies across clinical indications. *Semin Oncol.* Vol.37, No.5, (Oct 2010), pp. 499-507, ISSN: 1532-8708

Dummer, R.; Hauschild, A.; Becker, J.C.; Grob, J.J.; Schadendorf, D.; Tebbs, V.; Skalsky, J.; Kaehler, K.C.; Moosbauer, S.; Clark, R.; Meng, T.C. & Urosevic, M. (2008). An exploratory study of systemic administration of the toll-like receptor-7 agonist 852A in patients with refractory metastatic melanoma. *Clin Cancer Res,* Vol.14, No.3, (Feb 2008), pp. 856-864, ISSN: 1557-3265

Elias, E.G.; Zapas, J.L.; Beam, S.L. & Brown, S.D. (2005). GM-CSF and IL-2 combination as adjuvant therapy in cutaneous melanoma: early results of a phase II clinical trial. *Oncology (Williston Park),* Vol.19, No.(4 Suppl 2), (Apr 2005), pp. 15-18, ISSN: 0890-9091

Elias, E.G.; Zapas, J.L.; McCarron, E.C.; Beam, S.L.; Hasskamp, J.H. & Culpepper, W.J. (2008). Sequential administration of GM-CSF (Sargramostim) and IL-2 +/- autologous vaccine as adjuvant therapy in cutaneous melanoma: an interim report of a phase II clinical trial. *Cancer Biother Radiopharm,* Vol.23, No.3, (Jun 2008), pp. 285-291, ISSN: 1084-9785

Erdmann, M. & Schuler-Thurner, B. (2008). Dendritic cell vaccines in metastasized malignant melanoma. *G. Ital. Dermatol. Venereol.,* Vol.143, No.4, (Aug 2008), pp. 235-250, ISSN: 0026-4741

Escudier, B.; Dorval, T.; Chaput, N.;André, F.; Caby, M.-P.; Novault, S.; Flament, C.; Leboulaire, C.; Borg, C.; Amigorena, S.; Boccaccio, C.; Bonnerot, C.; Dhellin, O.; Movassagh, M.; Piperno, S.; Robert, C.; Serra, V.; Valente, N.; Le Pecq, J.-B.; Spatz, A.; Lantz, O.; Tursz, T.; Angevin, E. & Zitvogel, L. (2005). Vaccination of metastatic melanoma patients with autologous dendritic cell (DC) derived-exosomes: results of the first phase I clinical trial. *J Transl Med,* No.3, (March 2005), pp. 10, ISSN: 1479-5876

Esteller, M. (2007). Cancer epigenomics: DNA methylomes and histonemodification maps. *Nat Rev Genet,* Vol.8, No.4, (Apr 2007), pp. 286-298, ISSN: 1471-0064

Frankenburg, S.; Grinberg, I.; Bazak, Z.; Fingerut, L.; Pitcovski, J.; Gorodetsky, R.; Peretz, T.; Spira, R.M.; Skornik, Y. & Goldstein, R.S. (2007) Immunological activation following transcutaneous delivery of HR-gp100 protein. *Vaccine,* Vol.25, No. 23, (Jun 2007), pp. 4564-4570, ISSN: 0264-410X

Green, D.S.; Dalgleish, A.G.; Belonwu, N.; Fischer, M.D. & Bodman-Smith, M.D. (2008). Topical imiquimod and intralesional interleukin-2 increase activated lymphocytes and restore the Th1/Th2 balance in patients with metastatic melanoma. *Br. J. Dermatol.,* Vol.159, No.3, (Sep 2008), pp. 606-614, ISSN: 1365-2133

Hadnagy, A.; Beaulieu, R. & Balicki, D. (2008). Histone tail modifications and noncanonical functions of histones: perspectives in cancer epigenetics. *Mol Cancer Ther,* Vol.7, No.4, (Apr 2008), pp. 740-748, ISSN: 1538-8514

Hao, S.; Bai, O.; Yuan, J.; Qureshi, M. & Xiang J. (2006). Dendritic cell-derived exosomes stimulate stronger CD8+ CTL responses and antitumor immunity than tumor cell-derived exosomes. *Cell Mol Immunol,* Vol.3, No.3, (June 2006), pp. 205-211, ISSN: 1672-7681

Hofmann, M.A.; Kors, C., Audring, H.; Walden, P.; Sterry, W. & Trefzer, U. (2008). Phase 1 evaluation of intralesionally injected TLR9-agonist PF-3512676 in patients with basal cell carcinoma or metastatic melanoma. *J Immunother,* Vol.31, No.5, (Jun 2008), pp. 520-527, ISSN: 1524-9557

Howell, P.M. Jr; Liu, S.; Ren, S.; Behlen, C.; Fodstad, O. & Riker, A.I. (2009). Epigenetics in human melanoma. *Cancer Control,* Vol.16, No.3, (Jul 2009), pp. 200-218, ISSN: 1073-2748

Hsueh, E.C. & Morton, D.L. (2003). Antigen-based immunotherapy of melanoma: Canvaxin therapeutic polyvalent cancer vaccine. *Semin Cancer Biol,* Vol.13 (Dec 2003), pp. 401-407, ISSN: 1044-579X

Jones, P.A. & Baylin, S.B. (2007). The epigenomics of cancer. *Cell,* No.128, (Feb 2007), pp. 683-692

Kirkwood, J.M.; Ibrahim, J.G.; Sosman, J.A.; Sondak, V.K.; Agarwala, S.S.; Ernstoff, M.S. & Rao U. (2001). High-dose interferon a-2b significantly prolongs relapse-free and overall survival compared with the GM2-KLH/QS-21 vaccine in patients with resected stage IIB-III melanoma: results of Intergroup Trial E1694/S9512/C509801. *J Clin Oncol,* Vol.19, No.9, (May 2001), pp. 2370-2380, ISSN: 1527-7755

Kirkwood, J.M.; Manola, J.; Ibrahim, J.; Sondak, V.; Ernstoff, M.S. & Rao, U. (2004). A pooled analysis of ECOG and Intergroup trials of adjuvant high-dose interferon for melanoma. *Clin Cancer Res,* Vol.10, No.5, (March 2004), pp. 1670-1677, ISSN: 1557-3265

Lalou, C.; Scamuffa, N.; Mourah, S.; Plassa, F.; Podgorniak, M.-P.; Soufir, N.; Dumaz, N.; Calvo, F.; Seguin, N.B. & A.-M. Khatib (2010). Inhibition of the proprotein convertases represses the invasiveness of human primary melanoma cells with altered p53, CDKN2A and N-Ras genes. *PLoS One.* Vol.5, No.4, (Apr 2010), pp. e9992, ISSN: 1932-6203

Langer, L.F.; Clay, T.M. & Morse, M.A. (2007). Update on anti-CTLA-4 antibodies in clinical trials. *Expert Opin. Biol. Ther.,* Vol.7, No.8, (Aug 2007), pp. 1245-1256, ISSN: 1744-7682

Lee, J.R.; Shin, J.H.; Park, J.H.; Song, S.U. & Choi, G.S. (2007). Combined treatment with intratumoral injection of dendritic cells and topical application of imiquimod for murine melanoma. *Clin Exp Dermatol,* Vol.32, No.5, (Sep 2007), pp. 541-549, ISSN: 1365-2230

Lewis, J.J. (2004). Therapeutic cancer vaccines: using unique antigens. *Proc Natl Acad Sci USA* 2004; Vol.101, (Suppl 2), (Oct 2004), pp. 14653-14656, ISSN: 1091-6490

Lienard, D.; Avril, M.F.; Le Gal, F.A.; Baumgaertner, P.; Vermeulen, W.; Blom, A.; Geldhof, C.; Rimoldi, D.; Pagliusi, S.; Romero, P.; Dietrich, P.Y.; Corvaia, N. & Speiser, D.E. (2009). Vaccination of melanoma patients with Melan-A/Mart-1 peptide and Klebsiella outer membrane protein p40 as an adjuvant. *J Immunother,* Vol.32, No.8, (Oct 2009), pp. 875-878, ISSN: 1537-4513

Lyko, F. & Brown, R. (2005). DNA methyltransferase inhibitors and the development of epigenetic cancer therapies. *J Natl Cancer Inst,* Vol.97, No.20 (Oct 2005), pp. 1498-1506, ISSN: 1460-2105

Macatonia, S.E.; Knight, S.C.; Edwards, A.J.; Griffiths, S. & Fryer P. (1987). Localization of antigen on lymph node dendritic cells after exposure to the contact sensitizer fluorescein isothiocyanate. Functional and morphological studies. *J Exp Med,* Vol.166, No.6, (Dec 1987), pp. 1654–1667, ISSN: 1540-9538

Mackensen, A.; Meidenbauer, N.; Vogl, S.; Laumer, M.; Berger, J. & Andreesen, R. (2006). Phase I study of adoptive T-cell therapy using antigen-specific CD8+ T cells for the treatment of patients with metastatic melanoma. *J. Clin. Oncol.*, Vol.24, No.31, (Nov 2006), pp. 5060-5069, ISSN: 1527-7755

Marchi, L.H.; Paschoalin, T.; Travassos, L.R. & Rodrigues, E,G. (2011). Gene therapy with interleukin-10 receptor and interleukin-12 induces a protective interferon-γ-dependent response against B16F10-Nex2 melanoma. *Cancer Gene Ther,* Vol.18, No.2, (Feb 2011), pp. 110-122, ISSN: 0929-1903

Mayordomo, J.I.; Andres, R.; Isla, M.D.; Murillo, L.; Cajal, R.; Yubero, A.; Blasco, C.; Lasierra, P.; Palomera, L.; Fuertes, M.A.; Güemes, A.; Sousa, R.; Garcia-Prats, M.D.; Escudero, P.; Saenz, A.; Godino, J.; Marco, I.; Saez, B.; Visus, C.; Asin, L.; Valdivia, G.; Larrad, L. & Tres A. (2007). Results of a pilot trial of immunotherapy with dendritic cells pulsed with autologous tumor lysates in patients with advanced cancer. *Tumori,* Vol.93, No.1 (Jan-Feb 2007), pp. 26-30, ISSN: 0300-8916

Ménard, C.; Ghiringhelli, F.; Roux, S.; Chaput, N.; Mateus, C.; Grohmann, U.; Caillat-Zucman, S.; Zitvogel L. & Robert C. (2008). CTLA-4 blockade confers lymphocyte resistance to regulatory T-cells in advanced melanoma: surrogate marker of efficacy of tremelimumab? *Clin. Cancer Res,* Vol.14, No.16, (Aug 2008), pp. 5242-5249, ISSN: 1557-3265

Molnár, V.; Tamási, V.; Bakos, B.; Wiener, Z. & Falus, A. (2008). Changes in miRNA expression in solid tumors: an miRNA profiling in melanomas. *Semin Cancer Biol.* Vol.18, No.2, (April 2008), pp. 111-122, ISSN: 1044-579x

Motl, S.E. (2004). Technology evaluation: Canvaxin, John Wayne Cancer Institute/Cancer Vax. *Curr Opin Mol Ther,* Vol.6, No.1, (Feb 2004), pp. 104-111, ISSN: 1464-8431

Najar, H.M. & Dutz J.P. (2008) Topical CpG enhances the response of murine malignant melanoma to dacarbazine. *J Investig Dermatol,* Vol.128, No.9, (Sep 2008), pp. 2204-2210, ISSN: 1523-1747

Neagu, M.; Constantin, C. & Tanase, C. (2010) Immune-related biomarkers for diagnosis/prognosis and therapy monitoring of cutaneous melanoma. *Expert Rev Mol Diagn,* Vol.10, No.7, (Oct 2010), pp. 897-919, ISSN: 1473-7159

Phan, G.Q.; Weber, J.S. & Sondak, V.K. (2008). CTLA-4 blockade with monoclonal antibodies in patients with metastatic cancer:surgical issues. *Ann Surg Oncol,* Vol.15, No.11, (Nov 2008), pp. 3014-3021, ISSN: 1534-4681

Rabinovich, G.A.; Gabrilovich, D. & Sotomayor, E.M. (2007). Immunosuppressive strategies that are mediated by tumor cells. *Annu. Rev. Immunol,* Vol.25, (Apr 2007), pp. 267-296, ISSN: 0732-0582

Rigel, D.S. Trends in Dermatology: Melanoma Incidence. *Arch Dermatol.* Vol.146, No.3, (March 2010), pp. 318, ISSN: 0096-5359

Riker, A.I., Cormier, J., Panelli, M., Kammula, U.; Wang, E.; Abati, A.; Fetsch, P.; Lee, K.-H.; Steinberg, S.; Rosenberg, S.; Marincola, F. (1999). Immune selection after antigen-specific immunotherapy of melanoma. *Surgery,* Vol.126, No.2, (Aug 1999), pp. 112-120, ISSN: 0039-6060

Riker, A.I.; Jove, R. & Daud, A.I. (2006) Immunotherapy as part of a multidisciplinary approach to melanoma treatment. *Front Biosci,* No.11, (Jan 2006), pp. 1-14, ISSN: 1093-4715

Rivoltini, L.; Castelli, C.; Carrabba, M.; Mazzaferro, V.; Pilla, L.; Huber, V.; Coppa, J.; Gallino, G.; Scheibenbogen, C.; Squarcina, P.; Cova, A.; Camerini, R.; Lewis, J.J.; Srivastava, P.K. & Parmiani, G. (2003). Human tumor-derived heat shock protein 96 mediates in vitro activation and in vivo expansion of melanoma- and colon carcinoma-specificTcells. *J Immunol,* Vol.171, No.7, (Oct 2003), pp. 3467-3474, ISSN 1550-6606

Robert, C.; Thomas, L.; Bondarenko, I.; O'Day, S.; Weber, J.; Garbe, C.; Lebbe, C.; Baurain, J.F.; Testori, A.; Grob, J.J.; Davidson, N.; Richards, J.; Maio, M.; Hauschild, A.; Miller, W.H. Jr.; Gascon, P.; Lotem, M.; Harmankaya, K.; Ibrahim, R.; Francis, S.; Chen, T.T.; Humphrey, R.; Hoos, A., & Wolchok, J.D. (2011). Ipilimumab plus dacarbazine for previously untreated metastatic melanoma. *N Engl J Med,* Vol.364, No.26, (Jun 2011), pp. 2517-2526, ISSN: 1533-4406

Rosato, A.; Zambon, A.; Macino, B.; Mandruzzato, S.; Bronte, V.; Milan, G.; Zanovello, P. & D. Collavo (1996). Anti-L-selectin monoclonal antibody treatment in mice enhances tumor growth by preventing CTL sensitization in peripheral lymph nodes draining the tumor area. *Int J Cancer,* Vol.65, No.6, (March 1996), pp. 847–851, ISSN: 1097-0215

Rosenberg, S.A.; Yang, J.C. & Restifo, N.P. (2004). Cancer immunotherapy: moving beyond current vaccines. *Nat Med,* Vol.10, No.9 (Sep 2004), pp. 909-915, ISSN: 1546-170X

Rosenberg, S.A.; Yang, J.C.; Schwartzentruber, D.J.; Hwu, P.; Marincola, F.M.; Topalian, S.L.; Restifo, N.P.; Dudley, M.E.; Schwarz, S.L.; Spiess, P.J.; Parkhurst, M.R.; Kawakami, Y.; Seipp, C.A.; Einhorn, J.H. & White, D.E. (1998). Immunologic and therapeutic evaluation of a synthetic peptide vaccine for the treatment of patients with metastatic melanoma. *Nat Med* 1998; Vol.4, No.3, (March 1998), pp. 321–327, ISSN: 1078-8956

Salazar, L.G. & Disis, M.L. (2005). Cancer vaccines: the role of tumor burden in tipping the scale toward vaccine efficacy. *J Clin Oncol,* Vol.23, No.30 (Oct 2005), pp. 7397-7398, ISSN: 1527-7755

Satzger, I.; Mattern, A.; Kuettler, U.; Weinspach, D.; Voelker, B.; Kapp, A. & Gutzmer, R. (2010). MicroRNA-15b represents an independent prognostic parameter and is correlated with tumor cell proliferation and apoptosis in malignant melanoma. *Int J Cancer,* Vol.126, No.11, (Jun 2010), pp. 2553-2562, ISSN: 1097-0215

Schermelleh, L.; Spada, F.; Easwaran, H.P.; Zolghadr, K.; Margot, J.B.; Cardoso, M.C. & Leonhardt, H. (2005). Trapped in action: direct visualization of DNA methyltransferase activity in living cells. *Nat Methods,* Vol.2, No.10 (Oct 2005), pp. 751-756, ISSN: 1548-7105

Schwartzentruber, D.J.; Lawson, D.H.; Richards, J.M.; Conry, R.M.; Miller, D.M.; Treisman, J.; Gailani, F.; Riley, L.; Conlon, K.; Pockaj, B.; Kendra, K.L.; White, R.L.; Gonzalez, R.; Kuzel, T.M.; Curti, B.; Leming, P.D.; Whitman, E.D.; Balkissoon, J.; Reintgen, D.S.; Kaufman, H.; Marincola, F.M.; Merino, M.J.; Rosenberg, S.A.; Choyke, P.; Vena, D. & Hwu, P. (2011). gp100 peptide vaccine and interleukin-2 in patients with advanced melanoma. *N Engl J Med.,* Vol.364, No.22, (Jun 2011), pp. 2119-2127, ISSN: 1533-4406

Segura, M.F.; Hanniford, D.; Menendez, S.; Reavie, L.; Zou, X.; varez-Diaz, S.; Zakrzewski, J.; Blochin, E.; Rose, A.; Bogunovic, D.; Polsky, D.; Wei, J.; Lee, P.; Belitskaya-Levy, I.; Bhardwaj, N.; Osman, I. & Hernando, E. (2009). Aberrant miR-182 expression promotes melanoma metastasis by repressing FOXO3 and microphthalmia-associated transcription factor. *Proc Natl Acad Sci USA,* Vol.106, No.6, (Feb 2009), pp. 1814-1819, ISSN: 1091-6490

Selcuklu, S.D. & Spillane, C. (2008). Clinical approaches to epigenome therapeutics for cancer. *Epigenetics,* Vol.3, No.2, (March/April 2008), pp. 107-112, ISSN: 1559-2308

Setiadi, A.F.; Omilusik, K.; David, M.D.; Seipp, R.P.; Hartikainen, J.; Gopaul, R.; Choi, K.B. & Jefferies, W.A. (2008). Epigenetic Enhancement of Antigen Processing and Presentation Promotes Immune Recognition of Tumors. *Cancer Research,* Vol. 68, No. 23, (Dec 2008), pp. 9601-9607, ISSN: 1538-7445

Sigalotti, L.; Covre, A.; Fratta, E.; Parisi, G.; Colizzi, F.; Rizzo, A.; Danielli, R.; Hugues, JM Nicolay; Coral, S. & Maio, M. (2010). Epigenetics of human cutaneous melanoma: setting the stage for new therapeutic strategies. *Journal of Translational Medicine,* No.8, (Jun 2010), pp.56, ISSN: 1479-5876

Slingluff Jr, C.L.; Yamshchikov, G.V.; Hogan, K.T.; Hibbitts, S.C.; Petroni, G.R.; Bissonette, E.A.; Patterson, J.W.; Neese, P.Y.; Grosh, W.W.; Chianese-Bullock, MD K.A.; Czarkowski, A.; Rehm, P.K. & Parekh, J. (2008). Evaluation of the Sentinel Immunized Node for Immune Monitoring of Cancer Vaccines. *Ann Surg Oncol,* Vol.15, No.12, (Dec 2008), pp. 3538–3549, ISSN: 1534-4681

Slingluff, C.L.Jr; Petroni, G.R.; Olson, W.; Czarkowski, A.; Grosh, W.W.; Smolkin, M.; Chianese-Bullock, K.A.; Neese, P.Y.; Deacon, D.H.; Nail, C.; Merrill, P.; Fink, R.; Patterson, J.W. & Rehm, P.K. (2008). Helper T-cell responses and clinical activity of a melanoma vaccine with multiple peptides from MAGE and melanocytic differentiation antigens. *J Clin Oncol,* Vol.26, No.30,(Oct 2008), pp. 4973-4980, ISSN: 1527-7755

Sondak, V.K.; Sabel, M.S. & Mulé, J.J. (2006). Allogeneic and Autologous Melanoma Vaccines: Where Have We Been and Where Are We Going? *Clin Cancer Res,* Vol.12, No.7, (April 2006), pp. 2337s-2341s, ISSN: 1557-3265

Sondak, V.K.; Sosman, J.; Unger, J.; Liu, P.Y.; Thompson, J.; Tuthill, R.; Kempf, R. & L. Flaherty. (2004). Significant impact of HLA class I allele expression on outcome in melanoma patients treated with an allogeneic melanoma cell lysate vaccine: final analysis of SWOG-9035 (abstract). *J Clin Oncol,* 2004 ASCO Annual Meeting Proceedings (Post-Meeting Edition). Vol.22, No.14S (July 15 Supplement), pp. 7501, ISSN: 1527-7755

Sood, P.; Krek, A.; Zavolan, M.; Macino, G. & Rajewsky, N. (2006). Cell-type-specific signatures of microRNAs on target mRNA expression. *Proc Natl Acad Sci U S A,* Vol.103, No.8, (Feb 2006), pp. 2746-2751, ISSN: 1091-6490

Sosman, J.A.; Unger, J.M.; Liu, P.-Y.; Flaherty, L.E.; Park, M.S.; Kempf, R.A.; Thompson, J.A.; Terasaki, P.I. & Sondak, V.K. (2002). Adjuvant immunotherapy of resected, intermediate-thickness node-negative melanoma with an allogeneic tumor vaccine: impact of HLA class I antigen expression on outcome. *J Clin Oncol,* Vol.20, No.8, (April 2002), pp. 2067-2075, ISSN: 1527-7755

Stoeter, D.; de Liguori Carino, N.; Marshall, E.; Poston, G.J. & Wu A. (2008). Extensive necrosis of visceral melanoma metastases after immunotherapy. *World J Surg Oncol*, Vol.4, No.6, (March 2008), pp. 30, ISSN: 1477-7819

Su, D.M.; Zhang, Q.; Wang, X.; He, P.; Zhu, Y.J.; Zhao, J.; Rennert, O.M. & Y.A. Su (2009). Two types of human malignant melanoma cell lines revealed by expression patterns of mitochondrial and survival-apoptosis genes: implications for malignant melanoma therapy. *Mol. Cancer Ther.*, Vol.8, No.5, OF1-13 (May 2009), pp. ISSN: 1538-8514

Takeda, K.; Kaisho, T. & Akira, S. (2003). TOLL-LIKE RECEPTORS. *Annu. Rev. Immunol.*, Vol.21, (Apr 2003), pp. 335–376

Tarhini, A.; Lo, E. & Minor, D.R. (2010). Releasing the brake on the immune system: Ipilimumab in melanoma and other tumors. *Cancer Biother Radiopharm*, Vol.25, No.6, (Dec 2010), pp. 601-613, ISSN: 1557-8852

Ugurel, S.; Schrama, D.; Keller, G.; Schadendorf, D.; Bröcker, E.B.; Houben, R.; Zapatka, M.; Fink, W.; Kaufman, H.L. & Becker, J.C. (2008). Impact of the CCR5 gene polymorphism on the survival of metastatic melanoma patients receiving immunotherapy. *Cancer Immunol Immunother*, Vol.57, No.5, (May 2008), pp. 685-691, ISSN: 1432-0851

Varker KA, Kondadasula SV, Go MR Lesinski, G.B.; Ghosh-Berkebile, R.; Lehman, A.; Monk, J.P.; Olencki, T.; Kendra, K. & Carson III, W.E. (2006). Multiparametric flow cytometric analysis of signal transducer and activator of transcription 5 phosphorylation in immune cell subsets in vitro and following interleukin-2 immunotherapy. *Clin Cancer Res.*, Vol.12, No.19, (Oct 2006), pp. 5850-5858, ISSN: 1557-3265

Viaud, S.; Théry, C.; Ploix, S.; Tursz, T.; Lapierre, V.; Lantz, O.; Zitvogel, L. & Chaput, N. (2010). Dendritic Cell-Derived Exosomes for Cancer Immunotherapy:What's Next? *Cancer Res*, No.70, (Feb 2010), pp. 1281-1285, ISSN: 0008-5472

Viguier, M.; Lemaître, F.; Verola, O.; Cho, M-S.; Gorochov, G.; Dubertret, L.; Bachelez, H.; Kourilsky, P. & Ferradini, L. (2004). Foxp3 expressing CD4+CD25high regulatoryTcells are overrepresented in human metastatic melanoma lymph nodes and inhibit the function of infiltrating T cells. *J Immunol*, Vol.173, No.2, (July 2004), pp. 1444 -1453, ISSN: 1550-6606

Wang, W., Edington, H.D., Rao, U.N., Jukic, D.M., Land, S.R., Ferrone, S. & Kirkwood, J.M. (2007). Modulation of signal transducers and activators of transcription 1 and 3 signaling in melanoma by high-dose IFNalpha2b. *Clin. Cancer Res.*, Vol.13, No.5, (March 2007), pp. 1523-1531, ISSN: 1557-3265

Weber, J. (2008). Overcoming Immunologic Tolerance to Melanoma:Targeting CTLA-4 with Ipilimumab (MDX-010), *The Oncologist*, Vol.13(suppl 4), (Oct 2008), pp. 16–25, ISSN: 1549-490X

Wolf, I.H.; Kodama, K.; Cerroni, L. & Kerl, H. (2007). Nature of inflammatory infiltrate in superficial cutaneous malignancies during topical imiquimod treatment. *Am J Dermatopathol*, Vol.29, No.3, (Jun 2007), pp. 237-241, ISSN: 0193-1091

Yamshchikov GV, Barnd DL, Eastham S, Galavotti, H.; Patterson, J.W.; Deacon, D.H.; Teates, D.; Neese, P.; Grosh, W.W.; Petroni, G.; Engelhard, V.H. & Slingluff, C.L. Jr. (2001). Evaluation of peptide vaccine immunogenicity in draining lymph nodes and peripheral blood of melanoma patients. *Int J Cancer*, 2001 Jun 1;Vol.92, No.5, (Jun 2001), pp. 703-711, ISSN: 1097-0215

Yoo, C.B.; Jeong, S.; Egger, G.; Liang, G.; Phiasivongsa, P.; Tang, C.; Redkar, S. & Jones, P.A. (2007). Delivery of 5-aza-2'-deoxycytidine to cells using oligodeoxynucleotides. *Cancer Res*, Vol.67, No.13 (July 2007), pp. 6400-6408, ISSN: 0008-5472

Yoshizawa, H.; Chang, A.E. & Shu, S. (1991). Specific adoptive immunotherapy mediated by tumor-draining lymph node cells sequentially activated with anti-CD3 and IL-2. *J Immunol*, Vol.147, No.2, (July 1991), pp. 729–737, ISSN: 1550-6606

Yuan, J.; Gnjatic, S.; Li, H.; Powel, S.; Gallardo, H.F.; Ritter, E.; Ku, G.Y.; Jungbluth, A.A.; Segal, N.H.; Rasalan, T.S.; Manukian, G.; Xu, Y.; Roman, R.-A.; Terzulli, S.L.; Heywood, M.; Pogoriler, E.; Ritter, G.; Old, L.J.; Allison, J.P. & Wolchok, J.D. (2008). CTLA-4 blockade enhances polyfunctional NY-ESO-1 specific T cell responses in metastatic melanoma patients with clinical benefit. *PNAS*, Vol.105, No.51 (Dec 2008), pp. 20410–20415, ISSN: 1091-6490

Yurkovetsky, Z.R.; Kirkwood, J.M.; Edington, H.D.; Marrangoni, A.M.; Velikokhatnaya, L.; Winans, M.T.; Gorelik, E. & Lokshin, A.E. (2007). Multiplex analysis of serum cytokines in melanoma patients treated with interferon-alpha2b. *Clin. Cancer Res.*, Vol.13, No.8, (Apr 2007), pp. 2422-2428, ISSN: 1557-3265

Zhao, X.; Bose, A.; Komita, H.; Taylor, J.L.; Kawabe, M.; Chi, N.; Spokas, L.; Lowe, D.B.; Goldbach, C.; Alber, S.; Watkins, S.C.; Butterfield, L.H.; Kalinski, P.; Kirkwood, J.M. & Storkus, W.J. (2011). Intratumoral IL-12 gene therapy results in the crosspriming of Tc1 cells reactive against tumor-associated stromal antigens. *Mol Ther.*, Vol.19, No.4, (Apr 2011), pp. 805-814, ISSN: 1525-0024

Zimmerer, J.M.; Lesinski, G.B.; Ruppert, A.S.; Radmacher, M.D.; Noble, C.; Kendra, K.; Walker, M.J. & Carson III, W.E. (2008). Gene expression profiling reveals similarities between the in vitro and in vivo responses of immune effector cells to IFN-alpha. *Clin Cancer Res.*, Vol.14, No.18, (Sep 2008), pp. 5900-5906, ISSN: 1557-3265

6

Innate Immunity-Based Immunotherapy of Cancer

Kouji Maruyama et al.*
Experimental Animal Facility,
Shizuoka Cancer Center Research Institute,
Japan

1. Introduction

The immune system protects against invading pathogens and transformed cells, including cancer. Mammalian immune system is divided into two major categories, i.e., innate and adaptive immunity. Innate immunity consists of cellular and biochemical defense mechanisms that respond in the early phase after harmful events, such as encounters with microbes or transformed cells. The cellular components of innate immunity include dendritic cells (DCs), macrophages and monocytes, polynuclear cells (e.g. neutrophils and mast cells), natural killer (NK) cells, γδ T cells and natural killer T (NKT) cells. Adaptive immunity consists of T and B lymphocytes and their humoral mediators, including cytokines and antibodies, and achieves excellent antigen specificity by somatic rearrangement of the antigen receptor genes of each lymphocyte lineage; T cell receptor for T lymphocytes and immunoglobulin for B lymphocytes, respectively. Furthermore, another excellent characteristic of adaptive immunity is a "memory system" to maintain antigen-specific lymphocytes in a functionally quiescent or slowly cycling state for many years. The memory system enables host organisms to respond to the second and subsequent exposure to the same or related antigens in a more rapid and effective manner.

Dr. William Coley, an American bone surgeon, is credited with pioneering work in the field of cancer immunotherapy. In the 1890s, he noted that patients with sarcoma who developed bacterial infections after surgery had visible regression of their cancer. At first, Dr. Coley injected live cultures of streptococcus to produce erysipelas in cancer patients and assessed their responses (Bickels et al., 2002; MacCarthy, 2006). He found that the antitumor effects depended upon the toxins of the bacteria, and eventually developed mixed toxins of a Gram-positive and -negative bacterium called Coley toxins (also called "mixed bacterial vaccines"). A compilation of Dr. Coley's clinical observations indicated that in certain tumor

---

*Hidee Ishii[1], Sachiko Tai[1], Jinyan Cheng[2], Takatomo Satoh[2], Sachiko Karaki[2],
Shingo Akimoto[3] and Ken Yamaguchi[4]
[1]*Experimental Animal Facility, Shizuoka Cancer Center Research Institute,*
[2]*Advanced Analysis Technology Department, Corporate R&D Center, Olympus Corporation,*
[3]*Department of Pediatric Hematology and Oncology Research,*
National Medical Center for Children and Mothers Research Institute,
[4]*Shizuoka Cancer Center Hospital and Research Institute, Japan*

types, such as soft tissue sarcoma and lymphoma, the response is marked even by today's standards (Tsung & Norton, 2006). Following the pioneering works by Dr. Coley and his daughter, Dr. Helen Coley Nauts, efforts to treat cancer based on the function of the immune system, i.e., immunotherapy, have continued. As with Coley's toxins, the innate immune response against microbes could provoke anti-tumor effects as a secondary response. Although the exact molecular mechanisms of innate immune cells to recognize the components of microorganisms have not been fully understood, the substances such as bacteria-derived materials which evoke tumor immunity have been categorized as 'biological response modifier (BRM)'.

In Japan, several original BRMs have been developed since 1950's. Dr Chisato Maruyama noticed that there were few cancer patients in sanatoriums for tuberculosis or Hansen's disease, and he started research to apply extracts from *Mycobacterium tuberculosis* to cancer treatment. His preparation, named Specific Substance MARUYAMA (SSM, also called the "MARUYAMA vaccine") (Suzuki et al., 1986a; Suzuki et al., 1986b; Sasaki et al., 1990) was composed of deproteinized extracts, and contained lipoarabinomannan, a kind of polysaccharide, as the main component. SSM received much attention from the public as a miracle drug for cancer treatment before being approved by the Ministry of Health and Welfare of Japan at that time. SSM has not been approved to date as a anti-neoplastic drug, but its related preparation, referred to as Z-100 or Ancer, has been approved since 1991 as a drug for radiotherapy associated leucopenia. Ttwo other BRM drugs, krestin (PS-K, polysaccharide-protein complexes extracted from basidiomycetes, *Trametes versicolor*) (Akiyama et al., 1977; Mizushima et al., 1982) and picibanil (OK-432, a lyophilized preparation of attenuated group A *Streptococcus haemolyticus*) (Kai et al., 1979; Kataoka et al., 1979) were approved by the Ministry of Health and Welfare of Japan as anti-neoplastic drugs in 1975. Another example of Japanese BRMs is BCG-CWS, a cell wall skeleton preparation of *Mycobacterium bovis* bacillus Calmette-Guérin, a tuberculosis vaccine strain which is almost nonpathogenic yet retains the immunogenic properties of tuberculosis (Tsuji et al., 2000). BCG-CWS contains a peptidoglycan that is covalently linked to arabinogalactan and mycolic acids (Azuma et al., 1974). Although BCG-CWS has been clinically used for a long time (Hayashi et al., 2009; Kodama et al., 2009), it has not been approved by the Ministry of Health and Welfare of Japan.

One of the characteristics of classical BRMs is that they are crude products which are not fully purified. Their multiple components seem to be important for the induction of efficient anti-tumor effects as seen with Coley toxins.

2. Stimulators of innate immunity

2.1 Toll-like receptors (TLRs)

The cells of the innate immune system recognize infectious agents by receptors for characteristic components of pathogenic microorganisms. The structures of these components are highly conserved and are called pathogen-associated molecular patterns (PAMPs). The receptors for PAMPs, referred to as pattern recognition receptors (PRRs), are germline-encoded and highly conserved across species. The innate immune system detects various classes of pathogens and abnormal cells through PRRs, and serves as a first line of defense against microbes.

Toll, a gene involving to the establishment of dorsal-ventral pattern of Drosophila embryo (Hashimoto et al., 1988), other function in immune response against fungus in Drosophila adults (Lemaitre et al., 1996). In 1997, a cloning of human homologue of Drosophila Toll and its function as an antigen receptor was reported (Medzhitov et al., 1997). At present, 10 molecules have been identified in humans and are referred to as Toll-like receptors (TLRs) (Takeda et al., 2003; Iwasaki & Medzhitov, 2004). The identification of TLRs in mammalian species could give us clues to understand the molecular basis for the early phase events of host defense against microbial infection. In addition, accumulating evidence has shed light on the broad range of their roles in various biological processes. The TLR family is one of the most extensively characterized families of PRRs, and is also regarded as the most rapidly growing research field in immunology.

TLRs are type I transmembrane proteins containing repeated leucine-rich motifs in their extracellular domains similar to such motifs in other PRRs, and have a conserved intracellular motif (i.e. TIR domain, which initiates signal transduction). The typical microbial ligands for TLRs are summarized in Table 1. The initial step of signal transduction from TLRs is mediated through several adaptor molecules, including myeloid differentiation factor 88 (MyD88), Toll receptor-associated activator of interferon (TRIF), MyD88-adaptor-like/TIR-associated protein (MAL/TIRAP) and Toll receptor-associated molecule (TRAM), relayed to the inflammatory pathways involving NF-κB, Janus kinase (JNK)/p38 kinase and interferon regulatory factor (IRF) 3, 5 and 7. Finally, TLR signal transduction induces various transcripts, including cytokines such as tumor necrosis factor-α (TNF-α) and interferon (IFN)-inducible genes.

TLR1/TLR2/TLR6	Bacterial lipoproteins and lipotechoic acid, fungal zymosan
TLR3	Double stranded RNA
TLR4	Lipopolysaccharide (LPS) from Gram-negative bacteria
TLR5	Bacterial fragelin
TLR7/TLR8	Single-stranded RNA
TLR9	Unmethylated CpG motifs in DNA
TLR10	Unknown

Table 1. Typical ligands for human TLRs known as pathogen-associated molecular patterns (PAMPs)

2.1.1 Roles of TLRs in tissue homeostasis

In addition to their role in the host defense system, TLRs have been shown to be involved in various aspects of tissue homeostasis, including tissue repair and regeneration (van Noort & Bsibsi, 2009; Li et al., 2010). TLRs have also been reported to recognize various host-derived endogenous ligands, including cellular proteins such as heat shock proteins (Asea et al., 2002; Dybdahl et al., 2002; Ohashi et al., 2000; Roelofs et al., 2006; Vabulas et al., 2001; Vabulas et al., 2002a; Vabulas et al., 2002b) and high mobility group box1 (HMGB1) (Park et al., 2004; Park et al., 2006), uric acid crystal (Liu-Bryan et al., 2005a; Liu-Bryan et al., 2005b), surfactant protein A (Guillot et al., 2002), and products of the extracellular matrix, such as fibronectin (Okamura et al., 2001), heparan sulfate (Johnson et al., 2002), biglycan (Schaefer et al., 2005), fibrinogen (Smiley et al., 2001), oligosaccharides of hyaluronan and degraded hyaluronan products (Termeer et al., 2002; Jiang et al., 2005). These endogenous ligands, referred to as damage-associated molecular patterns (DAMPs), are released from dead or dying cells in injured or inflamed tissues, and trigger the activation of TLRs, leading to "sterile inflammation" (inflammation at the site without microbes).

TLRs have a cytoprotective role and prevent tissue injury under stress conditions in the lung and intestine. In bleomycin-induced lung injury, hyaluronan-TLR2/TLR4 interactions were shown to provide signals that initiate inflammatory responses, maintain epithelial cell integrity and promote recovery from acute lung injury (Jiang et al., 2005). In the dextran sulfate sodium-induced intestine injury model, TLR4 and MyD88 signaling have been shown to be required for optimal proliferation and protection against apoptosis in the injured intestine, and activation of TLRs by commensal microflora was shown to be critical for protection against gut injury and associated mortality (Rakoff-Nahoum et al., 2004; Fukata et al., 2006). The injury-promoting effects of TLR4 have been shown in hepatic, renal, cerebral, and cardiac ischemia-reperfusion experiments using TLR4-mutant or -deficient mice (Oyama et al., 2004; Tsung et al., 2005; Tang et al., 2007; Wu et al., 2007). Alcoholic liver injury has been shown to depend on TLR4 and LPS (Bjarnason et al., 1984; Adachi et al., 1995; Uesugi et al., 2001). In the central nervous system, TLRs have been shown to coordinate the protective response to axonal and crush injury of the brain and spinal cord (Babcock et al., 2006; Kigerl et al., 2007; Kim et al., 2007). Thus, TLRs are thought to control inflammation after tissue injury in positive and negative manners.

The involvement of TLRs in tissue/organ regeneration responses is exemplified by liver regeneration after partial hepatectomy (Seki et al., 2005). Regeneration responses consist of multiple biological functions, including cell proliferation, angiogenesis, reconstruction of extra cellular matrix, epithelialization. TLRs have been reported to regulate the compensatory proliferation of parenchymal cells after injury (Rakoff-Nahoum et al., 2004; Tsung et al., 2005; Pull et al., 2005; Campbell et al., 2006; Zhang & Schluesener, 2006), induce cyclooxygenases, chemokines, vascular endothelial growth factor (VEGF), and matrix metalloproteinases (Fukata et al., 2006; Rakoff-Nahoum et al., 2004; Pull et al., 2005), and activate mesenchymal stem cells (Pevsner-Fischer et al., 2007). Thus, TLRs are involved throughout the process of tissue repair and regeneration, indicating their critical role in tissue homeostasis. TLRs may have acquired dual roles in tissue homeostasis during the evolutionary process, i.e. to regulate inflammation and to promote regenerative processes. It seems reasonable that the same molecule mediates two important processes which sequentially take place at the same site; however, accumulating evidence has shown another aspect of TLR roles in carcinogenesis and cancer development.

2.1.2 TLRs and cancer

2.1.2.1 Anti-tumor effects induced by TLR signaling

BRMs derived from biological materials have been used in cancer immunotherapy, however, the detailed molecular mechanisms evoking tumor immunity have been obscure. During the past couple of decades, dozens of immunity-related molecules including PRRs have been identified, and their identifications greatly help us to understand the relationship between innate immunity and cancer. Among the above mentioned classical BRMs, the following TLRs have been shown to mediate their anti-tumor effects; TLR4 for Coley toxin

(Garay et al., 2007) and OK-432 (Hironaka et al., 2006; Okamoto et al., 2006), TLR2/TLR4 for BCG-CWS (Uehori et al., 2005), respectively. TLR agonists mediate anti-tumor activity by multiple mechanisms (Rakoff-Nahoum & Medzhitov, 2008). TLR agonists have been shown to directly kill both tumor cells and ancillary cells of the tumor microenvironment, such as vascular endothelium (Salaun et al., 2006; El Andaloussi et al., 2006; Haimovitz-Friedman et al., 1997; Nogueras et al., 2008). TLR activation may also lead to tumor regression directly or indirectly (TNF-mediated) by increasing vascular permeability (Garay et al., 2007), recruitment of leukocytes, activation of the tumor lytic activity of NK cells and cytotoxic T lymphocytes (CTL), and increasing the sensitivity of tumor cells to elimination mechanisms by effector molecules, such as TRAIL, TNF, and granzyme B/perforin (Smyth et al., 2006; Akazawa, 2007).

In cancer patients with a growing tumor, immune tolerance between the host immune system and tumor may have already been established. Agonists of TLRs induce intrinsic innate immune responses against microbial infection, leading to adaptive immune responses also to microbial pathogens. At the same time, the triggered innate immune response may also act to break the established tolerance between host and tumor, and induce an adaptive immune response against the tumor, mainly through activated antigen-presenting cell (APC) functions. Breaking the tolerance to tumor self-antigens is a property known as adjuvanticity. The mechanisms by which TLRs induce effective antitumor adaptive immune responses include the uptake, processing and presentation of tumor antigens, enhancement of survival, and induction of costimulatory molecules on professional APCs, induction of Th1 and CTL responses, and the inhibition of regulatory T cell activity (Garay et al., 2007; Smyth et al., 2006; Akazawa et al., 2007).

2.1.2.2 Positive effects of TLRs in cancer development

In the 19th century, Rudolf Virchow, one of the founding fathers of modern pathology, postulated a link between chronic inflammation and cancer (Kluwe et al., 2009). Chronic inflammatory diseases, including inflammatory bowel diseases, hepatitis and *Helicobacter pyroli* infection, have been shown to be associated with cancer development (Chen et al., 2007). Although the detailed mechanisms of tumor-promoting effects by chronic inflammation are far from understood, TLRs are likely candidates as mediators of the effects of the innate immune system on carcinogenesis (Kluwe et al., 2009).

The tumor-promoting effects of TLRs have been shown in studies using adoptively transferred tumor models. Lipopolysaccharide (LPS) enhanced tumor growth in a lung metastasis model of mouse mammary carcinoma cells (Pidgeon et al., 1999; Harmey et al., 2002) and mouse colon cancer cells (Luo et al., 2004). Direct injection of *Listeria monocytogenes*, a Gram-positive facultative intracellular bacterium, promoted tumor growth in a subcutaneous tumor model of hepatocarcinoma cells (Huang et al., 2007). In a study using the mouse mammary tumor cell line and its highly antigenic subline D2F2/E2, which stably expresses human ErbB-2, *Salmonella typhimurium* flagellin, a TLR5 ligand, showed complicated effects in the subcutaneous tumor setting; flagellin inhibited tumor growth only in the D2F2/E2 cells when administered 8-10 days after tumor inoculation, but it accelerated tumor growth in both cell lines when administered at the time of inoculation (Sfondrini et al., 2006) suggesting that the status of interactions between the tumor and its microenvironment and/or host immune system are critical for the effects of flagellin.

Furthermore, the combination of falagellin and TLR9 agonist, CpG containing oligodeoxynucleotide (CpG ODN) administered 8-10 days after tumor inoculation, abrogated D2F2/E2 tumor growth.

The involvement of TLR signaling in caricinogenesis has been shown in studies using TLR-deficient or its signaling molecule-deficient mice (Fukata et al., 2007; Rakoff-Nahoum & Medzhitov, 2007; Naugler et al., 2007). TLR4-deficient mice were protected from colon tumorigenesis in an azoxymethan-induced chronic inflammation model, and TLR4 signaling was suggested to be involved in tumorigenesis *via* cyclooxygenase-2 (Cox-2) expression and prostaglandin (PG) E_2 production, leading to the activation of EGFR signaling (Fukata et al., 2007). MyD88 deficiency resulted in decreased colon tumor development in mice with heterozygous mutation of the adenomatous polyposis coli gene (spontaneous model), and also in an azoxymethane-induced colon tumor model (Rakoff-Nahoum & Medzhitov, 2007). Significant reduction of tumor formation was observed in MyD88 or interleukin (IL)-6 deficient male but not female mice in a diethylnitrosamine-induced hepatocellular carcinoma model (Naugler et al., 2007).

A wide range of human cancer cells have been shown to express various TLRs (Sato et al., 2009). For example, nine TLRs are expressed in normal colon epithelial cells, and three TLRs (TLR2-4) are elevated in most colorectal cancer cell lines (Sfondrini et al., 2006). Four TLRs (TLR2-5) are expressed in both normal ovary epithelial cells and ovarian cancer cell lines (Zhou et al., 2009). The significance of the expression of multiple TLRs in a wide range of cancer cells is not fully understood; however, simultaneous activation of multiple TLR types might be able to enhance the biological response, as in the case of synergistic effects by combined TLR ligation reported for cytokine production in DCs (Whitmore et al., 2004; Roelofs et al., 2005; Warger et al., 2006; Gautier et al., 2005; Theiner et al., 2007; Zhu et al., 2008; Krummen et al., 2010) and macrophages (Sato et al., 2000; Ouyang et al., 2007). It is possible that tumor cells express multiple TLRs to recognize various DAMPs in their microenvironment, and thereby enhance the biological process triggered by TLR activation to produce favorable conditions for growth and survival. Furthermore, ligation of TLRs in tumor cells has also been shown to increase the production of immunosuppressive cytokines, such as interleukin (IL)-10 and transforming growth factor (TGF)-β (Sato et al., 2009), suggesting that tumor cells also utilize the TLR functions to escape from the tumor immunosurveillance.

2.1.3 TLRs as target molecules for drug development

In simple terms, TLR signaling pathway can be facilitated by agonistic agents to enhance the immune response, and inhibited by antagonistic agents to attenuate a hyper-immune reaction. The former can be applied to diseases including cancer and infectious diseases, and the latter to autoimmune diseases, excessive inflammation, and bacteria-induced pathological conditions, such as sepsis. TLR ligands and their related compounds which can bind to TLRs directly are the primary candidates as therapeutic agent. Most of the TLR-targeting drugs under development are agonistic agents, and a few antagonists for TLR4 seems to be developed as therapeutics for sepsis, such as Eritoran (Eisai Co. Ltd, Tokyo, Japan) (Rossignol et al., 2004). These drugs include various types of compounds, including single and double-stranded RNA, CpG ODN, small compounds, etc., but agonistic agents could be roughly divided into two categories in terms of their usage; an immunomodulatory agent and an adjuvant for vaccination. Agonists of TLRs produce their therapeutic efficacy *via* stimulation of APCs of innate immunity, such as DCs and macrophages, as an initial step, and then their activation/maturation trigger secondary immune responses, including the activation of effector cells of both innate and adaptive immunity, such as NK and T cells; therefore, TLR activation is an indirect stimulus of adaptive immunity. Antigens in vaccines are incorporated by APCs at first, and then presented to T lymphocytes to evoke specific adaptive immune responses. TLR agonists could be one of the best candidates for a vaccine adjuvant, because they are well characterized, and their extensive scientific backgrounds make it possible to produce novel compounds with favorable properties, such as less toxicity, stronger immunostimulatory effects, and longer half life. In the TLR-targeting drugs under development, more than half of compounds seem to be targeting TLR9 (Krishnan et al., 2009; Romagne, 2007), and the reasons for that could be their chemical nature (ready to synthesize and handle) and the economic benefit of DNA and its derivatives in addition to their features as strong inducers of Th1 immune responses.

2.1.4 TLR-targeting drugs for cancer

Here, the most advanced two examples of TLR-targeting drug development will be discussed; i.e. agonists for TLR9 and TLR7. A group, so-called antiviral TLRs, including TLR3 and TLR7-9 are predominantly localized intracellularly to endosomal membranes, and recognize nucleic acids and related compounds (Table 1).

2.1.4.1 TLR9 agonists: CpG ODN

TLR9 detects the unmethylated CpG dinucleotides prevalent in bacterial and viral DNA but not in vertebrate genomes (Krieg, 2007). TLR9 has been shown to have the narrowest expression profile among all the TLRs; among resting immune cells, B cells and plasmacytoid DCs (pDCs) seem to exclusively express TLR9 (Iwasaki & Medzhitov, 2004). pDCs are extremely important cells in host defense as they produce most of the type I IFN that is made in response to viral infection and that is essential to control viral replication and to promote the development of an immune response to eradicate infected cells and prevent recurrence (Liu, 2005). One of the most notable features of TLR9 activation is that strong Th1 responses are triggered. In synthetic CpG ODN used *in vivo* applications, including animal experiments and clinical trials, native phosphodiester backbones are replaced partially or fully with phosphorothioate backbones to improve stability.

In animal experiments, significant anti-tumor effects of TLR9 agonists have been demonstrated in a variety of settings; not only in monotherapy (Lonsdorf et al., 2003; Baines & Celis, 2003), but also in combination therapy with monoclonal antibody therapy (Buhtoiarov et al., 2006; Daftarian et al., 2004; Davila et al., 2003; Dercamp et al., 2005; Guiducci et al., 2005; Vicari et al., 2002; Wooldridge et al., 1997), cytokines, chemokines and related factors (Chaudhry et al., 2006; Ishii et al., 2003; Merad et al., 2002; Okano et al., 2005), TLR3 and TLR5 ligands (Sfondrini et al., 2006; Whitmore et al., 2004), EGFR-related signaling and angiogenesis inhibition (Damiano et al., 2006), radiotherapy (Mason et al., 2005), surgery (Ohashi et al., 2006; Weigel et al., 2003), cryotherapy (den Brok et al., 2006), and chemotherapy (Balsari et al., 2004; Pratesi et al., 2005; Taieb et al., 2006; van der Most et al., 2006; H. Wang et al. 2006; X.S. Wang et al., 2005; Weigel et al., 2003). TLR9 has been thought to be the only TLR for which a systemically administered specific agonist has shown substantial evidence of anti-tumor activity in human clinical trials (reviewed in Krieg, 2007). CPG 7909 (also called PF-3512676), a CpG ODN with a fully modified phosphorothioate backbone, has been thought to be one of the most promising drug candidates for cancer therapy.

Unfortunately, it has been announced that the sponsor pharmaceutical company made the decision to terminate phase III clinical trials of CPG 7907. In these phase III clinical trials, the efficacy of CPG 7909 had been tested in combination with gemcitabine/cisplatin or paclitaxel/carboplatin in patients with advanced non-small-cell lung cancer.

2.1.4.2 TLR7 agonists: Imiquimod

TLR7 recognizes single-stranded RNA, and acts as a potent activator of innate immune responses to viral infections (Diebold et al., 2004; Heil et al., 2004). Other than the natural ligands, several distinct classes of low-molecular-weight compounds have been shown to effectively and selectively activate this receptor (Hemmi et al., 2002; Lee et al., 2003). Imiquimod (also called Aldara, R-837, and S-28463), a member of the imidazoquinoline family, has antiviral activity in guinea pigs infected with herpes simplex virus (Harrison et al., 1988), and against arbovirus and cytomegalovirus (Akira & Hemmi, 2003). The first report on the anti-tumor activity of imiquimod was published in 1992, using subcutaneous tumor models of mouse colon carcinoma and mouse sarcoma and a lung metastasis model of mouse Lewis lung carcinoma (Sidky et al., 1992); however, the mechanism of imiquimod action as TLR agonist was totally unknown at that time. Subsequently, anti-tumor effects of imiquimod have been shown to be mediated by the induction of cytokines, including IFN-γ and IL-12 (Hemmi et al., 2002), the enhancement of the activation of tumor antigen-specific CTLs in vaccination studies (Prins et al., 2006; Rechtsteiner et al., 2005), and the activation of a myeloid DC subset with cytotoxic activity (Stary et al., 2007). Because of the intracellular localization of TLR7, small molecules such as imiquimod might have an advantage in terms of cellular uptake (Schön & Schön, 2008).

Imiquimod is a success story of TLR-targeting drugs. A topical cream formulation of imiquimod has been approved to treat actinic keratosis and external genital warts, and its additional indication for the treatment of superficial basal cell carcinoma was approved by the United States Food and Drug Administration in 2004. At present, 20 clinical oncology trials with imiquimod are ongoing (Maruyama et al., 2011). In these clinical trials, new target cancers are included such as basal cell carcinoma of different types/stages, melanoma, cancers of the breast, ovary, uterine cervix, and lung, glioblastoma, neuroblastoma, rhabdomyosarcoma, and osteogenic sarcoma. In addition, imiquimod is used as a vaccine adjuvant in 10 out of 20 trials. Vaccines in these clinical trials include DC-based vaccines, peptides or proteins of tumor associated antigens, human papilloma virus related DNA vaccines (Maruyama et al., 2011). Thus, imiquimod has already been established as a therapeutic product, and is under development as a vaccine adjuvant.

2.1.5 Perspectives: TLRs as double-edged swords in cancer therapy

TLRs have dual important roles in mammals; host defense from infection and maintaining tissue homeostasis by regulating inflammatory and tissue repair responses to damage. Antitumor effects of TLR agonists, including classical BRMs, depend on the former role of

TLRs in the immune systems. TLRs initiate innate immune responses, bridge the response from innate to adaptive immunity, and lead to the elimination of transformed cancer cells; however, cancer cells themselves utilize the latter role of TLRs in tissue homeostasis for their growth and survival by means of a variety of strategies; suppression of host immune responses by the production of various immunosuppressive factors, promotion of cell growth and angiogenesis, induction of cytoprotective and anti-apoptotic factors. These findings suggest that TLR signaling acts as a double-edged sword in cancer therapy. Administration routes and doses may be critical issues to develop TLR-targeting drugs for cancer treatment. Systemic administration of TLR agonists may include the risks of promoting growth and survival of tumor. On the other hand, local application, especially transcutaneous or intradermal administration could be a promising modality to lower the risks. In addition, the dose of the TLR agonist may be an important issue. It has been suggested that exceptionally high doses of TLR agonists appear to have an antitumor effect, whereas low doses of TLR agonists promote tumor growth (Kluwe et al., 2009). It is critical to know how we can dominantly use the unilateral antitumor edge of the TLR sword. Furthermore, another point to be tested in clinical studies may be the combinatorial usage of agonists for different types of TLRs, such as TLR4 agonist plus TLR9 agonist, as tested in animal experiments. As mentioned above, the mixed nature of classical BRMs seems to contribute to efficient antitumor effects. The evidence on the role of TLRs in tissue homeostasis has been obtained mainly from the studies focused on TLR2 and TLR4. For a better understanding of the role of TLRs in tissue homeostasis, carcinogenesis, and tumor progression, more research data on other types of TLR are necessary.

2.2 Fms-like tyrosine kinase 3 ligand (FL)

2.2.1 Cloning of FL as a ligand for fms-like tyrosine kinase-3 (Flt3-R)

FL is a transmembrane or soluble protein and is expressed by a variety of cells including hematopoietic and bone marrow stromal cells. In synergy with other cytokines and growth factors, FL stimulates proliferation and development of a wide range of hematopoietic cells including stem cells, myeloid and lymphoid progenitor cells, DCs and NK cells (Drexler & Quentmeier, 2004; Lyman & Jacobsen, 1998). FL was cloned as a ligand for Flt3-R, a tyrosine kinase receptor belongs to the class III receptor tyrosine kinase family structurally related to macrophage colony-stimulating factor receptor (c-fms) and to mast stem cell factor (also known as steel factor, stem cell factor, and c-kit ligand) receptor (c-kit) (Matthews et al., 1991; Rosnet et al., 1991a; Rosnet et al., 1991b). Lyman et al. isolated a murine Flt3L cDNA by screening an expression library with a fusion protein consisting of the extra cellular domain of the Flt3-R (Lyman et al., 1993). Hannum et al. purified FL from conditioned medium of a murine thymic stromal cell line using an affinity column made with Flt3-R extracellular domain (Hannum et al., 1994). Subsequently, a human counterpart of a murine FL was cloned using a mouse cDNA as a probe (Hannum et al., 1994; Lyman et al., 1994b). The mouse and human FL proteins are 72% identical at the amino acid level with a greater homology in the extracellular region than in the cytoplasmic domain.

Multiple isoforms of FL have been reported for mouse and human; the first one is a transmebrane protein which is a predominant isoform in human (Hannum et al., 1994; Lyman et al., 1993; Lyman et al., 1994b), and is converted to biologically active soluble form by proteolytic cleavage (Lyman et al., 1993). The second biologically active isoform, the most abundantly found in mouse (Lyman et al., 1995b), is a membrane bound form which lacks a normal transmembrane structure but has a hydrophobic amino acid stretch in N-terminus (Hannum et al., 1994; Lyman et al., 1995a). The third isoform identified in mouse and human is a soluble form generated by alternative splicing (Lyman et al., 1995a, Lyman et al., 1995b).

2.2.2 Biological activity of FL

It is known that FL is interactive between different species, mouse and human FL can be fully active on cells expressing either the mouse or human Flt3-R (Lyman et al., 1994a). Although physiological importance for the ubiquitous expression is not clear, FL is widely expressed in murine and human tissues, the transcripts have been detected almost every tissue tested (Hannum et al., 1994; Lyman et al., 1994b; Lyman et al., 1995a). In contrast to FL, its receptor Flt3-R seems to have a relatively limited expression profile. Flt3-R expression in hematopoietic system appear predominantly restricted to the progenitor/stem cell compartment (Drexler et al., 2004).

FL stimulates proliferation and development of a wide range of hematopoietic cells including hematopoietic stem cells, myeloid and lymphoid progenitor cells (reviewed in Drexler et al., 2004). In this section, effects of in vivo administered FL on DCs and NK cells will be discussed.

2.2.2.1 Effects of FL on DC development

DCs express CD45 and arise from BM progenitor cells; evidence suggests that DCs are derived from myeloid and lymphoid progenitor cells (Caux et al., 1995; Peters et al., 1996). Early studies of mouse in vivo experiments identified that FL as a cytokine that could affect DC proliferation (Maraskovsky et al., 1996; Pulendran et al., 1999). In vivo administration of FL in mouse results in a dramatic increase in the number of myeloid- and lymphoid-derived functional DC in BM, spleen, thymus, peripheral blood, and other tissues indicating an absolute increase in functionally mature DC (Maraskovsky et al., 1996). In contrast, polyethylene glycol-modified granulocyte-macrophage colony-stimulating factor (GM-CSF) into mice only expands the myeloid-related DC subset (Pulendran et al., 1999).

In human, two distinct classes of blood DC subsets, CD11c^{+} immature DCs and CD11c^{-} pDCs with different morphologies, phenotypes, and functional properties, have been identified (Liu, 2001). Blood CD11c^{+} DCs are considered to be myeloid derived, whereas pDCs, also known as type 1 interferon-producing cells as mentioned in section 5.1, are considered to be lymphoid related (Liu, 2001). Administration of FL to healthy volunteers significantly expands the number of circulating CD11c^{+} and CD11c^{-} DC subsets and DC precursors (Maraskovsky, 2000).

2.2.2.2 Effects of FL on NK cells

FL administered to mice increased number of NK cells (Brasel et al., 1996; Shaw et al., 1998). Brasel et al. reported that daily subcutaneous injection of recombinant FL (10 μg) for 10 days resulted in 2.5-fold increase in NK cell absolute number in spleen (Brasel et al., 1996). Shaw et al. also showed daily intraperitoneal administration of recombinant FL resulted in increase in the absolute number of $CD3^-$ $NK1.1^+$ NK cell especially in spleen and liver (Shaw et al., 1998). Similar effect of FL on NK expansion was reported by He et al. using intravenous injection of a plasmid expression vector for FL cDNA encoding extra cellular domain (He et al., 2000). These in vivo effects of FL on NK expansion was supported by the evidence obtained from mice lacking FL in which a marked deficiency of NK cells in the spleen was noted (McKenna et al., 2000). The ability of FL to expand NK cells in vivo has been confirmed by subsequent studies (Guimond et al., 2010; Péron et al., 1998; Smith et al., 2001).

In contrast to the mouse findings in vivo, few are available on the effect of FL on human NK cells in vivo. In a phase I clinical trial, FL was subcutaneously injected into cancer patients including Hodgkin disease, non-Hodgikin lymphoma, or advanced-stage breast cancer after autologous hematopoietic cell transplantation (Chen et al., 2005). Injection of FL was safe and well tolerated and significantly increased blood DC subsets without affecting other mature cell lineages including NK cells (Chen et al., 2005). According to the findings obtained, the activity of FL alone to induce cellular expansion is higher in DCs than that in NK cells. It appears necessary to combine FL with other cytokines to induce effective NK cell expansion in vivo especially in human.

2.2.3 Anti-tumor effects evoked by FL

The finding that FL administration resulted in dramatic expansion of DCs led to the studies to test anti-tumor effect of FL. Early study demonstrated that FL alone induced the regression of methylcholanthrene (MCA)-induced fibrosarcoma (Lynch et al., 1997). Subsequently, anti-tumor effect of systemically administered FL has been demonstrated in a lot of syngeneic murine tumor models of melanoma, lymphoma (Esche et al., 1998), Lewis lung carcinoma (Chakravarty et al., 1999), liver metastasis (Péron et al., 1998), mesothelioma (Fernandez et al., 1999), breast cancer (Chen et al., 1997), prostate cancer (Ciavarra et al., 2000). The anti-tumor effect of FL has been shown also in rat syngeneic colon cancer model (Favre-Felix et al., 2000) and xenograft model of human ovarian cancer (Silver et al., 2000). In these tumor models, NK cells seem to have a critical role in the anti-tumor effect induced by FL administration, because depletion of NK cells resulted in abrogation of anti-tumor effect (Fernandez et al., 1999; Péron et al., 1998; Silver et al., 2000). However, the anti-tumor effects induced by FL have also been shown to be T-cell mediated in several mouse models (Chen et al., 1997; Lynch et al., 1997). Fernandez et al. reported that in mice with MHC class I-negative tumors, adoptively transferred- or FL-expanded DCs promoted NK cell-dependent anti-tumor effects (Fernandez et al., 1999). Kelly et al. demonstrated that primary rejection of MHC-class I negative-CD70 expressing RMA-S tumor cells by NK cells efficiently evoked the subsequent development of tumor-specific cytotoxic and T helper type 1 responses to the parental MHC class I-sufficient RMA tumor cells (Kelly et al., 2002). Activated NK cells can facilitate adaptive immune responses via induction of DC maturation by secretion of cytokines and a cell-cell contact (Walzer et al., 2005). These findings suggest that interaction between NK cells and DCs induces not only anti-tumor effects by NK cells, but also adaptive anti-tumor immunity.

At present, limited information are available on clinical studies using FL administration. Marroquin et al. reported that FL administration resulted in a 19-fold increase in DC number in the peripheral blood of patients with melanoma and renal cancer, however, DC generated in vivo appeared only partially activated. This partial activation might account for the lack of enhanced immune responses to melanoma antigens and absence of clinical response in the patients even in combination with antigen immunization (Marroquin et al., 2002). Rini et al. reported that administration of FL either alone or in combination with interleukin-2 (IL-2), although capable of inducing expansion of circulating myeloid and plasmacytoid DCs in patients with metastatic renal cell carcinoma, lacks significant clinical activity (Rini et al., 2002). The above mentioned report by Chen et al. showed that FL administration significantly increased the frequency and absolute number of myeloid DCs, plasmacytoid DCs, and monocytes in the patients with Hodgkin disease, non-Hodgikin lymphoma, or advanced-stage breast cancer after autologous hematopoietic cell transplantation (Chen et al., 2005). In the clinical studies mentioned here, expected clinical responses were not obtained.

The clinical application of DCs for cancer vaccines, however, has been moderately successful (Rosenberg et al., 2004). In the clinical procedure to prepare DC vaccines, monocytes harvested from cancer patients by leukocyte apheresis are cultured in the presence of cytokines to generate DCs. The generated DCs are matured in vitro, treated with tumor antigens such as peptides and tumor lysates, and then injected into patients. The course to prepare DC vaccines needs a lot of times, efforts, and costs. If the in vivo expansion of DCs by FL could be induced effectively and appropriately, it is possible that there is no need to generate DC vaccines ex vivo. Furthermore, ability to expand NK cells is another important point in the clinical application of FL. In the clinical trial mentioned above (Chen et al., 2005), administration of FL to cancer patients did not result in apparent expansion of NK cells. Combination of FL with other cytokines like IL-15 may be the promising strategy to expand human NK cells in vivo (Yu et al., 1998).

2.3 Alpha-galactosylceramide (α-GalCer)

2.3.1 Isolation, identification, and synthesis of α-GalCer

Glycosphingolipid compounds, named agelasphins, were isolated from an extract of the Okinawan marine sponge, *Agelas mauritianus*, by Kirin Pharmaceuticals, and some of them were found to possess anti-tumor activity in mice (Natori et al., 1994; Tsuji, 2006). Because of the low contents of agelasphins in the marine sponge, and the difficulty of their scale-up synthesis, the structure of agelasphins was modified, and a novel compound, α-GalCer (also called KRN7000) was synthesized (Kobayashi et al., 1995). This glycolipid was shown to bind non-classical MHC molecule CD1d of human and mice (Gansert et al., 2003; Taniguchi & Nakayama, 2000), and activate natural killer T (NKT) cells of both species in vitro and in vivo when it is presented on CD1d molecule (Brossay et al., 1998; Burdin et al., 1998; Kawano et al., 1998; Spada et al., 1998) . To date, α-GalCer has been the most extensively studied ligand for CD1d molecules and stimulant for NKT cells.

2.3.2 NKT cells

NKT cells are a unique subpopulation of T cells which play important role in regulating immune responses by bridging innate and adaptive immune systems. The term 'NKT cells' was first used in 1995 (Makino et al., 1995) to define a subset of mouse T cells that share some characteristics with NK cells, particularly expression of the NK1.1 marker (Nkrp1c or CD161c). At present, the term NKT cells is well accepted and broadly applied to mice, humans, and other species (Godfrey et al., 2004). NKT cells express an antigen-specific T cell receptor (TCR), but unlike with conventional T cells that detect peptide antigens presented by MHC molecules, NKT cells recognize lipid antigens presented by CD1d molecule. NKT cells have been shown to involve wide spectrum of disorders including infectious diseases caused by bacteria, parasites, and virus, autoimmunity, and cancer (Terabe & Berzofsky, 2008).

Accumulating several lines of evidences which obtained from the late 80's to 90's had been integrated into the establishment of novel immune cell lineage 'NKT cells' (Bendelac et al., 1997; Bendelac et al., 2007; Godfrey et al., 2004; Godfrey et al., 2010; Macdonald., 2007; Taniguchi et al., 2003; Terabe. & Berzofsky, 2008). However, an ambiguous definition of NKT cells has caused confusion in our understanding of their biological roles. At present, it has been proposed to classify NKT cells into two types (Godfrey et al., 2010).

Type I NKT cells, also called invariant NKT cells or iNKT cells, are defined by their expression of the canonical invariant TCRα chain of Vα14Jα18 in mouse (Vα24Jα18 in human) with a limited number of TCRβ chains of Vβ8, Vβ7, and Vβ2 in mouse (Vβ11 in human). Type I NKT cells are detected with α-GalCer-loaded CD1d tetramers, however, other CD1d restricted T cells exist (Godfrey et al., 2004; Godfrey et al., 2010; Terabe & Berzofsky, 2007). On stimulation with α-GalCer, type I NKT cells produce a large amount of TH1 (IFN-γ) and Th2 (IL-4 and IL-13) cytokines. Although type I NKT cells have NK-like cytolytic activity, they are considered to be regulators of immune responses because they rapidly produce large amount of both Th1 and Th2 cytokines in autoimmune diseases, infectious diseases, and cancer. Another subset of CD1d-restricted NKT cells which does not respond to α-GalCer, seems to recognize a range of hydrophobic antigens including sulfatide (Jahng et al., 2004), lysophosphatidylcholine (Chang et al., 2008), and small aromatic (non-lipid) molecules (Van Rhijn et al., 2004). This NKT subset, called 'type II NKT cells', is present in humans and mice, and has been shown to be more heterogeneous than type I in both TCRα and TCRβ chain usage (Godfrey et al., 2004; Godfrey et al., 2010; Terabe & Berzofsky, 2007; Terabe & Berzofsky, 2008). In this chapter, the findings on type I NKT cells and their ligands will be discussed hereafter.

2.3.3 Anti-tumor effects of α-GalCer

Originally, a mother compound of α-GalCer, agelasphins, was selected from several glycosphingolipids extracted from marine sponge depending on their anti-tumor effects in mouse tumor models (Natori et al., 1994). Anti-tumor effect caused by α-GalCer injection has been shown in mouse tumor models (Kobayashi et al., 1995; Motoki et al., 1995; Morita et al., 1995). Subsequently, protective roles of NKT cells stimulated by α-GalCer were confirmed by liver and lung metastasis models in mice using B16 melanoma cells and Lewis lung carcinoma cells, respectively (Kawano et al., 1998). A complete inhibition of B16 melanoma metastasis in the liver was observed when α-GalCer-pulsed DCs were injected 7 days after transfer of tumor cells to mice where metastatic nodules were already formed (Toura et al., 1999). In addition, long-term administration of α-GalCer inhibited primary tumor formation in the tumor models of MCA-induced sarcoma, mammary carcinomas in Her-2/neu transgenic mice, and spontaneous sarcomas in p53 deficient mice (Hayakawa et al., 2003).

Anti-tumor effects of α-GalCer depend on the production of IFN–γ from activated type I NKT cells (Terabe & Berzofsky, 2007). Crowe et al. showed that IFN-γ production by NKT cells was essential for protection against tumor, and perforin production by effector cells, but not NKT cells, was also critical in MCA-induced sarcoma models (Crowe et al., 2002). Smyth et al. reported that both NK cells and NKT cells were essential and collaborate in host protection from MCA-induced sarcoma (Smyth et al., 2001), and sequential production of IFN-γ by NKT cells and NK cells was essential for the antimetastatic effect of α-GalCer in B16 melanoma metastasis models (Smyth et al., 2002).

In addition to the essential role of IFN-γ, IL-12 was shown to be critical for the anti-tumor effect of NKT cells. Kitamura et al. demonstrated that production of IFN-γ by NKT cells in response to α-GalCer required IL-12 produced by DCs and direct contact between NKT cells and DCs through CD40-CD40 ligand interactions (Kitamura et al., 1999). Hayakawa et al. showed that both CD28-CD80/CD86 and CD40-CD40 ligand costimulatory pathways are essential for α-GalCer-induced IFN-γ production by NKT cells (Hayakawa et al., 2001). Furthermore, administration of α-GalCer induced not only innate immune response, but also adaptive immune response. A single dose of α-GalCer rapidly stimulated the full maturation of DCs in NKTcell-dependent manner, and this maturation accounted for the induction of combined Th1 $CD4^+$ and $CD8^+$ T cell immunity to a coadministered antigen (Fujii et al., 2003).

Taken together, anti-tumor effects of α-GalCer are thought to be evoked by the following sequential processes; α-GalCer presented on CD1d of DCs is recognized by NKT cells, and up-regulates CD40 ligand on NKT cells. Activated DCs by CD40 and CD28 costimulatory pathways produce IL-12, and activate NKT cells by IL-12. IFN-γ produced by fully activated NKT cells trigger DC maturation, activation and recruitment of NK cells, Th1 $CD4^+$ and $CD8^+$ T cell leading to direct anti-tumor effects.

2.3.4 Clinical trials using α-GalCer in cancer patients

At present, a number of clinical trials of α-GalCer have been conducted in multiple institutes, and their results have been published since 2002. Early study of phase I clinical trial in which α-GalCer was injected intravenously reported that α-GalCer was well tolerated in cancer patients over a wide range of doses (Giaccone et al., 2002). Phase I studies of α-GalCer-pulsed DCs have been conducted in patients with various solid tumors and myeloma (Chang et al., 2005; Dhodapkar et al., 2004; Ishikawa et al., 2005; Nieda et al., 2004; Okai et al., 2002; Uchida et al., 2008). However, none of these clinical trials reported significant efficacy against tumors.

Recently, the research team of Chiba University in Japan reported the summary of their clinical trials (Motohashi et al., 2011). The research team has been well known by their pioneering works on α-GalCer, and has been conducted multiple clinical trials with enthusiasm (Ishikawa et al., 2005; Kunii et al., 2009; Kurosaki et al., 2011; Motohashi et al., 2006; Motohashi et al., 2009; Uchida et al., 2008; Yamasaki et al., 2011). The team conducted the α-GalCer-NKT cell-based clinical trials in patients with non-small cell lung cancer and head and neck squamous cell carcinoma (Motohashi et al., 2011). Alpha-GalCer-pulsed APCs seemed to produce better clinical outcomes in the patients with head and neck squamous cell carcinoma than in those with non-small cell lung cancer. The cells were injected into nasal submucosa of patients with head and neck squamous cell carcinoma, whereas intravenous injection was performed in the non-small cell lung cancer patients. Furthermore, the anti-tumor effect of α-GalCer-pulsed APCs seemed to be augmented by the combined adoptive transfer of α-GalCer-activated NKT cells. Thus, clinical efficacy of α-GalCer-based immunotherapy may depend on the tumor type and treatment settings. Further efforts are necessary to develop an effective treatment modality.

3. Conclusion

In cancer patients with a growing tumor, immune tolerance between the host immune system and tumor may have already been established. Agents mentioned in this chapter induce inherent innate immune responses intrinsically against microbial infection. The anti-tumor effect *via* activation of innate immune system may depend on the action to break the established tolerance between host and tumor leading to adaptive immune responses (Figure.1). In other words, the activation of innate immune system acts like as a 'reset

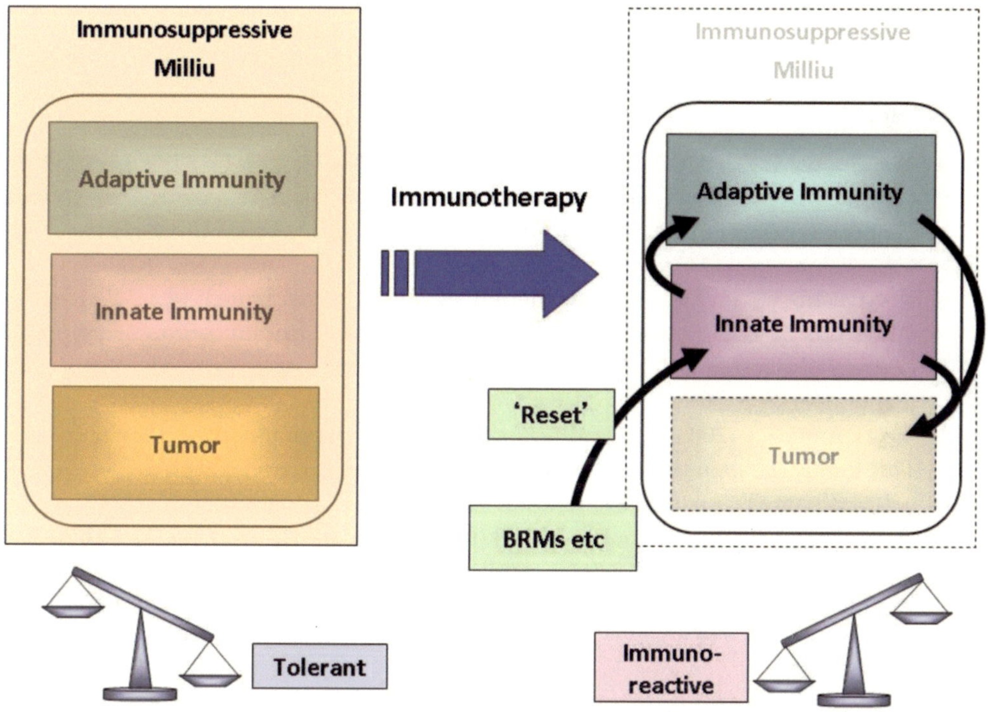

Fig. 1. In the cancer patients with a growing tumor, immune tolerance between host immune system and tumor may have already been established. Stimulants of innate immunity such as biological response modifiers (BRMs) or ligands for toll-like receptors induce inherent innate immune responses intrinsically against microbial infection. The anti-tumor effect *via* activation of innate immune system may depend on the action to break the established tolerance between host and tumor leading to adaptive immune responses.

button' in cancer patients to restart the immune responses. Administration of cytokines such as FL which induce expansion of immune cells can potentiate subsequent immune responses, and it may be the ideal pretreatment for cancer patients with immunosuppressive status. With regards to TLRs agonist, FL, and α-GalCer, the efforts to develop them as vaccine adjuvant have already been started. At present, the efficacy of a prophylactic vaccination against human papillomavirus has been established in the prevention of cervical cancer. Although tough and long-lasting works and huge research fund are required to perform clinical trials, one of the most promising immunotherapeutic modalities for cancer may be cancer prevention. Above mentioned three agents may be excellent vaccine adjuvants to enhance tumor immunity in cancer prevention. Further research efforts are required to establish more effective immunotherapy which will also achieve a better quality of life for cancer patients.

4. Acknowledgment

The authors wish to thank Dr. Masatoshi Kusuhara, Dr. Ken-ichi Urakami, Dr. Vincent Zangiacomi, and Ms. Yoko Masuda of Regional Resources Division of Shizuoka Cancer Center Research Institute, and Dr. Christophe Borg and Dr. Zohair Selmani of INSERM UMR 645, Besançon, France, for their kind collaborations.

5. References

Adachi, Y., Moore, L.E., Bradford, B.U., Gao, W. & Thurman, R.G. (1995). Antibiotics prevent liver injury in rats following long-term exposure to ethanol. *Gastroenterology*, Vol.108, No.1, (January), pp. 218–224.

Akiyama, J., Kawamura, T., Gotohda, E., Yamada, Y., Hosokawa, M., Kodama, T. & Kobayashi, H. (1977). Immunochemotherapy of transplanted KMT-17 tumor in WKA rats by combination of cyclophosphamide and immunostimulatory protein-bound polysaccharide isolated from basidiomycetes. *Cancer Research.*, Vol.37, No.9, (September), pp. 3042-3045.

Akira, S. & Hemmi, H. (2003). Recognition of pathogen-associated molecular patterns by TLR family. *Immunology Letters*, Vol.85, No.2, (January), pp. 85-95.

Akazawa, T., Ebihara, T., Okuno, M., Okuda, Y., Shingai, M., Tsujimura, K., Takahashi, T., Ikawa, M., Okabe, M., Inoue, N., Okamoto-Tanaka, M., Ishizaki, H., Miyoshi, J., Matsumoto, M. & Seya, T. (2007). Antitumor NK activation induced by the Toll-like receptor 3-TICAM-1 (TRIF) pathway in myeloid dendritic cells. *Proceedings of the National Academy of Sciences of the United States of America*, Vol.104, No.1, (January), pp. 252-257.

Asea, A., Rehli, M., Kabingu, E., Boch, J.A., Bare, O., Auron, P.E., Stevenson, M.A. & Calderwood, S.K. (2002). Novel signal transduction pathway utilized by extracellular HSP70: role of toll-like receptor (TLR) 2 and TLR4. *The Journal of Biological Chemistry*, Vol.277, No.17, (April), 15028–15034.

Azuma, I., Ribi, E.E., Meyer, T.J. & Zbar, B. (1974). Biologically active components from mycobacterial cell walls. I. Isolation and composition of cell wall skeleton and component P3. *Journal of the National Cancer Institute*, Vol.52, No.1, (January), pp. 95–101.

Babcock, A.A., Wirenfeldt, M., Holm, T., Nielsen, H.H., Dissing-Olesen, L., Toft-Hansen, H., Millward, J.M., Landmann, R., Rivest, S., Finsen, B. & Owens, T. (2006). Toll-like receptor 2 signaling in response to brain injury: an innate bridge to neuroinflammation. *The Journal of Neuroscience*, Vol.26, No.49, (December), pp. 12826-12837.

Baines, J. & Celis, E. (2003). Immune-mediated tumor regression induced by CpG-containing oligodeoxynucleotides. *Clinical Cancer Research*, Vol.9, No.7, (July), pp. 2693–2700.

Balsari, A., Tortoreto, M., Besusso, D., Petrangolini, G., Sfondrini, L., Maggi, R., Ménard, S. & Pratesi, G. (2004). Combination of a CpG-oligodeoxynucleotide and a topoisomerase I inhibitor in the therapy of human tumour xenografts. *European Journal of Cancer*, Vol.40, No.8, (May), pp. 1275–1281.

Bendelac, A., Rivera, M.N., Park, S.H. & Roark, J.H. (1997). Mouse CD1-specific NK1 T cells: development, specificity, and function. *Annual Review of Immunology*, Vol.15, (April), pp. 535-562.

Bendelac, A., Savage, P.B. & Teyton, L. (2007). The biology of NKT cells. *Annual Review of Immunology*, Vol.25, (April), pp. 297-336.

Bickels, J., Kollender, Y., Merinsky, O. & Meller, I. (2002). Coley's toxin: historical perspective. *The Israel Medical Association Journal*, Vol.4, (June), pp. 471-472.

Bjarnason, I., Peters, T.J. & Wise, R.J. (1984). The leaky gut of alcoholism: possible route of entry for toxic compounds. *Lancet*, Vol.1, No.8370, (January), pp. 179–182.

Brasel, K., McKenna, H.J., Morrissey, P.J., Charrier, K., Morris, A.E., Lee, C.C., Williams, D.E. & Lyman, S.D. (1996). Hematologic effects of flt3 ligand in vivo in mice. *Blood*, Vol.88, No.6, (September), pp. 2004-2012.

Brossay, L., Chioda, M., Burdin, N., Koezuka, Y., Casorati, G., Dellabona, P. & Kronenberg, M. (1998). CD1d-mediated recognition of an alpha-galactosylceramide by natural killer T cells is highly conserved through mammalian evolution. *The Jounal of Experimental Medicine* , Vol.188, No.8, (October), pp. 1521-1528.

Buhtoiarov, I.N., Lum, H.D., Berke, G., Sondel, P.M. & Rakhmilevich, A.L. (2006). Synergistic activation of macrophages via CD40 and TLR9 results in T cell independent antitumor effects. *The Journal of Immunology*, Vol.176, No.1, (January), pp. 309–318.

Burdin, N., Brossay, L., Koezuka, Y., Smiley, S.T., Grusby, M.J., Gui, M., Taniguchi, M., Hayakawa, K. & Kronenberg, M. (1998). Selective ability of mouse CD1 to present glycolipids: alpha-galactosylceramide specifically stimulates V alpha 14+ NK T lymphocytes. *The Journal of Immunology*, Vol.161, No.7, (October), pp. 3271–3281.

Campbell, J.S., Riehle, K.J., Brooling, J.T., Bauer, R.L., Mitchell, C. & Fausto, N. (2006). Proinflammatory cytokine production in liver regeneration is Myd88-dependent, but independent of Cd14, Tlr2, and Tlr4. *The Journal of Immunology*, Vol.176, No.4, (February), pp. 2522-2528.

Caux, C., Liu, Y.J. & Banchereau, J. (1995). Recent advances in the study of dendritic cells and follicular dendritic cells. *Immunology Today*, Vol.16, No.1, (January), pp. 2-4.

Chakravarty, P.K., Alfieri, A., Thomas, E.K., Beri, V., Tanaka, K.E., Vikram, B. & Guha, C. (1999). Flt3-ligand administration after radiation therapy prolongs survival in a murine model of metastatic lung cancer. *Cancer Research*, Vol.59, No.24, (December), pp. 6028-6032.

Chang, D.H., Deng, H., Matthews, P., Krasovsky, J., Ragupathi, G., Spisek, R., Mazumder, A., Vesole, D.H., Jagannath, S. & Dhodapkar, M.V. (2008). Inflammation-associated lysophospholipids as ligands for CD1d-restricted T cells in human cancer. *Blood*, Vol.112, No.4, (August), pp. 1308-1316.

Chang, D.H., Osman, K., Connolly, J., Kukreja, A., Krasovsky, J., Pack, M., Hutchinson, A., Geller, M., Liu, N., Annable, R., Shay, J., Kirchhoff, K., Nishi, N., Ando, Y., Hayashi, K., Hassoun, H., Steinman, R.M. & Dhodapkar, M.V. (2005). Sustained expansion of NKT cells and antigen-specific T cells after injection of alpha-galactosyl-ceramide loaded mature dendritic cells in cancer patients. *The Journal of Experimental Medicine*, Vol.201, No.9, (May), pp. 1503-1517.

Chaudhry, U.I., Kingham, T.P., Plitas, G., Katz, S.C., Raab, J.R. & DeMatteo, R.P. (2006). Combined stimulation with interleukin-18 and CpG induces murine natural killer dendritic cells to produce IFN-gamma and inhibit tumor growth. *Cancer Resesrch*, Vol.66, No.2, (November), pp. 10497–10504.

Chen, K., Braun, S., Lyman, S., Fan, Y., Traycoff, C.M., Wiebke, E.A., Gaddy, J., Sledge, G., Broxmeyer, H.E. & Cornetta, K. (1997). Antitumor activity and immunotherapeutic properties of Flt3-ligand in a murine breast cancer model. *Cancer Research*, Vol.57, No.16, (August), pp. 3511-3516.

Chen, K., Huang, J., Gong, W., Iribarren, P., Dunlop, N.M. & Wang J.M. (2007). Toll-like receptors in inflammation, infection and cancer. *International Immunopharmacology*, Vol.7, No.10, (October), pp. 1271-1285.

Chen, W., Chan, A.S., Dawson, A.J., Liang, X., Blazar, B.R. & Miller, J.S. (2005). FLT3 ligand administration after hematopoietic cell transplantation increases circulating dendritic cell precursors that can be activated by CpG oligodeoxynucleotides to enhance T-cell and natural killer cell function. *Biology of Blood and Marrow Transplantation*, Vol.11, No.1, (January), pp. 23-34.

Ciavarra, R.P., Somers, K.D., Brown, R.R., Glass, W.F., Consolvo, P.J., Wright, G.L. & Schellhammer, P.F. (2000). Flt3-ligand induces transient tumor regression in an ectopic treatment model of major histocompatibility complex-negative prostate cancer. *Cancer Research*, Vol.60, No,8, (April), pp. 2081-2084.

Crowe, N.Y., Smyth, M.J. & Godfrey, D.I. (2002). A critical role for natural killer T cells in immunosurveillance of methylcholanthrene-induced sarcomas. *The Journal of Experimental Medicine*, Vol.196, No.1, (July), pp. 119-127.

Daftarian, P., Song, G.Y., Ali, S., Faynsod, M., Longmate, J., Diamond, D.J. & Ellenhorn, J.D. (2004). Two distinct pathways of immuno-modulation improve potency of p53 immunization in rejecting established tumors. *Cancer Research*, Vol.64, No.15, (August), pp. 5407–5414.

Damiano, V., Caputo, R., Bianco, R., D'Armiento, F.P., Leonardi, A., De Placido, S., Bianco, A.R., Agrawal, S., Ciardiello, F. & Tortora, G. (2006). Novel toll-like receptor 9 agonist induces epidermal growth factor receptor (EGFR) inhibition and synergistic antitumor activity with EGFR inhibitors. *Clinical Cancer Research*, Vol.12, No.2, (January), pp. 577–583.

Davila, E., Kennedy, R. & Celis, E. (2003). Generation of antitumor immunity by cytotoxic T lymphocyte epitope peptide vaccination, CpG-oligodeoxynucleotide adjuvant, and CTLA4 blockade. *Cancer Research*, Vol.63, No.12, (June), pp. 3281–3288.

den Brok, M.H., Sutmuller, R.P., Nierkens, S., Bennink, E.J., Toonen, L.W., Figdor, C.G., Ruers, T.J. & Adema, G.J. (2006). Synergy between in situ cryoablation and TLR9 stimulation results in a highly effective in vivo dendritic cell vaccine. *Cancer Research*, Vol.66, No.14, (July), pp. 7285–7292.

Dercamp, C., Chemin, K., Caux, C., Trinchieri, G. & Vicari, A.P. (2005). Distinct and overlapping roles of interleukin-10 and CD25+ regulatory T cells in the inhibition of antitumor CD8 T-cell responses. *Cancer Research*, Vol.65, No. 18, (September), pp. 8479–8486.

Dhodapkar, K.M., Cirignano, B., Chamian, F., Zagzag, D., Miller, D.C., Finlay, J.L. & Steinman, R.M. (2004). Invariant natural killer T cells are preserved in patients with glioma and exhibit antitumor lytic activity following dendritic cell-mediated expansion. *International Journal of Cancer*, Vol.109, No.6, (May), pp. 893-899.

Diebold, S.S., Kaisho, T., Hemmi, H., Akira, S. & Reis e Sousa, C. (2004). Innate antiviral responses by means of TLR7-mediated recognition of single-stranded RNA. *Science*, Vol.303, No.5683, (March), pp. 1529-1531.

Drexler, H.G. & Quentmeier, H. (2004). FLT3: receptor and ligand. *Growth Factors*, Vol.22, No.2, (June), pp. 71-73.

Dybdahl, B., Wahba, A., Lien, E., Flo, T.H., Waage, A., Qureshi, N., Sellevold, O.F., Espevik, T. & Sundan, A. (2002). Inflammatory response after open heart surgery: release of heat-shock protein 70 and signaling through Toll-like receptor-4. *Circulation*, Vol.105, No.6, (February), pp. 685–690.

El Andaloussi, A., Sonabend, A.M., Han, Y. & Lesniak, M.S. (2006). Stimulation of TLR9 with CpG ODN enhances apoptosis of glioma and prolongs the survival of mice with experimental brain tumors. *Glia*, Vol.54, No.6, (November). pp. 526-535.

Esche, C., Subbotin, V.M., Maliszewski, C., Lotze, M.T., Shurin, M.R. (1998). FLT3 ligand administration inhibits tumor growth in murine melanoma and lymphoma. *Cancer Research*, Vol.58, No.3, (February), pp. 380-383.

Favre-Felix, N., Martin, M., Maraskovsky, E., Fromentin, A., Moutet, M., Solary, E., Martin, F. & Bonnotte, B. (2000). Flt3 ligand lessens the growth of tumors obtained after colon cancer cell injection in rats but does not restore tumor-suppressed dendritic cell function. *International Journal of Cancer*, Vol.86, No.6, (June), pp. 827-834.

Fernandez, N.C., Lozier, A., Flament, C., Ricciardi-Castagnoli, P., Bellet, D., Suter, M., Perricaudet, M., Tursz, T., Maraskovsky, E. & Zitvogel, L. (1999). Dendritic cells directly trigger NK cell functions: cross-talk relevant in innate anti-tumor immune responses in vivo. *Nature Medicine*, Vol.5, No.4, (April), pp. 405-411.

Fujii, S., Shimizu, K., Smith, C., Bonifaz, L. & Steinman, R.M. (2003). Activation of natural killer T cells by alpha-galactosylceramide rapidly induces the full maturation of dendritic cells in vivo and thereby acts as an adjuvant for combined CD4 and CD8 T cell immunity to a coadministered protein. *The Journal of Experimental Medicine*, Vol.198, No.2, (July), pp. 267-279.

Fukata, M., Chen, A., Klepper, A., Krishnareddy, S., Vamadevan, A.S., Thomas, L.S., Xu, R., Inoue, H., Arditi, M., Dannenberg, A.J. & Abreu, M.T. (2006). Cox-2 is regulated by Toll-like receptor-4 (TLR4) signaling: Role in proliferation and apoptosis in the intestine. *Gastroenterology*, Vol.131, No.3, (September), 862–877.

Fukata, M., Chen, A., Vamadevan, A.S., Cohen, J., Breglio, K., Krishnareddy, S., Hsu, D., Xu, R., Harpaz, N., Dannenberg, A.J., Subbaramaiah, K., Cooper, H.S., Itzkowitz, S.H. & Abreu, M.T. (2007). Toll-like receptor-4 promotes the development of colitis-associated colorectal tumors. *Gastroenterology*, Vol.133, No.6, (December), pp. 1869–1881.

Gansert, J.L., Kiessler, V., Engele, M., Wittke, F., Rollinghoff, M., Krensky, A.M., Porcelli, S.A., Modlin, R.L. and Stenger, S. (2003). Human NKT cells express granulysin and exhibit antimycobacterial activity. *The Journal of Immunology*, Vol.170, No.6, (March), pp. 3154–3161.

Garay, R., Viens, P., Bauer, J., Normier, G., Bardou, M., Jeannin, J.F. & Chiavaroli, C. (2007). Cancer relapse under chemotherapy: why TLR2/4 receptor agonists can help. *European Journal of Pharmacology*, Vol.563, No.1-3, (June), pp. 1-17.

Gautier, G., Humbert, M., Deauvieau, F., Scuiller, M., Hiscott, J., Bates, E.E., Trinchieri, G., Caux, C. & Garrone, P. (2005). A type I interferon autocrine-paracrine loop is involved in Toll-like receptor-induced interleukin-12p70 secretion by dendritic cells. *The Journal of Experimantal Medicine*, Vol.201, No.9, (May), 1435–1446.

Giaccone, G., Punt, C.J., Ando, Y., Ruijter, R., Nishi, N., Peters, M., von Blomberg, B.M., Scheper, R.J., van der Vliet, H.J., van den Eertwegh, A.J., Roelvink, M., Beijnen, J., Zwierzina, H. & Pinedo, H.M. (2002). A phase I study of the natural killer T-cell ligand alpha-galactosylceramide (KRN7000) in patients with solid tumors. *Clinical Cancer Research*, Vol.8, No.12, (December), pp. 3702-3709.

Guiducci, C., Vicari, A.P., Sangaletti, S., Trinchieri, G. & Colombo M.P. (2005). Redirecting in vivo elicited tumor infiltrating macrophages and dendritic cells towards tumor rejection. *Cancer Research*, Vol.65, No.8, (April), 3437–3446.

Guillot, L., Balloy, V., McCormack, F.X., Golenbock, D.T., Chignard, M. & Si-Tahar, M. (2002). Cutting edge: the immunostimulatory activity of the lung surfactant protein-A involves Toll-like receptor 4. *The Journal of Immunology*, Vol.168, No.12, (June), pp. 5989–5992.

Guimond, M., Freud, A.G., Mao, H.C., Yu, J., Blaser, B.W., Leong, J.W., Vandeusen, J.B., Dorrance, A., Zhang, J., Mackall, C.L. & Caligiuri, M.A. (2010). In vivo role of Flt3 ligand and dendritic cells in NK cell homeostasis. *The Journal of Immunology*, Vol.184, No.6, (February), pp. 2769-2775.

Godfrey, D.I., MacDonald, H.R., Kronenberg, M., Smyth, M.J. & Van Kaer, L. (2004). NKT cells: what's in a name? *Nature Review of Immunology*, Vol.4, No.3, (March), pp. 231-237.

Godfrey, D.I., Stankovic, S. & Baxter, A.G. (2010). Raising the NKT cell family. *Nature Immunology*, Vol.11, No.3, (March), pp. 197-206.

Haimovitz-Friedman, A., Cordon-Cardo, C., Bayoumy, S., Garzotto, M., McLoughlin, M., Gallily, R., Edwards, C.K. 3rd., Schuchman, E.H., Fuks, Z. & Kolesnick, R. (1997). Lipopolysaccharide induces disseminated endothelial apoptosis requiring ceramide generation. *The Journal of Experimental Medicine*, Vol.186, No.11, (December), pp. 1831-1841.

Hannum. C., Culpepper. J., Campbell, D., McClanahan, T., Zurawski, S., Bazan, J.F., Kastelein, R., Hudak, S., Wagner, J., Mattson, J., Luh, J., Duda, G., Martina, N., Peterson, D., Menon, S., Shanafelt, A.M., Muench, A.M., Kelner, G., Namikawa, R., Rennick, D., Roncarolo, M-G., Zlotnik, A., Rosnet, O., Dubreuil, P., Birnbaum, D. & Lee, F. (1994). Ligand for FLT3/FLK2 receptor tyrosine kinase regulates growth of haematopoietic stem cells and is encoded by variant RNAs. *Nature*, Vol.368, No.6472, (April), pp. 643-648.

Harmey, J.H., Bucana, C.D., Lu, W., Byrne, A.M., McDonnell, S., Lynch, C., Bouchier-Hayes, D. & Dong, Z. (2002). Lipopolysaccharide-induced metastatic growth is associated with increased angiogenesis, vascular permeability and tumor cell invasion. *International Journal of Cancer*, Vol.101, No.5, (October), pp. 415–422.

Harrison, C.J., Jenski, L., Voychehovski, T. & Bernstein, D.I. (1988). Modification of immunological responses and clinical disease during topical R-837 treatment of genital HSV-2 infection. *Antiviral Research*, Vol.10, No.4-5, (December), pp. 209-223.

Hashimoto, C., Hudson, K.L. & Anderson, K.V. (1988). The Toll gene of Drosophila, required for dorsal-ventral embryonic polarity, appears to encode a transmembrane protein. *Cell*, Vol.52, No.2, (January), pp. 269-279.

Hayakawa, Y., Rovero, S., Forni, G. & Smyth, M.J. (2003). Alpha-galactosylceramide (KRN7000) suppression of chemical- and oncogene-dependent carcinogenesis. *Proceedings of the National Academy of Sciences of the United States of America*, Vol.100, No.16, (August), pp. 9464-9469.

Hayakawa, Y., Takeda, K., Yagita, H., Van Kaer, L., Saiki, I. & Okumura K. (2001). Differential regulation of Th1 and Th2 functions of NKT cells by CD28 and CD40 costimulatory pathways. *The Journal of Immunology*, Vol.166, No.10, (May), pp. 6012-6018.

Hayashi, A., Nishida, Y., Yoshii, S., Kim, S.Y., Uda, H. & Hamasaki, T. (2009). Immunotherapy of ovarian cancer with cell wall skeleton of Mycobacterium bovis Bacillus Calmette-Guérin: effect of lymphadenectomy. *Cancer Science*, Vol.100, No.10, (October), pp. 1991-1995.

He, Y., Pimenov, A.A., Nayak, J.V., Plowey, J., Falo, L.D. Jr. & Huang, L. (2000). Intravenous injection of naked DNA encoding secreted flt3 ligand dramatically increases the number of dendritic cells and natural killer cells in vivo. *Human Gene Therapy*. Vol.11, No.4, (March), pp. 547-554.

Heil, F., Hemmi, H., Hochrein, H., Ampenberger, F., Kirschning, C., Akira, S., Lipford, G., Wagner, H. & Bauer, S. (2004). Species-specific recognition of single-stranded RNA via toll-like receptor 7 and 8. *Science*, Vol.303, No.5663, (March), pp. 1526-1529.

Hemmi, H., Kaisho, T., Takeuchi, O., Sato, S., Sanjo, H., Hoshino, K., Horiuchi, T., Tomizawa, H., Takeda, K. & Akira, S. (2002). Small anti-viral compounds activate immune cells via the TLR7 MyD88-dependent signaling pathway. *Nature Immunology*, Vol.3, No.2, (February), pp. 196-200.

Hironaka, K., Yamaguchi, Y., Okita, R., Okawaki, M. & Nagamine, I. (2006). Essential requirement of toll-like receptor 4 expression on CD11c+ cells for locoregional immunotherapy of malignant ascites using a streptococcal preparation OK-432. *Anticancer Research*, Vol.26, No.5B, (September-October), pp. 3701-3707.

Huang, B., Zhao, J., Shen, S., Li, H., He, K.L., Shen, G.X., Mayer, L., Unkeless, J., Li, D., Yuan, Y., Zhang, G.M., Xiong, H. & Feng, Z.H. (2007). Listeria monocytogenes promotes tumor growth via tumor cell toll-like receptor 2 signaling. *Cancer Research*, Vol. 67, No.9, (May), pp. 4346–4352.

Ishii, K.J., Kawakami, K., Gursel, I., Conover, J., Joshi, B.H., Klinman, D.M. & Puri, R.K. (2003). Antitumor therapy with bacterial DNA and toxin: complete regression of established tumor induced by liposomal CpG oligodeoxynucleotides plus interleukin-13 cytotoxin. *Clinical Cancer Research*, Vol.9, No.17, (December), pp. 6516–6522.

Ishikawa, A., Motohashi, S., Ishikawa, E., Fuchida, H., Higashino, K., Otsuji, M., Iizasa, T., Nakayama, T., Taniguchi, M. & Fujisawa, T. (2005). A phase I study of alpha-galactosylceramide (KRN7000)-pulsed dendritic cells in patients with advanced and recurrent non-small cell lung cancer. *Clinical Cancer Research*, Vol.11, No.5, (March), pp. 1910-1917.

Iwasaki, A. & Medzhitov, R. (2004). Toll-like receptor control of the adaptive immune responses. *Nature Immunology*, Vol.5, No.10, (October), pp. 987-995.

Jahng, A., Maricic, I., Aguilera, C., Cardell, S., Halder, R.C. & Kumar, V. (2004). Prevention of autoimmunity by targeting a distinct, noninvariant CD1d-reactive T cell population reactive to sulfatide. *The Journal of Experimental Medicine*, Vol.199, No.7, (April), pp. 947-957.

Jiang, D., Liang, J., Fan, J., Yu, S., Chen, S., Luo, Y., Prestwich, G.D., Mascarenhas, M.M., Garg, H.G., Quinn, D.A., Homer, R.J., Goldstein, D.R., Bucala, R., Lee, P.J., Medzhitov, R. & Noble, P.W. (2005). Regulation of lung injury and repair by Toll-like receptors and hyaluronan. *Nature Medicine*, Vol.11, No.11, (November), pp. 1173–1179.

Johnson, G.B., Brunn, G.J., Kodaira, Y. & Platt, J.L. (2002). Receptor-mediated monitoring of tissue well-being via detection of soluble heparan sulfate by Toll-like receptor 4. *The Journal of Immunology*, Vol.168, No.10, (May), pp. 5233–5239.

Kai, S., Tanaka, J., Nomoto, K. & Torisu, M. (1979). Studies on the immunopotentiating effects of a streptococcal preparation, OK-432. I. Enhancement of T cell-mediated immune responses of mice. *Clinical & Experimental Immunology*, Vol.37, No.1, (July), pp. 98-105.

Kataoka, T., Oh-hashi, F. & Sakurai, Y. (1979). Immunotherapeutic response of concanavalin A-bound L1210 vaccine enhanced by a streptococcal immunopotentiator, OK-432. *Cancer Research*, Vol.39, No.7, Part 1, (July), pp. 2807-2810.

Kawano, T., Cui, J., Koezuka, Y., Toura, I., Kaneko, Y., Sato, H., Kondo, E., Harada, M., Koseki, H., Nakayama, T., Tanaka, Y. & Taniguchi, M. (1998). Natural killer-like nonspecific tumor cell lysis mediated by specific ligand-activated Valpha14 NKT cells. *Proceedings of the National Academy of Sciences of the United States of America*, Vol.95, No.10, (May), pp. 5690-5693.

Kelly, J.M., Darcy, P.K., Markby, J.L., Godfrey, D.I., Takeda, K., Yagita, H. & Smyth, M.J. (2002). Induction of tumor-specific T cell memory by NK cell-mediated tumor rejection. *Nature Immunology*, Vol.3, No.1, (January), pp. 83-90.

Kigerl, K.A., Lai, W., Rivest, S., Hart, R.P., Satoskar, A.R. & Popovich, P.G. (2007). Toll-like receptor (TLR)-2 and TLR-4 regulate inflammation, gliosis, and myelin sparing after spinal cord injury. *Journal of Neurochemistry*, Vol.102, No.1, (July), pp. 37-50.

Kim, D., Kim, M.A., Cho, I.H., Kim, M.S., Lee, S., Jo, E.K., Choi, S.Y., Park, K., Kim, J.S., Akira, S., Na, H.S., Oh, S.B. & Lee, S.J. (2007). A critical role of toll-like receptor 2 in nerve injury-induced spinal cord glial cell activation and pain hypersensitivity. *The Journal of Biological Chemistry*, Vol.282, No.20, (May), pp. 14975-14983.

Kitamura, H., Iwakabe, K., Yahata, T., Nishimura, S., Ohta, A., Ohmi, Y., Sato, M., Takeda, K., Okumura, K., Van Kaer, L., Kawano, T., Taniguchi, M. & Nishimura, T. (1999). The natural killer T (NKT) cell ligand alpha-galactosylceramide demonstrates its immunopotentiating effect by inducing interleukin (IL)-12 production by dendritic cells and IL-12 receptor expression on NKT cells. *The Journal of Experimental Medicine*, Vol.189, No.7, (April), pp. 1121-1128.

Kluwe, J., Mencin, A. & Schwabe, R.F. (2009). Toll-like receptors, wound healing, and carcinogenesis. *Journal of Molecular Medicine*, Vol.87, No.2, (February), pp. 125-138.

Kobayashi, E., Motoki, K., Uchida, T., Fukushima, H. & Koezuka, Y. (1995). KRN7000, a novel immunomodulator, and its antitumor activities. *Oncology Research*, Vol.7, No.10-11, pp. 529-534.

Kodama. K., Higashiyama, M., Takami, K., Oda, K., Okami, J., Maeda, J., Akazawa, T., Matsumoto, M., Seya, T., Wada, M. & Toyoshima, K. (2009). Innate immune therapy with a Bacillus Calmette-Guérin cell wall skeleton after radical surgery for non-small cell lung cancer: a case-control study. *Surgery Today*, Vol.39, No.3, pp. 194-200.

Krieg, A.M. (2007). Development of TLR9 agonists for cancer therapy. *The Journal of Clinical Investigation*, Vol.117, No.5, (May), pp. 1184-1194.

Krishnan, J., Lee, G. & Choi, S. (2009). Drugs targeting Toll-like receptors. *Archives of Pharmcal Research*, Vol.32, No.11, (November), pp. 1485-1502.

Krummen, M., Balkow, S., Shen, L., Heinz, S., Loquai, C., Probst, H.C. & Grabbe, S. (2010). Release of IL-12 by dendritic cells activated by TLR ligation is dependent on MyD88 signaling, whereas TRIF signaling is indispensable for TLR synergy. *Journal of Leukocyte Biology*, Vol.88, No.1, (July), pp. 189-199.

Kunii, N., Horiguchi, S., Motohashi, S., Yamamoto, H., Ueno, N., Yamamoto, S., Sakurai, D., Taniguchi, M., Nakayama, T. & Okamoto, Y. (2009). Combination therapy of in vitro-expanded natural killer T cells and alpha-galactosylceramide-pulsed antigen-presenting cells in patients with recurrent head and neck carcinoma. *Cancer Science*, Vol.100, No.6, (June), pp. 1092-1098.

Kurosaki, M., Horiguchi, S., Yamasaki, K., Uchida, Y., Motohashi, S., Nakayama, T., Sugimoto, A. & Okamoto, Y. (2011). Migration and immunological reaction after the administration of αGalCer-pulsed antigen-presenting cells into the submucosa of patients with head and neck cancer. *Cancer Immunology, Immunotherapy*, Vol.60, No.2, (February), pp. 207-215.

Lee, J., Chuang, T.H., Redecke, V., She, L., Pitha, P.M., Carson, D.A., Raz, E. & Cottam, H.B. (2003). Molecular basis for the immunostimulatory activity of guanine nucleoside analogs: activation of Toll-like receptor 7. *Proceedings of the National Academy of Sciences of the United States of America*, Vol.100, No.11, (May), pp. 6646-6651.

Lemaitre, B., Nicolas, E., Michaut, L., Reichhart, J.M. & Hoffmann, J.A. (1996). The dorsoventral regulatory gene cassette spätzle/Toll/cactus controls the potent antifungal response in Drosophila adults. *Cell*, Vol.86. No.6, (September), 973-983.

Li, X., Jiang, S. & Tapping, R.I. (2010). Toll-like receptor signaling in cell proliferation and survival. *Cytokine*, Vol.49, No.1, (January), pp. 1-9.

Liu, Y.J. (2001). Dendritic cell subsets and lineages, and their functions in innate and adaptive immunity. *Cell.*, Vol.106, No.3, (August), pp. 259-262.

Liu Y.J. (2005). IPC: professional type 1 interferon-producing cells and plasmacytoid dendritic cell precursors. *Annual Review of Immunology*, Vol.23, (April), pp. 275-306.

Liu-Bryan, R., Scott, P., Sydlaske, A., Rose, D.M. & Terkeltaub, R. (2005a). Innate immunity conferred by Toll-like receptors 2 and 4 and myeloid differentiation factor 88 expression is pivotal to monosodium urate monohydrate crystal-induced inflammation. *Arthritis & Rheumatism*, Vol.52, No.9, (September), pp. 2936–2946.

Liu-Bryan, R., Pritzker, K., Firestein, G.S. & Terkeltaub, R. (2005b). TLR2 signaling in chondrocytes drives calcium pyrophosphate dihydrate and monosodium urate crystal-induced nitric oxide generation. *The Journal of Immunology*, Vol.174, No.8, (April), pp. 5016–5023.

Lonsdorf, A.F., Kuekrek, H., Stern, B.V., Boehm, B.O., Lehmann, P.V. & Tary-Lehmann, M. (2003). Intratumor CpG-oligodeoxynucleotide injection induces protective antitumor T cell immunity. *The Journal of Immunology*, Vol.171, No.8, (October), pp. 3941–3946.

Luo, J.L., Maeda, S., Hsu, L.C., Yagita, H. & Karin, M. (2004). Inhibition of NF-kappaB in cancer cells converts inflammation-induced tumor growth mediated by TNFalpha to TRAIL-mediated tumor regression. *Cancer Cell*, Vol.6, No.3, (September), pp. 297–305.

Lyman, S.D., Brasel, K., Rousseau, A.M. & Williams, D.E. (1994a). The flt3 ligand: a hematopoietic stem cell factor whose activities are distinct from steel factor. *Stem Cells*, Vol.12, Supplement 1, pp. 99-110.

Lyman, S.D. & Jacobsen, S.E. (1998). c-kit ligand and Flt3 ligand: stem/progenitor cell factors with overlapping yet distinct activities. *Blood*, Vol.91, No.4, (February), pp. 1101-1134.

Lyman, S.D., James, L., Escobar, S., Downey, H., de Vries, P., Brasel, K., Stocking, K., Beckmann, M.P., Copeland, N.G., Cleveland, L.S., Jenkins, N.A., Belmont, J.W. & Davison, B.L. (1995a). Identification of soluble and membranebound isoforms of the murine flt3 ligand generated by alternative splicing of mRNAs. *Oncogene*, Vol.10, No.1, (January), pp. 149-157.

Lyman, S.D., James, L., Johnson, L., Brasel, K., de Vries, P., Escobar, S.S., Downey H., Splett, R.R., Beckmann, M.P. & McKenna, H.J. (1994b). Cloning of the human homologue of the murine flt3 ligand: a growth factor for early hematopoietic progenitor cells. *Blood*, Vol.83, No.10, (May), pp. 2795-2801.

Lyman, S.D., James, L., Vanden Bos, T., de Vries, P., Brasel, K., Gliniak, B., Hollingsworth, L.T., Picha, K.S., McKenna, H.J., Splett, R.R., Fletcher, F.A., Maraskovsky, E., Farrah, T., Foxworthe, D., Williams, D.E. & Beckmann, M.P. (1993). Molecular cloning of a ligand for the flt3/flk-2 tyrosine kinase receptor: a proliferative factor for primitive hematopoietic cells. *Cell*, Vol.75, No.6, (December), pp. 1157-1167.

Lyman, S.D., Stocking, K., Davison, B., Fletcher, F., Johnson, L. & Escobar, S. (1995b). Structural analysis of human and murine flt3 ligand genomic loci. *Oncogene*. Vol.11, No.6, (September), pp. 1165-1172.

Lynch, D.H., Andreasen, A., Maraskovsky, E., Whitmore, J., Miller, R.E. & Schuh, J.C. (1997). Flt3 ligand induces tumor regression and antitumor immune responses in vivo. *Nature Medicine*, Vol.3, No.6, (June), pp. 625-631.

Macdonald, H.R. (2007). NKT cells: In the beginning... *European Journal of Immunology*, Vol.37, Supplement 1, S111-115.

Makino, Y., Kanno, R., Ito, T., Higashino, K. & Taniguchi, M. (1995). Predominant expression of invariant V alpha 14+ TCR alpha chain in NK1.1+ T cell populations. *International Immunology*, Vol.7, No.7, (July), pp. 1157-1161.

Maraskovsky, E., Brasel, K., Teepe, M., Roux, E.R., Lyman, S.D., Shortman, K. & McKenna, H.J. (1996). Dramatic increase in the numbers of functionally mature dendritic cells in Flt3 ligand-treated mice: multiple dendritic cell subpopulations identified. *The Journal of Experimental Medicine*, Vol.184, No.5, (November), pp. 1953-1962.

Maraskovsky, E., Daro, E., Roux, E., Teepe, M., Maliszewski, C.R., Hoek, J., Caron, D., Lebsack, M.E. & McKenna, H.J. (2000). In vivo generation of human dendritic cell subsets by Flt3 ligand. *Blood*, Vol.96, No.3, (August), pp. 878-884.

Marroquin, C.E., Westwood, J.A., Lapointe, R., Mixon, A., Wunderlich, J.R., Caron, D., Rosenberg, S.A. & Hwu, P. (2002). Mobilization of dendritic cell precursors in patients with cancer by flt3 ligand allows the generation of higher yields of cultured dendritic cells. *Journal of Immunotherapy*, Vol.25, No.3, (May-June), pp. 278-288.

Maruyama, K., Selmani, Z., Ishii, H. & Yamaguchi, K. (2011). Innate immunity and cancer therapy. *International Immunopharmacology*, Vol.11, No.3, (March), pp. 350-357.

Mason, K.A., Ariga, H., Neal, R., Valdecanas, D., Hunter, N., Krieg, A.M., Whisnant, J.K. & Milas, L. (2005). Targeting toll-like receptor 9 with CpG oligodeoxynucleotides enhances tumor response to fractionated radiotherapy. *Clinical Cancer Research*, Vol.11, No.1, (January), pp. 361-369.

Matthews, W., Jordan, C.T., Wiegand, G.W., Pardoll, D. & Lemischka, I.R. (1991). A receptor tyrosine kinase specific to hematopoietic stem and progenitor cell-enriched populations. *Cell*, Vol.65, No.7, (June), pp. 1143-1152.

McCarthy, E.F. (2006). The toxins of William B. Coley and the treatment of bone and soft-tissue sarcomas. *The Iowa Orthopaedic Journal*, Vol.26, pp. 154-158.

McKenna, H.J., Stocking, K.L., Miller, R.E., Brasel, K., De Smedt, T., Maraskovsky, E., Maliszewski, C.R., Lynch, D.H., Smith, J., Pulendran, B., Roux, E.R, Teepe, M., Lyman, S.D. & Peschon, J.J. (2000). Mice lacking flt3 ligand have deficient hematopoiesis affecting hematopoietic progenitor cells, dendritic cells, and natural killer cells. *Blood*, Vol.95, No.11, (June), pp. 3489-3497.

Medzhitov, R., Preston-Hurlburt, P. & Janeway, C.A. Jr. (1997). A human homologue of the Drosophila Toll protein signals activation of adaptive immunity. *Nature*, Vol.388, No.6640, (July), pp. 394-397.

Merad, M., Sugie, T., Engleman, E.G. & Fong, L. (2002). In vivo manipulation of dendritic cells to induce therapeutic immunity. *Blood*, Vol.99, No.5, (March), pp. 1676–1682.

Mizushima, Y., Yuhki, N., Hosokawa, M., & Kobayashi, H. (1982). Diminution of cyclophosphamide-induced suppression of antitumor immunity by an immunomodulator PS-K and combined therapeutic effects of PS-K and cyclophosphamide on transplanted tumor in rats. *Cancer Research*, Vol.42, No.12, (December), pp. 5176-5180.

Morita, M., Motoki, K., Akimoto, K., Natori, T., Sakai, T., Sawa, E., Yamaji, K., Koezuka, Y., Kobayashi, E. & Fukushima, H. (1995). Structure-activity relationship of alpha-galactosylceramides against B16-bearing mice. *Journal of Medicinal Chemistry*, Vol.38, No.12, (June), pp. 2176-2187.

Motohashi, S., Ishikawa, A., Ishikawa, E., Otsuji, M., Iizasa, T., Hanaoka, H., Shimizu, N., Horiguchi, S., Okamoto, Y., Fujii, S., Taniguchi, M., Fujisawa, T. & Nakayama, T. (2006). A phase I study of in vitro expanded natural killer T cells in patients with advanced and recurrent non-small cell lung cancer. *Clinical Cancer Research*, Vol. 12, No.20, (October), pp. 6079-6086.

Motohashi, S., Nagato, K., Kunii, N., Yamamoto, H., Yamasaki, K., Okita, K., Hanaoka, H., Shimizu, N., Suzuki, M., Yoshino, I., Taniguchi, M., Fujisawa, T. & Nakayama, T. (2009). A phase I-II study of alpha-galactosylceramide-pulsed IL-2/GM-CSF-cultured peripheral blood mononuclear cells in patients with advanced and recurrent non-small cell lung cancer. *The Journal of Immunology*, Vol.182, No.4, (February), pp. 2492-2501.

Motohashi, S., Okamoto, Y., Yoshino, I. & Nakayama, T. (2011). Anti-tumor immune responses induced by iNKT cell-based immunotherapy for lung cancer and head and neck cancer. *Clinical Immunology*, Vol.140, No.2, (August), pp. 167-176.

Motoki, K., Morita, M., Kobayashi, E., Uchida, T., Akimoto, K., Fukushima, H. & Koezuka, Y. (1995). Immunostimulatory and antitumor activities of monoglycosylceramides having various sugar moieties. *Biological & Pharmaceutical Bulletin*, Vol.18, No.11, (November), pp. 1487-1491.

Natori, T., Morita, M., Akimoto, K. & Koezuka, Y. (1994). Agelasphins, novel antitumor and immunostimulatory cerebrosides from the marine sponge Agelas mauritianus. *Tetrahedron*, Vol.50, No.9, (February), pp. 2771–2784.

Naugler, W.E., Sakurai, T., Kim, S., Maeda, S., Kim, K., Elsharkawy, A.M. & Karin, M. (2007). Gender disparity in liver cancer due to sex differences in MyD88-dependent IL-6 production. *Science*, Vol.317, No.5834, (July), pp. 121-124.

Nieda, M., Okai, M., Tazbirkova, A., Lin, H., Yamaura, A., Ide, K., Abraham, R., Juji, T., Macfarlane, D.J. & Nicol, A.J. (2004). Therapeutic activation of Valpha24+Vbeta11+ NKT cells in human subjects results in highly coordinated secondary activation of acquired and innate immunity. *Blood*, Vol.103, No.2, (January), pp. 383-389.

Nogueras, S., Merino, A., Ojeda, R., Carracedo, J., Rodriguez, M., Martin-Malo, A., Ramírez, R. & Aljama, P. (2008). Coupling of endothelial injury and repair: an analysis using an in vivo experimental model. *American Journal of Physiology Heart and Circulatory Physiology*, Vol.294, No.2, (February), pp. H708-713.

Ohashi, K., Burkart, V., Flohe, S. & Kolb, H. (2000). Cutting edge: heat shock protein 60 is a putative endogenous ligand of the toll-like receptor-4 complex. *The Journal of Immunology*, Vol.164, No.2, (January), 558–561.

Ohashi, K., Kobayashi, G., Fang, S., Zhu, X., Antonia, S.J., Krieg, A.M. & Sandler, A.D. (2006) Surgical excision combined with autologous whole tumor cell vaccination is an effective therapy for murine neuroblastoma. *Journal of Pediatric Surgery*, Vol.41, No.8, (August), pp. 1361–1368.

Okai, M., Nieda, M., Tazbirkova, A., Horley, D., Kikuchi, A., Durrant, S., Takahashi, T., Boyd, A., Abraham, R., Yagita, H., Juji, T. & Nicol, A. (2002). Human peripheral blood Valpha24+ Vbeta11+ NKT cells expand following administration of alpha-galactosylceramide-pulsed dendritic cells. *Vox Sanguinis*, Vol.83, No.3, (October), pp. 250-253.

Okamoto, M., Oshikawa, T., Tano, T., Ahmed, S.U., Kan, S., Sasai, A., Akashi, S., Miyake, K., Moriya, Y., Ryoma, Y., Saito, M. & Sato, M. (2006). Mechanism of anticancer host response induced by OK-432, a streptococcal preparation, mediated by phagocytosis and Toll-like receptor 4 signaling. *Journal of Immunotherapy*, Vol.29, No.1, (January-February), pp. 78-86.

Okamura, Y., Watari, M., Jerud, E.S., Young, D.W., Ishizaka, S.T., Rose, J., Chow, J.C. & Strauss, J.F. (2001). The extra domain A of fibronectin activates Toll-like receptor 4. *The Journal of Biological Chemistry*, Vol.276, No.13, (March), pp. 10229–10233.

Okano, F., Merad, M., Furumoto, K. & Engleman, E.G. (2005). In vivo manipulation of dendritic cells overcomes tolerance to unmodified tumor-associated self antigens and induces potent antitumor immunity. *The Journal of Immunology*, Vol.174, No.5, (March), pp. 2645–2652.

Ouyang, X., Negishi, H., Takeda, R., Fujita, Y., Taniguchi, T. & Honda, K. (2007). Cooperation between MyD88 and TRIF pathways in TLR synergy via IRF5 activation. *Biochemical Biophysical Research Communications*, Vol.354, No.4, (March), pp. 1045-1051.

Oyama, J., Blais, C. Jr., Liu, X., Pu, M., Kobzik, L., Kelly, R.A. & Bourcier, T. (2004). Reduced myocardial ischemiareperfusion injury in toll-like receptor 4-deficient mice. *Circulation*, Vol.109, No.6, (February), 784–789.

Park, J.S., Gamboni-Robertson, F., He, Q., Svetkauskaite, D., Kim, J.Y., Strassheim, D., Sohn, J.W., Yamada, S., Maruyama, I., Banerjee, A., Ishizaka, A. & Abraham, E. (2006). High mobility group box 1 protein interacts with multiple Toll-like receptors. *American Journal of Cell Physiology*, Vol.290, No.3, (March), C917–924.

Park, J.S., Svetkauskaite, D., He, Q., Kim, J.Y., Strassheim, D., Ishizaka, A. & Abraham, E. (2004). Involvement of toll-like receptors 2 and 4 in cellular activation by high mobility group box 1 protein. *The Journal of Biological Chemistry*, Vol.279, No.9, (February), 7370–7377.

Péron, J.M., Esche, C., Subbotin, V.M., Maliszewski, C., Lotze, M.T. & Shurin, M.R. (1998). FLT3-ligand administration inhibits liver metastases: role of NK cells. *The Journal of Immunology*, Vol.161, No.11, (December), pp. 6164-6170.

Peters, J.H., Gieseler, R., Thiele, B. & Steinbach, F. (1996). Dendritic cells: from ontogenetic orphans to myelomonocytic descendants. *Immunology Today*, Vol.17, No.6, (June), pp. 273-278.

Pevsner-Fischer, M., Morad, V., Cohen-Sfady, M., Rousso-Noori, L., Zanin-Zhorov, A., Cohen, S., Cohen, I.R. & Zipori, D. (2007). Toll-like receptors and their ligands control mesenchymal stem cell functions. *Blood*, Vol.109, No.4, (February), pp. 1422-1432.

Pidgeon, G.P., Harmey, J.H., Kay, E., Da Costa, M., Redmond, H.P. & Bouchier-Hayes, D.J. (1999). The role of endotoxin/lipopolysaccharide in surgically induced tumour growth in a murine model of metastatic disease. *British Journal of Cancer*, Vol.81, No.8, (December), pp. 1311–1317.

Pratesi, G., Petrangolini, G., Tortoreto, M., Addis, A., Belluco, S., Rossini, A., Selleri, S., Rumio, C., Menard, S. & Balsari, A. (2005). Therapeutic synergism of gemcitabine and CpG-oligodeoxynucleotides in an orthotopic human pancreatic carcinoma xenograft. *Cancer Research*, Vol.65, No.14, (July), pp. 6388–6393.

Pulendran, B., Smith, J.L., Caspary, G., Brasel, K., Pettit, D., Maraskovsky, E. & Maliszewski, C.R. (1999). Distinct dendritic cell subsets differentially regulate the class of immune response in vivo. *Proceedings of the National Academy of Sciences of the United States of America*, Vol.96, No.3, (February), pp. 1036-1041.

Pull, S.L., Doherty, J.M., Mills, J.C., Gordon, J.I. & Stappenbeck, T.S. (2005). Activated macrophages are an adaptive element of the colonic epithelial progenitor niche necessary for regenerative responses to injury. *Proceedings of the National Academy of Sciences of the United States of America*, Vol.102, No.1, (January), pp. 99-104.

Prins, R.M., Craft, N., Bruhn, K.W., Khan-Farooqi, H., Koya, R.C., Stripecke, R., Miller, J.F. & Liau, L.M. (2006). The TLR-7 agonist, imiquimod, enhances dendritic cell survival and promotes tumor antigen-specific T cell priming: relation to central nervous system antitumor immunity. *The Journal of Immunology*, Vol.176, No.1, (January), pp. 157–164.

Rakoff-Nahoum, S. & Medzhitov, R. (2007). Regulation of spontaneous intestinal tumorigenesis through the adaptor protein MyD88. *Science*, Vol.317, No.5834, (July), pp. 124–127.

Rakoff-Nahoum, S. & Medzhitov, R. (2008). Role of toll-like receptors in tissue repair and tumorigenesis. *Biochemistry* (Mosc), Vol.73, No.5, (May), pp. 555-561.

Rakoff-Nahoum, S., Paglino, J., Eslami-Varzaneh, F., Edberg, S. & Medzhitov, R. (2004). Recognition of commensal microflora by toll-like receptors is required for intestinal homeostasis. *Cell*, Vol.118, No.2, (July), pp. 229–241.

Rechtsteiner, G., Warger, T., Osterloh, P., Schild, H. & Radsak, M.P. (2005). Cutting edge: priming of CTL by transcutaneous peptide immunization with imiquimod. *The Journal of Immunology*, Vol.174, No.5, (March), pp. 2476–2480.

Rini, B.I., Paintal, A., Vogelzang, N.J., Gajewski, T.F. & Stadler, W.M. (2002). Flt-3 ligand and sequential FL/interleukin-2 in patients with metastatic renal carcinoma: clinical and biologic activity. *The Journal of Immunotherapy*, Vol.25, No.3, (May-June), pp. 269-277.

Roelofs, M.F., Joosten, L.A., Abdollahi-Roodsaz, S., van Lieshout, A.W., Sprong, T., van den Hoogen, F.H., van den Berg, W.B. & Radstake, T.R. (2005). The expression of Toll-like receptors 3 and 7 in rheumatoid arthritis synovium is increased and costimulation of Toll-like receptors 3, 4, and 7/8 results in synergistic cytokine production by dendritic cells. *Arthritis & Rheumatism,* Vol.52, No.8, (August), pp. 2313–2322.

Roelofs, M.F., Boelens, W.C., Joosten, L.A., Abdollahi-Roodsaz, S., Geurts, J., Wunderink, L.U., Schreurs, B.W., van den Berg, W.B. & Radstake, T.R. (2006). Identification of small heat shock protein B8 (HSP22) as a novel TLR4 ligand and potential involvement in the pathogenesis of rheumatoid arthritis. *The Journal of Immunology,* Vol.176, No.11, (June), pp. 7021–7027.

Romagne, F. (2007). Current and future drugs targeting one class of innate immunity receptors: the Toll-like receptors. *Drug Discovery Today,* Vol.12, No.1-2, (January), pp. 80-87.

Rosenberg, S.A., Yang, J.C. & Restifo, N.P. (2004). Cancer immunotherapy: moving beyond current vaccines. *Nature Medicine,* Vol.10, No.9, (September). pp. 909-915.

Rosnet, O., Marchetto, S., deLapeyriere, O. & Birnbaum, D. (1991a). Murine Flt3, a gene encoding a novel tyrosine kinase receptor of the PDGFR/CSF1R family. *Oncogene,* Vol.9, No.9, (September), pp. 1641-1650.

Rosnet, O., Matteï, M.G., Marchetto, S. & Birnbaum, D. (1991b). Isolation and chromosomal localization of a novel FMS-like tyrosine kinase gene. *Genomics,* Vol.9, No.9, (February), pp. 380-385.

Rossignol, D.P., Wasan, K.M., Choo, E., Yau, E., Wong, N., Rose, J., Moran, J. & Lynn, M. (2004). Safety, pharmacokinetics, pharmacodynamics, and plasma lipoprotein distribution of eritoran (E5564) during continuous intravenous infusion into healthy volunteers. *Antimicrobial Agents and Chemotherapy,* Vol.48, No.9, (September), pp. 3233-3240.

Salaun, B., Coste, I., Rissoa, M.C., Lebecque S.J. & Renno, T. (2006). TLR3 can directly trigger apoptosis in human cancer cells. *The Journal of Immunology,* Vol.176, No.8, (April), pp. 4894-4901.

Sasaki, H., Schmitt, D., Hayashi, Y., Pollard, R.B. & Suzuki, F. (1990). Induction of interleukin 3 and tumor resistance by SSM, a cancer immunotherapeutic agent extracted from Mycobacterium tuberculosis. *Cancer Research.* Vol.50, No.13, (July), pp. 4032-4037.

Sato, S., Nomura, F., Kawai, T., Takeuchi, O., Mühlradt, P.F., Takeda, K. & Akira, S. (2000). Synergy and cross-tolerance between toll-like receptor (TLR) 2- and TLR4-mediated signaling pathways. *The Journal of Immunology,* Vol.165, No.12, (December), 7096-7101.

Sato, Y., Goto, Y., Narita, N. & Hoon, D.S. (2009). Cancer cells expressing Toll-like receptors and the tumor microenvironment. *Cancer Microenvironment,* Suppl. 1, (September), pp. 205-214.

Schaefer, L., Babelova, A., Kiss, E., Hausser, H.J., Baliova, M., Krzyzankova, M., Marsche, G., Young, M.F., Mihalik, D., Götte, M., Malle, E., Schaefer, R.M. & Gröne, H.J. (2005). The matrix component biglycan is proinflammatory and signals through Toll-like receptors 4 and 2 in macrophages. *The Journal of Clinical Investigation*, Vol.115, No.8, (August), pp. 2223–2233.

Schön, M.P. & Schön, M. (2008). TLR7 and TLR8 as targets in cancer therapy. *Oncogene*, Vol.27, No.2, (January), pp. 190–199.

Seki, E., Tsutsui, H., Iimuro, Y., Naka, T., Son, G., Akira, S., Kishimoto, T., Nakanishi, K. & Fujimoto, J. (2005). Contribution of Toll-like receptor/myeloid differentiation factor 88 signaling to murine liver regeneration. *Hepatology*, Vol.41, No.3, (March), pp. 443–450.

Sfondrini, L., Rossini, A., Besusso, D., Merlo, A., Tagliabue, E., Mènard, S. & Balsari, A. (2006). Antitumor activity of the TLR-5 ligand flagellin in mouse models of cancer. *The Journal of Immunology*, Vol.76, No.11, (June), pp. 6624-6630.

Shaw, S.G., Maung, A.A., Steptoe, R.J., Thomson, A.W. & Vujanovic, N.L. (1998). Expansion of functional NK cells in multiple tissue compartments of mice treated with Flt3-ligand: implications for anti-cancer and anti-viral therapy. *The Journal of Immunology*, Vol.161, No.6, (September), pp. 2817-2824.

Sidky, Y.A., Borden, E.C., Weeks, C.E., Reiter, M.J., Hatcher, J.F. & Bryan, G.T. (1992). Inhibition of murine tumor growth by an interferon-inducing imidazoquinolinamine. *Cancer Research*, Vol.52, No.13, (July), pp. 3528-3533.

Silver, D.F., Hempling, R.E., Piver, M.S. & Repasky, E.A. (2000). Flt-3 ligand inhibits growth of human ovarian tumors engrafted in severe combined immunodeficient mice. *Gynecologic Oncology* , Vol.77, No.3, (June), pp. 377-382.

Smiley, S.T., King, J.A. & Hancock, W.W. (2001). Fibrinogen stimulates macrophage chemokine secretion through toll-like receptor 4. *The Journal of Immunology*, Vol.167, No.5, (September), pp. 2887–2894.

Smith, J.R., Thackray, A.M. & Bujdoso, R. (2001). Reduced herpes simplex virus type 1 latency in Flt-3 ligand-treated mice is associated with enhanced numbers of natural killer and dendritic cells. *Immunology*, Vol.102, No.3, (March), pp. 352-358.

Smyth, M.J., Crowe, N.Y. & Godfrey, D.I. (2001). NK cells and NKT cells collaborate in host protection from methylcholanthrene-induced fibrosarcoma. *International Immunology*, Vol.13, No.4, (April), pp. 459-463.

Smyth, M.J., Crowe, N.Y., Pellicci, D.G., Kyparissoudis, K., Kelly, J.M., Takeda, K., Yagita, H. & Godfrey, D.I. (2002). Sequential production of interferon-gamma by NK1.1+ T cells and natural killer cells is essential for the antimetastatic effect of alpha-galactosylceramide. *Blood*, Vol.99, No.4, (February), pp. 1259-1266.

Smyth, M.J., Dunn, G.P. & Schreiber, R.D. (2006). Cancer immunosurveillance and immunoediting: the roles of immunity in suppressing tumor development and shaping tumor immunogenicity. *Advances in Immunology*, Vol.90, pp. 1-50.

Spada, F.M., Koezuka, Y. & Porcelli, S.A. (1998). CD1d-restricted recognition of synthetic glycolipid antigens by human natural killer T cells. *The Journal of Experimental Medicine*, Vol.188, No.8, (October), pp. 1529–1534.

Stary, G., Bangert, C., Tauber, M., Strohal, R., Kopp, T. & Stingl, G. (2007). Tumoricidal activity of TLR7/8-activated inflammatory dendritic cells. *The Journal of Experimental Medicine*, Vol.204, No.6, (June), pp. 1441–1451.

Suzuki, F., Brutkiewicz, R.R. & Pollard, R.B. (1986a). Importance of Lyt 1+ T-cells in the antitumor activity of an immunomodulator, SSM, extracted from human-type Tubercle bacilli. *Journal of the National Cancer Institute*, Vol.77, No.2, (August), pp. 441-447.

Suzuki, F., Brutkiewicz, R.R. & Pollard, R.B. (1986b). Lack of correlation between antitumor response and serum interferon levels in mice treated with SSM, an immunotherapeutic anticancer agent. *British Journal of Cancer*, Vol.53, No.4, (April). pp. 567-570.

Taieb, J., Chaput, N., Schartz, N., Roux, S., Novault, S., Ménard, C., Ghiringhelli, F., Terme, M., Carpentier, A.F., Darrasse-Jèze, G., Lemonnier, F. & Zitvogel, L. (2006). Chemoimmunotherapy of tumors: cyclophosphamide synergizes with exosome based vaccines. *The Journal of Immunology*, Vol.176, No.5, (March), pp. 2722–2729.

Takeda, K., Kaisho, T. & Akira, S. (2003). Toll-like receptors. *Annual Review of Immunology*, Vol.21, 335-376.

Tang, S.C., Arumugam, T.V., Xu, X., Cheng, A., Mughal, M.R., Jo, D.G., Lathia, J.D., Siler, D.A., Chigurupati, S., Ouyang, X., Magnus, T., Camandola, S. & Mattson, M.P. (2007). Pivotal role for neuronal Toll-like receptors in ischemic brain injury and functional deficits. *Proceedings of the National Academy of Sciences of the United States of America*, Vol.104, No.34, (August), pp. 13798–13803.

Taniguchi, M., Harada, M., Kojo, S., Nakayama, T. & Wakao, H. (2003). The regulatory role of Valpha14 NKT cells in innate and acquired immune response. *Annual Review of Immunology*, Vol.21, (April), pp. 483-513.

Taniguchi, M. & Nakayama, T. (2000). Recognition and function of Valpha14 NKT cells. *Seminars in Immunology*, Vol.12, No.6, (December), pp. 543–550.

Terabe, M. & Berzofsky, J.A. (2007). NKT cells in immunoregulation of tumor immunity: a new immunoregulatory axis. *Trends in Immunology*, Vol.28, No.11, (November), pp. 491-496.

Terabe, M. & Berzofsky, J.A. (2008). The role of NKT cells in tumor immunity. Advances in Cancer Research, Vol.101, pp. 277-348.

Termeer, C., Benedix, F., Sleeman, J., Fieber, C., Voith, U., Ahrens, T., Miyake, K., Freudenberg, M., Galanos, C. & Simon, J.C. (2002). Oligosaccharides of Hyaluronan activate dendritic cells via toll-like receptor 4. *The Journal of Experimental Medicine*, Vol.195, No.1, (January), pp. 99–111.

Theiner, G., Rossner, S., Dalpke, A., Bode, K., Berger, T., Gessner, A. & Lutz, M.B. (2007). TLR9 cooperates with TLR4 to increase IL-12 release by murine dendritic cells. *Molecular Immunology*, Vol.45, No.1, (January), pp. 244–252.

Toura, I., Kawano, T., Akutsu, Y., Nakayama, T., Ochiai, T. & Taniguchi, M. (1999). Cutting edge: inhibition of experimental tumor metastasis by dendritic cells pulsed with alpha-galactosylceramide. *The Journal of Immunology*, Vol.163, No.5, (September), pp. 2387-2391.

Tsuji, M. (2006). Glycolipids and phospholipids as natural CD1d-binding NKT cell ligands. *Cellular and Molecular Life Sciences*, Vol.63, No.16, (August), pp. 1889-1898.

Tsuji, S., Matsumoto, M., Takeuchi, O., Akira, S., Azuma, I., Hayashi, A., Toyoshima, K. & Seya, T. (2000). Maturation of human dendritic cells by cell wall skeleton of

Mycobacterium bovis bacillus Calmette-Guérin: involvement of toll-like receptors. *Infection and Immunity*, Vol.68, No.12, (December), pp. 6883-6890.

Tsung, A., Sahai, R., Tanaka, H., Nakao, A., Fink, M.P., Lotze, M.T., Yang, H., Li, J., Tracey, K.J., Geller, D.A. & Billiar, T.R. (2005). The nuclear factor HMGB1 mediates hepatic injury after murine liver ischemiareperfusion. *The Journal of Experimental Medicine*, Vol.201, No.7, (April), pp. 1135–1143.

Tsung, K. & Norton, J.A. (2006). Lessons from Coley's Toxin. Surgical Oncology, Vol. 15, No.1, (July), pp. 25-28.

Uchida, T., Horiguchi, S., Tanaka, Y., Yamamoto, H., Kunii, N., Motohashi, S., Taniguchi, M., Nakayama, T. & Okamoto, Y. (2008). Phase I study of alpha-galactosylceramide-pulsed antigen presenting cells administration to the nasal submucosa in unresectable or recurrent head and neck cancer. *Cancer Immunology, Immunotherapy*, Vol.57, No.3, (March), pp. 337-345.

Uehori, J., Fukase, K., Akazawa, T., Uematsu, S., Akira, S., Funami, K., Shingai, M., Matsumoto, M., Azuma, I., Toyoshima, K., Kusumoto, S. & Seya, T. (2005). Dendritic cell maturation induced by muramyl dipeptide (MDP) derivatives: monoacylated MDP confers TLR2/TLR4 activation. *The Journal of Immunology*, Vol.174, No.11, (June), pp. 7096-7103.

Uesugi, T., Froh, M., Arteel, G.E., Bradford, B.U. & Thurman, R.G. (2001). Toll-like receptor 4 is involved in the mechanism of early alcohol-induced liver injury in mice. *Hepatology*, Vol.34, No.1, (July), pp. 101–108.

Vabulas, R.M., Ahmad-Nejad, P., da Costa, C., Miethke, T., Kirschning, C.J., Häcker, H. & Wagner, H. (2001). Endocytosed HSP60s use toll-like receptor 2 (TLR2) and TLR4 to activate the Toll/interleukin-1 receptor signaling pathway in innate immune cells. *The Journal of Biological Chemistry*, Vol.276, No.33, (August), pp. 31332–31339.

Vabulas, R.M., Ahmad-Nejad, P., Ghose, S., Kirschning, C.J., Issels, D. & Wagner, H. (2002a). HSP70 as endogenous stimulus of the Toll/interleukin-1 receptor signal pathway. *The Journal of Biological Chemistry*, Vol.277, No.17, (April), pp. 15107–15112.

Vabulas, R.M., Braedel, S., Hilf, N., Singh-Jasuja, H., Herter, S., Ahmad-Nejad, P., Kirschning, C.J., Da Costa, C., Rammensee, H.G., Wagner, H. & Schild, H. (2002b). The endoplasmic reticulum-resident heat shock protein Gp96 activates dendritic cells via the Toll-like receptor 2/4 pathway. *The Journal of Biological Chemistry*; Vol.277, No.23, (June), pp. 20847–20853.

van der Most, R.G., Himbeck, R., Aarons, S., Carter, S.J., Larma, I., Robinson, C., Currie, A. & Lake, R.A. (2006). Antitumor efficacy of the novel chemotherapeutic agent coramsine is potentiated by cotreatment with CpG-containing oligodeoxynucleotides. *Journal of Immunotherapy*, Vol.29, No.2, (March-April), pp. 134–142.

van Noort, J.M. & Bsibsi, M. (2009). Toll-like receptors in the CNS: implications for neurodegeneration and repair. *Progress in Brain Research*, Vol.175, pp. 139-48.

Vicari, A.P., Chiodoni, C., Vaure, C., Aït-Yahia, S., Dercamp, C., Matsos, F., Reynard, O., Taverne, C., Merle, P., Colombo, M.P., O'Garra, A., Trinchieri, G. & Caux, C. (2002). Reversal of tumor-induced dendritic cell paralysis by CpG immunostimulatory oligonucleotide and anti-interleukin 10 receptor antibody. *The Journal of Experimental Medicine*, Vol.196, No.4, (August), pp. 541–549.

Van Rhijn, I., Young, D.C., Im, J.S., Levery, S.B., Illarionov, P.A., Besra, G.S., Porcelli, S.A., Gumperz, J., Cheng, T.Y. & Moody, D.B. (2004). CD1d-restricted T cell activation by nonlipidic small molecules. *Proceedings of the National Academy of Sciences of the United States of America*, Vol.101, No.37, (September), pp. 13578-13583.

Walzer, T., Dalod, M., Robbins, S.H., Zitvogel, L. & Vivier, E. (2005). Natural-killer cells and dendritic cells: "l'union fait la force". *Blood*, Vol.106, No.7, (October), pp. 2252-2258.

Wang, H., Rayburn, E.R., Wang, W., Kandimalla, E.R., Agrawal, S. & Zhang, R. (2006). Chemotherapy and chemosensitization of non-small cell lung cancer with a novel immunomodulatory oligonucleotide targeting Toll-like receptor 9. *Molecular Cancer Therapeutics*, Vol.5, No.6, (June), pp. 1585–1592.

Wang, X.S., Sheng, Z., Ruan, Y.B., Guang, Y. & Yang, M.L. (2005). CpG oligodeoxynucleotides inhibit tumor growth and reverse the immunosuppression caused by the therapy with 5-fluorouracil in murine hepatoma. *World Journal of Gastroenterology*, Vol.11, No. 8, (February), pp. 1220–1224.

Warger, T., Osterloh, P., Rechtsteiner, G., Fassbender, M., Heib, V., Schmid, B., Schmitt, E., Schild, H. & Radsak, M.P. (2006). Synergistic activation of dendritic cells by combined Toll-like receptor ligation induces superior CTL responses in vivo. *Blood*, Vol.108, No.2, (July), pp. 544–550.

Weigel, B.J., Rodeberg, D.A., Krieg, A.M. & Blazar, B.R. (2003). CpG oligodeoxynucleotides potentiate the antitumor effects of chemotherapy or tumor resection in an orthotopic murine model of rhabdomyosarcoma. *Clinical Cancer Research*, Vol.9, No.8, (August), pp. 3105–3114.

Whitmore, M.M., DeVeer, M.J., Edling, A., Oates, R.K., Simons, B., Lindner, D. & Williams, B.R. (2004). Synergistic activation of innate immunity by double-stranded RNA and CpG DNA promotes enhanced antitumor activity. *Cancer Resesrch*, Vol.64, No.16, (August), pp. 5850–5860.

Wooldridge, J.E., Ballas, Z., Krieg, A.M. & Weiner, G.J. (1997). Immunostimulatory oligodeoxynucleotides containing CpG motifs enhance the efficacy of monoclonal antibody therapy of lymphoma. *Blood*, Vol.89, No.8, (April), pp. 2994–2998.

Wu, H., Chen, G., Wyburn, K.R., Yin, J., Bertolino, P., Eris, J.M., Alexander, S.I., Sharland, A.F. & Chadban, S.J. (2007). TLR4 activation mediates kidney ischemia/reperfusion injury. *The Journal of Clinical Investigation*, Vol.117, No.10, (October), pp. 2847–2859.

Yamasaki, K., Horiguchi, S., Kurosaki, M., Kunii, N., Nagato, K., Hanaoka, H., Shimizu, N., Ueno, N., Yamamoto, S., Taniguchi, M., Motohashi, S., Nakayama, T. & Okamoto, Y. (2011). Induction of NKT cell-specific immune responses in cancer tissues after NKT cell-targeted adoptive immunotherapy. *Clinical Immunology*, Vol.138, No.6, (June), pp. 255-265.

Yu, H., Fehniger, T.A., Fuchshuber, P., Thiel, K.S., Vivier, E., Carson, W.E. & Caligiuri, M.A. (1998). Flt3 ligand promotes the generation of a distinct CD34(+) human natural killer cell progenitor that responds to interleukin-15. *Blood*, Vol.92, No.10, (November), pp. 3647-3657.

Zhang, Z. & Schluesener, H.J. (2006). Mammalian toll-like receptors: from endogenous ligands to tissue regeneration. *Cellular and Molecular Life Sciences*, Vol.63, No.24, (December), pp. 2901-2907.

Zhou, M., McFarland-Mancini, M.M., Funk, H.M., Husseinzadeh, N., Mounajjed, T. & Drew, A.F. (2009). Toll-like receptor expression in normal ovary and ovarian tumors. *Cancer Immunology, Immunotherapy*, Vol.5, No.9, (September), pp. 1375-1385.

Zhu, Q., Egelston, C., Vivekanandhan, A., Uematsu, S., Akira, S., Klinman, D., Belyakov, I. & Berzofsky, J. (2008). Toll-like receptor ligands synergize through distinct dendritic cell pathways to induce T cell responses: implications for vaccines. *Proceedings of the National Academy of Sciences of the United States of America*, Vol.105, No.42, (October), pp. 16260–16265.

7

The Potential Use of Triterpene Compounds in Dendritic Cells-Based Immunotherapy

Masao Takei[1], Akemi Umeyama[3] and Je-Jung Lee[1,2]
[1]Research Center for Cancer Immunotherapy, Chonnam National University Hwasun Hospital, 160 Ilsim-ri, Hwasun-eup, Hwsaun-gun, Jeollanam-do,
[2]Department of Hematology-Oncology, Chonnam National University Medical School, Gwangiu,
[3]Faculty of Pharmaceutical Sciences, Tokushima University, Yamashiro-cho, Tokushima,
[1,2]South Korea
[3]Japan

1. Introduction

The immune system is confronted with antigens and proteins that have not been previously encountered by the body. Dendritic cells are professional antigen-presenting cells and play a key role in the induction of these immune responses (Banchereau and Steinman, 1998; Lanzavecchia and Sallustoa, 2001; Mellman and Steinman, 2001). Dendritic cells orchestrate a variety of immune responses by stimulating the differentiation of naïve CD4+ T cells into helper T effectors such as Th1, Th2, Treg cells and Th17 cells and several factors determine the direction of T cell polarization (Romagnani 1994; Kuchroo et al. 1995; Lederer et al. 1996; Tao et al. 1997; Forster et al. 1999; Lezz et al. 1999; Tanaka et al. 2000; O'gara, 20001; Steinman and Dhodapkar, 2001). The cytokine profile present during an immune reaction is an important element in directing the response to T cell polarization. A maturation process, IL-12 production, the up-regulation of MHC and costimulatory molecules, is critical for initiation of primary T cell response. Th1 responses predominate in organ-specific autoimmune disorders, acute allograft rejection and in some chronic inflammatory disorders (Trinchieri and Scott, 1994). Although different dendritic cells subsets may have some intrinsic potential to preferentially induce Th1, Th2, Treg cells or Th17 cells, dendritic cells also display considerable functional plasticity in response to signals from microbes and the local microenvironment (Steinman, 2007). Numerous stimuli can mediate dendritic cells maturation, the best characterized being Toll-like receptor (TLR) ligands and signals such as CD40L delivered by T cells and innate lymphocytes (Hermann et al. 1998). TLRs are expressed mainly on macrophages and dendritic cells, triggering results in the development of effector dendritic cells that promote Th1 responses (Okamoto and Sato, 2003). Recently, several studies proposed the significance of TLR signaling in the induction of anti-cancer immunity. In addition to their essential role in T cell priming, dendritic cells are also involved in innate immunity through the production of cytokines and the activation of NK or NKT cells. Thus, dendritic cells play a pivotal role in orchestrating the immune response.

The hooks of *Uncaria* sp. are contained in Choto-san as the main component herb. Choto-san has been used for hypertension and dementia, and well used as an important of many Chinese prescriptions in China, Korea and Japan. Uncarinic acid (URC) and Ursolic acid are isolated from *Uncaria rhynchophylla* and phytochemically classified as triterpene. A number of alkaloids have been reported as antihypertensive principles from the genus *Uncaria*. URC showed potent inhibitory activity against phospholipase Cγ1 and inhibited the growth of cancer cells at high doses (Lee et al. 2000). Ursolic acid augments the inhibitory effects of anticancer drugs on growth of human tumor cells and triggers apoptosis in cancer cells. Triterpene have been identified as a unique class of natural products possessing diverse biological activities. Terpenes also contain pharmacologically active substance. Recently, we have reported that numerous terpenes induce the differentiation of dendritic cells from human monocytes, and drive Th1 and Th2 differentiation (Takei et al. 2005, 2007, 2008). For immunotherapeutic applications, it appears crucial to identify factors that might affect the differentiation and function of dendritic cells. Although various terpene compounds have pharmacological activity, relatively little is known in regards to the influences URC and Ursolic acid exert on the initiation of specific immune response at the level of dendritic cells. Therefore, to further understand the cellular basis of immunological with abnormalities associated URC and Ursolic acid exposure, we investigated the ability of URC and Ursolic acid on human dendritic cells differentiation (surface molecule), function (cytokines production) and their activation (NF-κB translocation to the nucleus) in detail. Some terpene compounds may lead to the development of effective immunotherapy for cancer.

2. Monocyte-derived dendritic cells phenotype

In order to study the direct effect of URC and Ursolic acid on the function of human monocyte dendritic cells, immature monocyte-derived dendritic cells were exposed to URC and Ursolic acid, and phenotypic and functional dendritic cells maturation was analyzed. URC and Ursolic acid were prepared as previously described (Lee et al. 2000). The purity of URC and Ursolic acid was > 99%. URC and Ursolic acid was dissolved in dimethyl sulfoxide. The concentration of dimethyl sulfoxide in the culture medium was 0.1%, which had no effect on the culture and the production of cytokines under the conditions used in this study. The endotoxin in URC and Ursolic acid was removed using End Trap 5/1 (Profos AG, Regensburg, Germany). Endotoxin levels in URC and Ursolic acid were below 0.05 EU/ml. Human monocytes were cultured with GM-CSF and IL-4 for 6 days under standard conditions, followed by an additional 2 days in the presence of URC and Ursolic acid. Under these conditions, we found that CD1a, CD38, CD40, CD54, CD80, CD83, CD86 and HLA-DR expression levels on URC-primed dendritic cells and Ursolic acid-primed dendritic cells were slightly enhanced. Typical data of phenotypes are shown in Fig.1. The viability of cells treated with a concentration of 0.1 μM URC and 1.0 μM Ursolic acid was >95%. URC and Ursolic acid were kept at 0.1 or 1.0 μM, respectively, for subsequent experiments. As a positive control, human monocytes were cultured with GM-CSF and IL-4 for 6 days, followed by another 2 days in the presence of LPS or TNF-α. LPS and TNF-α are a known dendritic cells maturation-enhancing factors. The expression of co-stimulatory molecules and maturation markers including CD38, CD80, CD83, CD86 and HLA-DR on LPS (100 ng/ml)-primed dendritic cells or TNF-α (25 ng/ml)-primed dendritic cells was higher than URC-primed dendritic cells and Ursolic acid-primed dendritic cells (Fig. 1). Immature dendritic cells (with medium) were generated by cultivating human monocytes with GM-

CSF and IL-4 for 8 days served as a control. The expression level of CD14 as expressed by MFI on day 8 was found to be low or undetectable in some samples. Type 1 interferons' are (IFNs) are important in immune responses against tumors. When human monocyte-derived dendritic cells were stimulated with URC in the presence of IFN-γ (100 ng/ml), the expression of co-stimulatory molecules and maturation markers on URC-primed dendritic cells was significantly increased by IFN-γ administration (data not shown). Immature dendritic cells are efficient in capturing Ag and have a high level of endocytosis. To determine whether mechanisms of Ag capture could also be modulated by URC and Ursolic acid, the endocytic activity was measured in immature dendritic cells, URC-, Ursolic acid-, LPS- and TNF-α-primed dendritic cells. FITC-dextran uptake mediated by URC-, Ursolic acid-, LPS- and TNF-α-primed dendritic cells was lower than immature dendritic cells (data not shown). These results suggested that dendritic cells differentiated by URC and Ursolic acid have down-regulated their endocytic capacity.

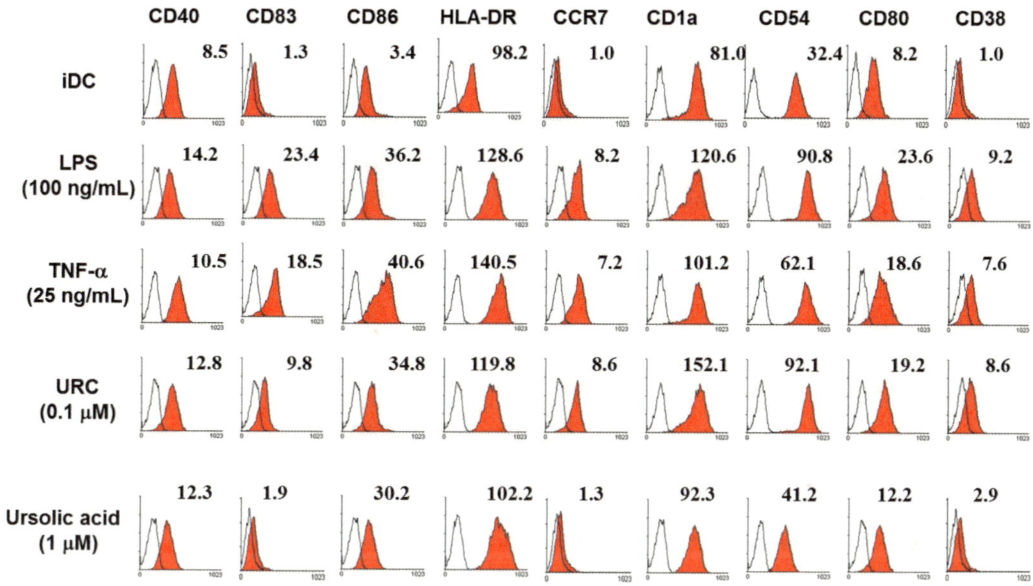

Fig. 1. Phenotype of dendritic cells differentiated with URC, Ursolic acid, LPS or TNF-α. Dendritic cells were generated by stimulating immature dendritic cells with URC (0.1 μM), Ursolic acid (1 μM), LPS (100 ng/ml) or TNF-α (25 ng/ml) and then were stained with FITC-conjugated Ab or PE-conjugated Ab against CD1a, CD38, CD40, CD54, CD80, CD83, CD86, HLA-DR and CCR-7 as described previously (Takei et al. 2005). Antibodies were overlayed with their isotype control. Data are one experiment representative of four independent experiments.

2.1 Immunostimulatory capacity in an allogeneic mixed lymphocyte reaction

The ability to induce allogeneic T cell proliferation is a functional hallmark of dendritic cells *in vitro*. Change in the surface marker expression is also reflected at a functional level, when analyzing the allostimulatory capacity of dendritic cells in an allogeneic mixed lymphocyte reaction. Efficiency in an allogeneic mixed lymphocyte reaction for URC-primed dendritic cells and Ursolic acid-primed dendritic cells were enhanced in a dose-dependent manner (data not shown). URC-, Ursolic acid- and LPS-primed dendritic cells was demonstrated a higher stimulatory efficiency in an allogeneic mixed lymphocyte reaction than immature dendritic cells and TNF-γ-primed dendritic cells (Fig. 2). Simultaneous dendritic cells stimulation with URC in the presence of IFN-γ (100 ng/ml) appeared to enhance this effect (data not shown). URC-primed dendritic cells and Ursolic acid-primed dendritic cells resulted in enhancement of T cell proliferation, indicating that URC and Ursolic acid potentiate the Ag-presenting activity of dendritic cells in an allogeneic mixed lymphocyte reaction.

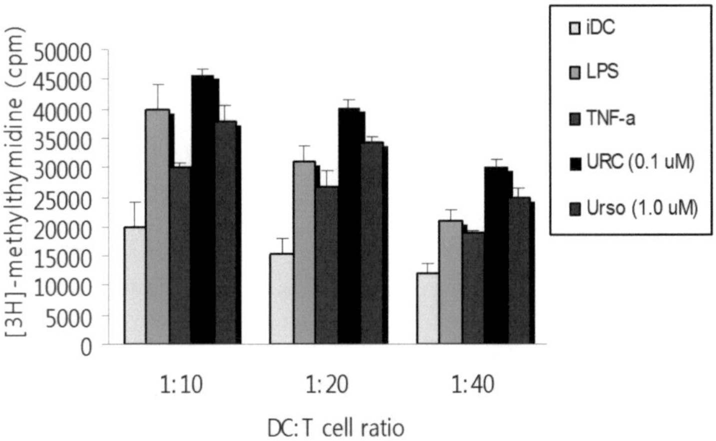

Fig. 2. Allogeneic T cell stimulatory capacity of dendritic cells differentiated with URC, Ursolic acid, LPS or TNF-α. Naïve T cells were co-cultured with gradually increasing doses of dendritic cells and on day 5, [^{3}H] methylthymidine was added 16 h. before measurement of the proliferation responses. Data are the mean cpm ± S.E.M. of five independent experiments. *$P < 0.05$ compared with immature dendritic cells.

2.2 IL-10 and IL-12p70 release by activated dendritic cells

Since dendritic cells serve as the professional antigen-presenting cells and their secretion of immunoregulatory and proinflammatory cytokines plays a crucial role in T cell priming, we then investigated whether cytokine production by human monocyte-derived dendritic cells was affected by treatment with URC and Ursolic acid. IL-10 is a pleiotropic cytokine known to have inhibitory effects on the accessory functions of dendritic cells and appears to play a central role in preventing overly pathological Th1 or Th2 responses in a variety of settings. In contrast, the level of IL-12 production by myeloid dendritic cells during activation of naïve T cells is a major factor driving the development of Th1 cells. Therefore, we measured IL-10 and IL-12p70 productions in immature dendritic cells (with medium) and in dendritic cells matured for 2 days in the presence of the above factors after stimulation by CD40 L-transfected for 24 h. Measurements of cytokines production were determined by ELISA kit. Major enhancements of IL-12p70 production were caused by URC and Ursolic acid, and this production was dose-dependent manner (Fig.3A and data not shown). Dendritic cells matured with URC in the presence of IFN-γ (100 ng/ml) produced even higher levels of IL-12p70 upon CD40 ligation (data not shown). In contrast, the production of IL-10 by URC-,

Ursolic acid-, LPS- or TNF-α-primed dendritic cells was low. On the other hand, the production of IL-10 and IL-12p70 by immature dendritic cells was low (Fig.3A and B).

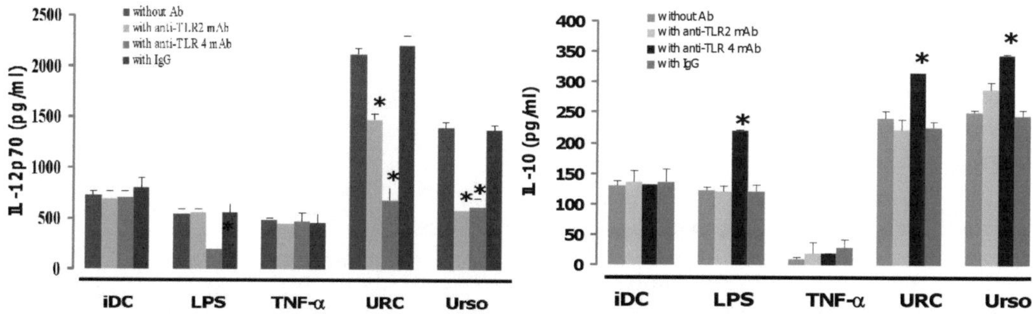

Fig. 3. The production of IL-12p70 by URC-primed dendritic cells and Ursolic acid-primed dendritic cells was inhibited by anti-TLR2 mAb and anti-TLR4 mAb. Dendritic cells were generated by stimulating immature dendritic cells with URC (0.1 μM), Ursolic acid (1 μM), LPS (100 ng/ml) or TNF-α (25 ng/ml). Cells ($4x10^4$ cells/well) were stimulated with the CD40 L-transfected J558 cells ($5x10^4$ cell/well) for 24 h., the production of IL-12p70 (A), and IL-10 (B) was measured by ELISA in culture supernatants. iDC: immature dendritic cells. Data are the mean ± S.E.M. of five independent experiments. *P< 0.05 compared without mAb.

2.2.1 Effects of anti-TLR 2 mAb and anti-TLR4 mAb on cytokine production by URC-primed dendritic cells and Ursolic acid-primed dendritic cells

Dendritic cells activation is mediated by a member of the Toll-like family of receptor and TLR agonists are potent activators of innate immune responses. TLR signaling results in the differentiation of dendritic cells from human monocytes which, in turn, prime an effective Th1 response as recent studies that focused on the molecular mechanisms underlying Th1/Th2 development. We evaluated the role for TLRs in the development of Th1 cells in naïve T cells co-cultured with URC and Ursolic acid. Before stimulation with URC and Ursolic acid, monocyte-derived dendritic cells were incubated in the presence of the TLR2 mAb (10 μg/ml), TLR4 mAb (10 μg/ml) or an isotype control (IgG1). Then, dendritic cells were stimulated with CD40 L -transfected J558 cells for 24 h. The anti-TLR2 mAb and anti-TLR4 mAb inhibited the production of IL-12p70 by URC-primed dendritic cells and Ursolic acid-primed dendritic cells by50-70% (Fig.3A). On the other hand, the production of IL-12p70 by LPS-primed dendrite cells was inhibited by the anti-TLR4 mAb, whereas the anti-TLR2 mAb was not inhibited the production of IL-12p70 by LPS-primed dendritic (Fig.3A). mAb did not inhibit the the production of IL-10 induced by URC-, Ursolic acid- and LPS-primed dendritic cells (Fig.3B). In contrast, the response to TNF-α was not influenced in the presence of the anti-TLR2 mAb and anti-TLR4 mAb did not inhibit (Fig.3A and B). The production of IL-12p70 by URC in combination with IFN-γ was not influenced by adding, whereas the production of IL-10 was not influenced by the anti-TLR4 mAb (data not shown). The production of IL-10 and IL-12p70 by URC-, Ursolic acid-, LPS- or TNF-α-primed dendritic cells was not influenced when IgG1 was added instead of anti-TLR 2 mAb or anti-TLR4 mAb (Fig.3A and B).

It was left undermined whether TLR2 and TLR4 express on URC-primed dendritic cells and Ursolic acid-primed dendritic cells. To address this question, we examined expression of TLR2 and TLR4 on URC-primed dendritic cells and Ursolic acid-primed dendritic cells. Total cellular RNA was extracted using RNeasy Mini kits (Qiagen GmbH, Germany), according to manufacturer's recommendations. Using RT-PCR, we found that URC-primed dendritic cells and Ursolic acid-primed dendritic cells expressed significant levels of mRNA coding for both TLR2 and TLR4 (data not shown). These data are compatible with URC and Ursolic acid activation of dendritic cells via TLRs.

2.2.2 NF-κB activation and TLR expression

Dendritic cells activation and maturation driven by TLR agonist such as LPS has been clearly associated to NF-κB activation. To determine whether URC and Ursolic acid uses similar activation pathways, we monitored thier ability to activate of the NF-κB translocation into the nucleus. EMES was performed with the Gel Shift assay system (Promega, El, USA). Dendritic cells were cultured in the presence of URC and Ursolic acid for 30 min, 1 h. and 2 h., and nuclear extracts were analyzed for NF-κB content. As shown in Fig.4A, URC was able to induce NF-κB translocation and activation. Similar results were obtained with Ursolic acid-primed dendritic cells and LPS-primed dendritic cells (data not shown and Fig.4A). The expression of TLR2 and TLR4 on monocytes, immature dendritic cells, URC-, Ursolic acid- and LPS-primed dendritic cells was further analyzed by real-time quantitative RT-PCR, because of their different selective expression on dendritic cells. Monocytes and immature dendritic cells expressed the highest levels of TLR2 and TLR4 on the cell population examined. mRNA expression of these two receptors was dramatically down-regulated upon differentiation of monocytes into dendritic cells after 8 days of culture with GM-CSF, IL-4 plus LPS, URC and Ursolic acid (Fig.4B and C). URC-primed dendritic cells and Ursolic acid-primed dendritic cells expressed considerable levels of TLR2 and TLR4. In URC-primed dendritic cells and Ursolic acid-primed dendritic cells, TLR4 expression seemed to be more prominent than TLR2 (Fig.4B and C). The expression of TLR4 on URC-primed dendritic cells and Ursolic acid-primed dendritic cells was higher than that of LPS-primed dendritic cells. Interestingly, we found that upon URC, Ursolic acid and LPS stimulation, mRNA expression of TLR2 and TLR4 was down-regulated with overall mRNA transcript detection levels being lower than in immature dendritic cells. It has been reported that monocyte-derived immature dendritic cells down-regulate TLR2 and TLR4 upon maturation with the corresponding cognate ligand LPS (Ismaili et al. 2002). Our experimental data support their observation showing that LPS in human dendritic cells and monocytes express different mRNA TLR transcripts. One might speculate that URC- and Ursolic acid-induced regulation of TLR2 and TLR4 expression may be involved in positively or negatively modulating the recognition of URC and Ursolic acid motifs by TLR2 and TLR4. URC, Ursolic acid and LPS were, in part, involved in down-regulation of human. These data suggest that URC and Ursolic acid might activate by dendritic cells via a TLR4 and/or TLR2 signaling. Our experiments showed that common pathways are activated by URC, Ursolic acid and LPS, as they modulate TLR expression. An important immunomodulatory property of TLR agonists is their capacity to enhance IL-12 production of dendritic cells and other innate immune cells. TLR signaling frequently generate dendritic cells and enhances the production of IL-12, a major Th-1-inducing cytokine (Okamoto and Sato, 2003). It suggests that dendritic cells activated by TLR2 and TLR4 stimulation may induce T cell differentiation toward Th1 by presenting antigens to T cells while promoting a Th1-leading situation in the local environment. Ability to promote Th1-type responses plays a key protective role in immunity to tumor. Interestingly, anti-TLR2 mAb and anti-TLR4 mAb enhanced the production of IL-10 by URC-primed dendritic cells and Ursolic acid-primed dendritic cells, and induced T cell differentiation towards Th2. IL-10 can promote Th2 responses that may be inhibitory for Th1 responses and negatively influences the ability of the differentiation of dendritic cells from human monocytes to produce IL-12p70. IL-10 might play a key role in the Th1/Th2 response by inhibiting IL-12p70. Therefore, our results suggest that the development of the Th1/2 response, at least in part, is controlled by the production of IL-12p70 via TLR2 and/or TLR4 signaling on dendritic cells. URC-primed dendritic cells and Ursolic acid-primed dendritic cells provide stronger costimulatory signals and/or the proinflammatory cytokines needed for T cell activation depending on TLR2 and/or TLR4, and induced Th1 development.

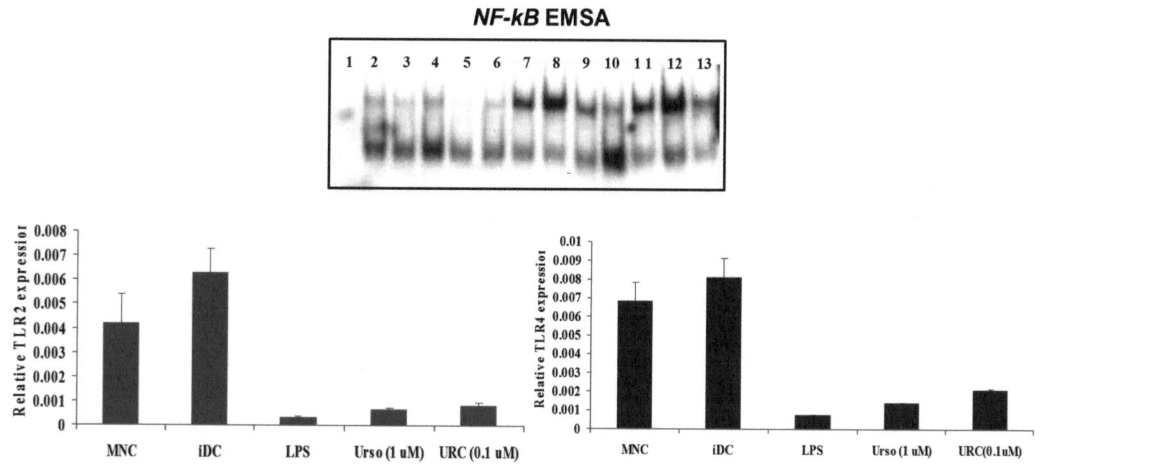

Fig. 4. URC induces NF-κB activation and modulates TLR2 and TLR4. (A) DC were stimulated with URC (0.5 μM), LPS (100 ng/ml) or medium for 30 min, 1 h. and 2 h., and nuclear extracts were analyzed for their NF-κB binding activity using EMSA. 1: Competition (x 100 cold) negative control 2: immature dendritic cells (0 min), 3: immature dendritic cells (30 min) 4: immature dendritic cells (1 h) 5: immature dendritic cells (2 h) 6: LPS (0 min) 7: LPS (30 min) 8: LPS (1 h) 9: LPS (2 h) 10: URC (0 min) 11: URC (30 min) 12: URC (1 h) 13: URC (2 h). (B) Relative TLR expression during the differentiation of dendritic cells. Monocytes were cultured with GM-CSF and IL-4 to differentiate to immature dendritic cells for 8 days. Maturation of dendritic cells was induced by URC (0.1 μM), Ursolic acid (1 μM) or LPS (1 μg/ml). Cells were collected at indicated time; mRNA were extracted and converted to cDNA. The cDNA were subjected to Realtime SYBR Green quantitative PCR using gene-specific primers pair for TLR2, TLR4 and β-actin. Relative gene expression was calculated using $2^{-\Delta\Delta Ct}$ method. Left panel: Relative TLR4 expression during differentiation of dendritic cells by LPS in comparison to stimulation of dendritic cells with URC or Ursolic acid. Right panel: Relative TLR2 expression during differentiation of DC by LPS in comparison to stimulation of dendritic cells with URC or Ursolic acid. Data are the mean ± S.E.M. of three independent experiments. *$P < 0.05$ compared with immature dendritic cells (iDC).

2.3 URC-primed dendritic cells and Ursolic acid-primed dendritic cells promote the differentiation of naïve T cells into Th1 cells

Given that the nature of cytokines secreted by dendritic cells are known to govern the type of T response observed, we evaluated the nature of primary allogeneic T cell responses stimulated by URC-primed dendritic cells and Ursolic acid-primed dendritic cells. Allogeneic URC-, Ursolic acid-, LPS- or TNF-α-primed dendritic cells induced as substantial increase in the secretion of IFN-γ by T cells (Fig.5A), but had little effect on IL-4 secretion (Fig.5B). Very consistently, the production of IL-4 and IL-10 are coherently dependent on the factors used to drive dendritic cells-maturation. In contrast, the production of IFN-γ and IL-4 induced by naïve T cells co-cultured with immature dendritic cells was low (Fig.5A and B). This Th1 response was confirmed by flow cytometry (data not shown).

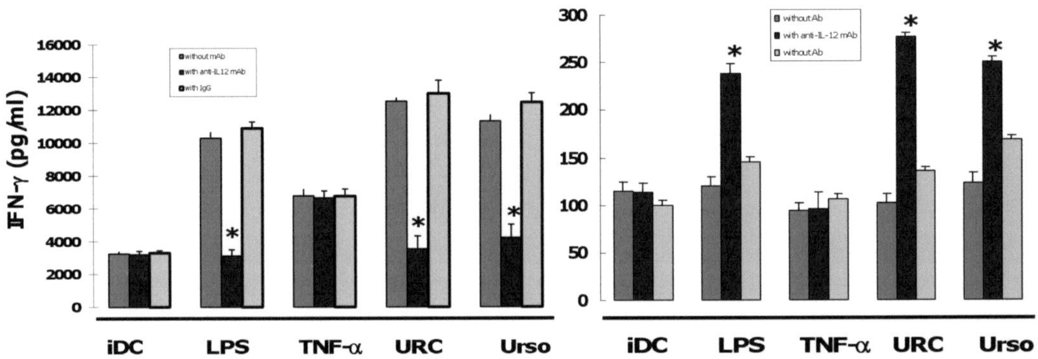

Fig. 5. Effect of anti-IL-12 mAb on polarization of naïve T cells by dendritic cells. Dendritic cells were co-cultured with naïve T cells days in the presence of control Ab or anti-IL-12 mAb (10 μg/ml). After 9 days of expansion in IL-2, T cells were counted and re-stimulated for 24 h with Dynabeads CD3/CD28. After 24 h, IFN-γ (A) or IL-4 (B) was measured by ELISA in culture supernatants. iDC: immature dendritic cells. Data are the mean ± S.E.M. of five independent experiments. *P< 0.05 compared without mAb.

To analyze the contribution of dendritic cells-derived IL-12p70 on the development of Th1 cells, we tested the effect of a neutralizing anti-IL-12 mAb in co-cultures of dendritic cells with naïve T cells. In naïve T cells co-cultured with URC-, Ursolic acid-, LPS- or TNF-α-primed dendritic cells, neutralization of IL-12 increased the development of IL-4 producing T cells and dramatically decreased the development of IFN-γ producing T cells (Fig.5A and B). In contrast, the production of IFN-γ and IL-4 by naïve T cells co-cultured with URC-, Ursolic acid-, LPS- or TNF-α-primed dendritic cells was not influenced when IgG1 was used instead of anti-IL-12 mAb (Fig.5A and B). Even higher production of IFN-γ by T cells was induced by dendritic cells matured with URC in the presence of IFN-γ (data not shown). Anti-IL-12 neutralizing Abs decreased IFN-γ secretion, confirming both the presence of bioactive IL-12 and its direct role in IFN-γ induction in this culture system. Th1 and Th2 development depend on the route of immunization, the nature and the concentration of Ag and the balance between IL-4 and IL-12 at priming. Our data showed that LPS-, URC- or Ursolic acid-primed dendritic cells polarized T cells into Th1 via high IL-12p70 secretion upon CD40-L (T cells engagement) stimulation and demonstrated that the production of

IFN-γ by naïve T cells co-cultured with URC-primed dendritic cells and Ursolic acid-primed dendritic cells was affected by the presence of a neutralizing anti-IL-12 mAb. The production of IL-12p70 by dendritic cells is a major inducer of IFN-γ. The reduced induction of IFN-γ after incubation with anti-IL-12 mAb indicates that IFN-γ induction is largely dependent on endogenous IL-12. Therefore, the data suggest that the effect of URC and Ursolic acid on the production of IL-12p70 by dendritic cells and strengthening of the Th1 response by naïve T cells might contribute to a potential antitumor effect of URC and Ursolic acid. The rational for selecting IL-12 production as a potency assay for dendritic cells generated for human therapy is based on IL-12 properties, and its confirmed role in host defense against pathogens and cancer. The generation of effective antitumor immunity involves the production of Th1 cytokines such as IL-12 and IFN-γ that might facilitate the induction and/or activation of tumor Ag-specific CD4 and CD8 cells. IL-12p70 is the cytokine responsible for antitumor responses of T lymphocytes. The understanding of mechanism controlling IL-12 induction by adjuvant in general and URC and Ursolic acid, in particular, may contribute to improving cellular immune responses in human therapies. It seems that TNF-α-primed dendritic cells drive the differentiation of naïve T cells towards Th1 cells via an unknown factor, because TNF-α-primed dendritic cells did not increase the IL-12 production upon adding CD40-L.

2.4 Cytotoxicity of CD8+T cells against T2 target cells

Dendritic cells are professional APC that are required for the initiation of immune responses. In the immunotherapy against malignant diseases, it has been suggested that the induction of tumor antigen-specific CTL is most important for eliminating tumor cells. Antitumor immunity has classically been measured by the quantity of tumor-antigen-specific CD8+ T cells. In this context, it is important to know whether URC-primed dendritic cells and Ursolic acid-primed dendritic cells enhanced specific CTL responses. We compared the CTL responses of autologus CD8+T cells supported by dendritic cells differentiated with URC or TNF-α. In an 8 h. to measure CTL apoptosis by tumor cells, T2 cells loaded with WT-1 peptides strongly induced DNA fragmentation of CTL that were generated with URC-primed dendritic cells pulsed with WT-1 peptides (Fig.6A). Details of the method used in these assay have been described previously (Takei et al. 2004, Mailliard and Lotz 2001, Nakano et al. 1998). As expected from their Th-1-polarizing effect, percentage of DNA fragmentation was dependent on the increased number of CTL cells. Similar results were obtained with a ^{51}Cr release assay to measure lysis of target cells (Fig.6B). URC-primed dendritic cells induced a stronger CTL response than immature dendritic cells or TNF-α-primed dendritic cells. On the other hand, percentage of DNA fragmentation in JAM assay and ^{51}Cr release were low or undetectable when T2 loaded with HIV-1 peptide (unrelated peptide) and T2 (without peptides) were used as the target cells (negative control) (Fig.6A and B). Dendritic cells activated with TLR agonists, especially TLR4 and TLR8 agonists stimulate IL-12-producing human myeloid dendritic cells, which activate CD8 CTL against tumors. Moreover, Kawasaki et al. (2000) have reported that TLR4 mediates LPS-mimetic signal transduction by anti-cancer agents Taxol, a plant-derived diterpene, in mice but not human. More recently, synthetic ligands for TLR4, TLR7 or TLR9 have been through preclinical evaluation and clinical trials against cancer. Therefore, that suggests that URC might be a promising agent for the treatment of cancer. The effects of dendritic cells matured with Ursolic acid in the CTL responses are not known yet. However, we expect to obtain similar results with URC-primed dendritic cells, because dendritic cells matured with Ursolica cid enhanced the differentiation of naïve T cells towards the Th1 type.

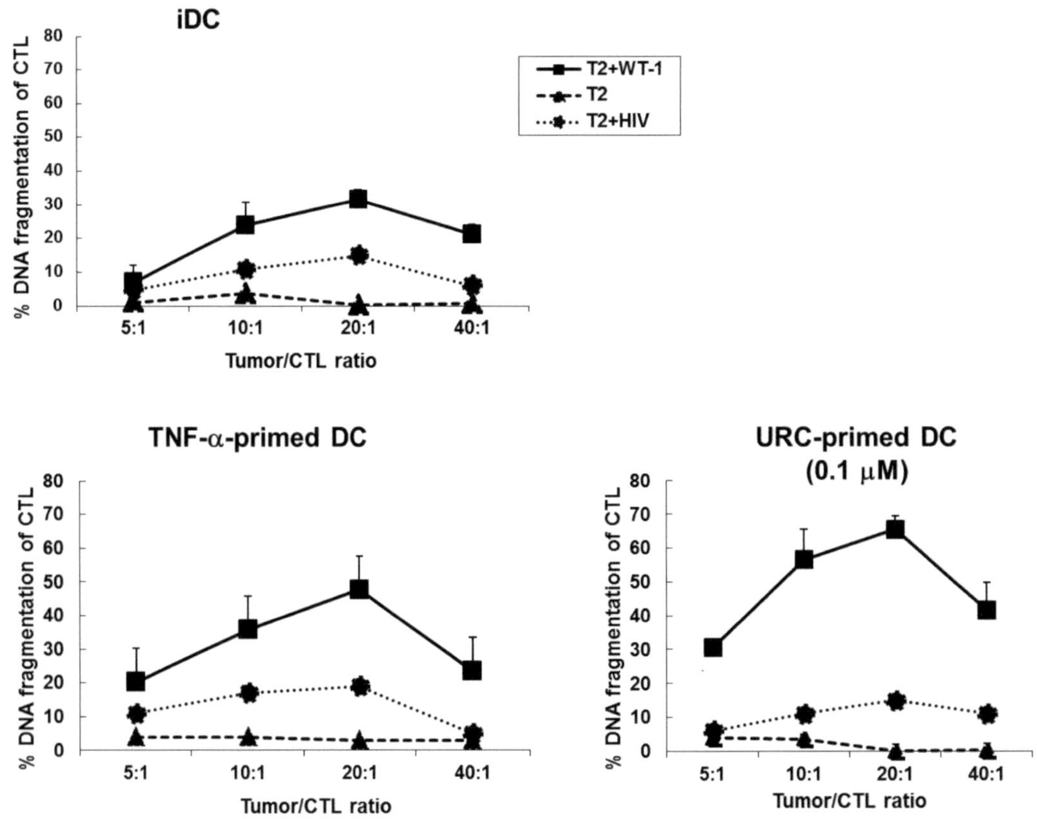

Fig. 6. Autologus CD8+T cells incubated with URC-primed dendritic cells showed higher cytolytic activity against T2 target cells loaded with WT-1 peptide at a high effector-to-target ratio than against T2 target cell without WT-1 peptide. (A) The CTL were labeled with [^{3}H]-methylthymidine and served as the target for tumor cell lines. T2 cells induced more DNA fragmentation of CTL that were generated with URC-primed dendritic cells pulsed with WT-1 peptides than those that were generated with immature dendritic cells or TNF-α-primed DC pulsed with WT-1 peptides. (B) Specific lysis was measured by ^{51}Cr release assay. Data are the mean ± S.E.M. of three independent experiments. *$P< 0.05$ compared with T2.

2.5 URC-primed dendritic cells and Ursolic acid-primed dendritic cells are capable of migration *in vitro*

The ability of dendritic cells to migrate to local lymph nodes and their subsequent presentation of antigen to T cells play an essential role in the initiation of adaptive immunity. In tissues, mature dendritic cells must be responsive to lymph node derived signals, but must also be able to down-regulate tissue anchoring proteins including Ecadherin that would otherwise detrimental dendritic cells migration and antigen presentation to naïve T cells. Migration to the secondary lymphoid organs and subsequent antigen presentation requires dendritic cells maturation, a process that is associated with up-regulation of co-stimulatory molecules. We investigated the migratory capacity of URC-primed dendritic cells and Ursolic acid-primed dendritic cells toward CCL19 and CCL21. URC-primed dendritic cells and Ursolic acid-primed dendritic cells had migration in response to CCL19 and CCL21 (Fig.7), and slightly up-regulated the expression of CCR7 and CD38 on URC-primed dendritic cells and Ursolic acid-primed dendritic cells (Fig.1). Expression of CCR7 seems also to be important for other aspects of dendritic cells biology, in particular in enhancing chemotaxis and trans-endothelial passage in response to CCL19 and CCL21. Recently, it has been reported that expression of CD38 on dendritic cells is essential for their coordinated migration to the T cell area of draining lymph node and increase dendritic cells function (Trepiakas et al. 2009). These results suggest that URC-primed dendritic cells and Ursolic acid-primed dendritic cells migrate *in vivo* and is a promising approach for the treatment of cancer. In most clinical trials using dendritic cells-based immunotherapy, immature monocyte-derived dendritic cells pulsed with tumor antigen peptides were used. Recent studies showed that mature dendritic cells could be a better antitumor adjuvant. However, there is no clear answer yet.

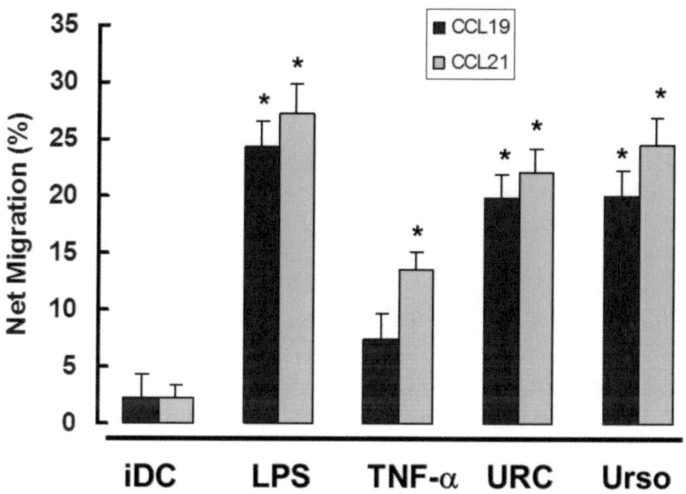

Fig. 7. Chemotaxis in response to CCL19 and CCL21 by URC-, Ursolic acid-, LPS- or TNF-α-primed dendritic cells. URC-, Ursolic acid-, LPS- or TNF-α-primed dendritic cells were prepared and recovered, and their migratory abilities in response to CCL19 (500 ng/ml) and CCL21 (500 ng/ml) were determined *in vitro*. Data are the mean ± S.E.M. of three independent experiments. *P< 0.05 compared with immature dendritic cells (iDC).

3. In conclusion

We described in this chapter a very promising and cost effective dendritic cells maturation factor consisting of URC and Ursolic acid, both mature dendritic cells which meet the dendritic cells criteria important for efficient immunotherapy, including the capacity to migrate and the production of IL-12p70 upon CD40 triggering. Although based on *in vitro* results, URC and Ursolica cid may be used in dendritic cells-based vaccine for cancer immunotherapy. Several mechanisms have been proposed to explain the apparent adjuvant effects of TLR agonists on atitumor immunity. TLR trigger the secretion of critical cytokines, and TLR can stimulate the proliferation of CD4+ T cells and CD8+ T cells. Moreover, TLR signaling frequently enhances the production of IL-12 in dendritic cells. Thus, it is strongly suggested that dendritic cells matured with TLR stimulation may induce T cell differentiation toward Th1 by presenting antigens to T cells while promoting a Th1-leading situation in the local environment. Several TLR agonists have been developed as anticancer drugs. We expect to be able to correlate the in vitro dendritic cells product attributes with *in vivo* immunologic and clinical end point.

4. Acknowledgments

Reprinted from European Journal Pharmacology, 643, Jung T-Y., Nguyen Pham T.N., Umeyama A., Shoji N., Hashimoto T., Lee J-J., Takei M., Ursolic acid isolated from *Uncaria rhynchophylla* activates human dendritic cells via TLR2 and/or TLR4 and induces the production IFN-γ by CD4+ naïve T cells, 297-303, Copyright (2010), with permission from Elsevier.

Reprinted from Biomarker Insights, 6, Kim S-K., Nguyen Pham T.N., Jin C-J., Umeyama A., Shoji N., Hashimoto T., Lee J-J., Takei M., Uncarinic acid C isolated from *Uncaria rhynchophylla* induces differentiation of Th1-promoting dendritic cells through TLR4 signaling, 1-12, Copyright (2011), with permission from Libertas Academica.

Reprinted from Cellular Immunology, 266, Bae W-K., Umeyama A., Shoji N., Hashimoto T., Lee J-J., Takei M., 104-110, Copyright (2010), with permission from Elsevier.

5. References

Banchereau J, Steinman, RM. (1998) Dendritic cells and the control of immunity. Nature 106, 245-252.

Forster R, Schube lA, Breitfeld D. (1999) CCR7 coordinates the primary immune response by establishing functional microenvironments in secondary lymphoid organ, Cell 99, 23-33.

Hermann P, Rubio M, Nakajima T, Delespesse G., Sarfati M. (1998) IFN-γ priming of human monocytes differentially regulates Gram positive and Gram negative bacteria-induced IL-10 release and selectively enhances IL-12p70, CD80 and MHC class I expression. J Immunol 161, 2011-2018.

Ismaili J, Rennesson J, Aksoy E. (2002) Monophosphoryl lipid A activates both human dendritic cells and T cells. J Immunol 68, 926-932.

Kawasaki K, Akashi S, Shimazu R, Yoshida T, Miyake K, Nishijima M. (2000) Mouse Tool-like receptor 4. MD-2 complex mediates lipopolysaccharide-mimetic signal transduction by Taxol. J Biol Chem 275, 2251-2254.

Kuchroo VK, Dasa MP, Brown AM. (1995) B7-1 and B7-2 costimulatory molecules activate differentially the Th1/Th2 development pathways: application to autoimmune disease therapy. Cell 80, 707-713.

Lanzavecchia A, Sallustoa AF. (2001) Regulation of T cell immunity by dendritic cells. Cell 106, 263-266.

Lederer JA, Perez VL, Desroches L, Kim S, Abbas A., Lichtman AH. (1996) Cytokine transcriptional events during helper T cell subset differentiation. J Exp Med 184, 397-406.

Lee JS, Kim J, Kim BY, Lee HS, Ahn JS, Chang YS. (2000) Inhibition of phospholipase Cγ1 and cancer cell proliferation by triterpene ester from *Uncaria rhynchophylla*. J Nat Prod 63, 753-756.

Lezz G., Scotet E, Scheidegger D, Lanzavecchia A. (1999) The interplay between the duration of TCR and cytokine signaling determines T cell polarization. Eur J Immunol 29, 4092-4101.

Mailliard RB, Lotz MT. (2001) Dendritic cells prolong tumor-specific T-cell survival and effector function after interaction with tumor targets. Clin Cancer Res 7, 980-988.

Mellman I, Steinman RM. (2001) Dendritic cells: specialized and regulated antigen processing machines. Cell 106, 2555-2558.

Nakano M, Shichijo S, Imaizumi T, Itho K. (1998) A gene encoding antigen peptides of human sequamous cell carcinoma recognized by cytotoxic T lymphocytes. J Exp Med 187: 277-283.

O'garra AC. (2001) cytokines induce the development of functionally heterogeneous T helper cell subsets. Immunity 8, 275-278.

Okamoto M, Sato M. (2003) Toll-like receptor signaling in anti-cancer immunity. J Med Invest 50, 9-24.

Romagnani S. (1994) Lymphokine production by human T cells in disease state. Annu Rev Immunol 12, 227-257.

Steinman RM, Dhodapkar M. (2001) Active immunization against cancer with dendritic cells: the near future. Int J Cancer 95, 459-473.

Steinman RM. (2007) A brief history of T(H)17, the first major revision in the T(H)1/T(H)2 hypothesis of T cell-mediated tissue damage. Nature Medicine 13, 139-145.

Takei M, Umeyam A, Hashimoto T. (2005) Epicubenol and Ferruginol induce DC from human monocytes and differentiate IL-10-producing regulatory T cells in vitro. Bioche Biophy Res Commun 337, 730-738.

Takei M, Umeyama A, Shoji N, Hashimoto T. (2007) Diterpenes inhibit IL-12 production by DC and enhance Th2 cells polarization. Bioche Biophy Res Commun 355, 603-610.

Takei M, Umeyama A, Shoji N, Hashimoto T. (2008) Diterpene, 16-phyllocladanol enhances Th1 polarization induced by LPS-primed DC, but not TNF-α-primed DC. Bioche Biophy Res Commun 370, 6-10.

Tanaka H, Demeure CE, Rubio M, Delespesse G., Sarfati M. (2000) Human monocyte-derived dendritic cells induce naïve T cell differentiation into T helper cell type 2 (Th2) or Th1/Th2 effectors: role of stimulator/responder ratio. J Exp Med 192, 403-411.

Tao, X., Grant, S., Constant, K., Bottomly, K., 1997, Induction of IL-4 producing CD4+ T cells by antigenic peptides altered for TCR binding. J Immunol 158, 4237-4244.

Trepiakas R, Pedersen AE, Met, O, Svane IM. (2009) Addition of interferon-alpha to a standard maturation cocktail induces CD38 up-regulation and increases dendritic cell function. Vaccine 27, 2213-2219.

Trinchieri G., Scott P. (1994) The role of interleukin 12 in the immune response, disease and therapy. Immunol Today 15, 460-463.

8

The Novel Use of Zwitterionic Bacterial Components and Polysaccharides in Immunotherapy of Cancer and Immunosuppressed Cancer Patients

A.S. Abdulamir[1,2], R.R. Hafidh[1,3] and F. Abubaker[1,4]
[1]*Institute of Bioscience, University Putra Malaysia, Serdang,*
[2]*Microbiology Department, College of Medicine, Alnahrain University, Baghdad,*
[3]*Microbiology Department, College of Medicine, Baghdad University,*
[4]*Faculty of Food Science and Technology, University Putra Malaysia, Serdang,*
[1,4]*Malaysia*
[2,3]*Iraq*

1. Introduction

The recognition of pathogenic antigens as foreign particles by adaptive immune cells induces T and B lymphocytes to start defensive humoral and cellular reaction. Latest research revealed that proteins and some lipids are the main molecules inducing protective T cell responses during microbial infections while polysaccharides which are important components of microbial pathogens and many vaccines were not regarded as important antigens. However, research regarding the role of the adaptive immune system by polysaccharides gained interest only recently. Traditionally, polysaccharides were considered to be T cell-independent antigens that did not directly activate T cells or induce protective immune responses, but chemically modified polysaccharides, namely zwitterionic polysaccharides (ZPSs) were recently found highly immunogenic. Therefore, in this chapter we will discuss the role of zwittrionized polysaccharides in immune reaction induction and their immunostimulatory effect in cancer patients. Several studies were conducted to use ZPSs to induce vigorous immune response and to establish immunostimulatory or immunomodulatroy effect which can be used in cancer immunotherapy. Bacterial ZPSs that are naturally zwitterionic or those that were artificially zwitterionized were recently identified as potent immune regulators. The immunomodulatory effect of ZPSs requires antigen processing and presentation by antigen presenting cells, the activation of CD4 T cells and subpopulations of CD8 T cells and the modulation of host cytokine responses.

In addition, a recent model research done by our team will be presented in this chapter. This research introduced, in a breakthrough approach, zwitterionic motifs experimentally into polysaccharides of pneumo-23 vaccine converting these polysaccharides into effective immunostimulatory agent in immunosuppressed cancer patients. This study intended to assess the in vitro immunostimulatory effect of zwitterionized penumoccocal vaccine compared with the nonzwitterionized commercial pneumo-23 vaccine. The in vitro immunostimulatory potential of zwitterionized penumoccocal vaccine was clearly observed in cancer immunosuppressed patients as well as, to a lesser extent, healthy control subjects, stimulating the synthesis of core cytokines of T-helper 1, and primarily inducing CD4+ and CD8+T cells. These studies collectively open the door wide for a new field for effective cancer immunotherapy.

2. The role of ZPS in eliciting immune response

The majority of the natural polysaccharide molecules consist of anionic sugar molecules which fail to activate T cells, and do not induce B-cell antibody isotype switching (Tzianabos et al., 1992). However, it was identified that a small group of bacterial polysaccharides carries both positive and negative charges in the same repeating sugar molecules which were accordingly called zwitterionic polysaccharides (ZPSs) (Baumann et al., 1992; Tzianabos et al., 1992; Coyne et al., 2000; Kalka-Moll, et al., 2001). Unlike most of bacterial polysaccharides, zwitterionic PS possess both positive and negative ions, which in turn found to be able to trigger T cell-dependent immune response, initiate class switching and affinity maturation of immunoglobulins, and induce long-term memory immunity (Gallorini et al., 2007; Cobb & Kasper, 2005; Wack et al., 2008; Richard & Amyes, 2004). Polysaccharides with both positively and negatively charged sugar molecules, unlike negatively charged polysaccharides, are able to stimulate both CD4 and CD8 T cells as well as antigen presenting cells of the adaptive immune system. This feature shows that molecules other than proteinaceous antigens are capable of activating conventional αβT cells.

However, development of specific T-Cell receptor (TCR) transgenic mouse models are required to understand the selection and development of ZPS-specific T cells. These cells may be more enriched in the mucosae as ZPS-producing bacteria such as *Bacteroides fragilis* (*B. fragilis*) and *Streptococcus. Pneumoniae* (*S. pneomoniae*) are contained within the commensal flora of the gut and upper respiratory track, respectively. ZPSs display an extended right-handed helix structure in which two repeating sugar units per turn form grooves with positive charges exposed on the outer surface (Wang et al., 2000). Due to this unique structure, ZPSs possess immunomodulatory activities, unlike other polysaccharides. Experimental studies in rats and mice have shown that intraperitoneal challenges with ZPSs induced vigorous pathogenic conditions, such as intra-abdominal abscesses which never happen in response to traditional polysaccharides (Tzianabos et al., 2000; Mazmanian et al., 2005). When ZPSs are accidently introduced into a sterile area, such as the peritoneal cavity during intra-abdominal surgical procedures when abdominal contents can spill into the peritoneal cavity, or by intraperitoneal inoculation with ZPS and a sterile cecal adjutant, a rapid recruitment of ZPS-specific, proinflammatory CD4 T cells may be induced. This recruitment of CD4 T cells together with other innate cells results in the generation of intra-abdominal abscess, a defensive mechanism of the body to contain the infection. Recent studies have shown that ZPS-mediated intraabdominal abscess induction depends on ZPS processing and presentation on MHC class-II molecules by APCs for recognition and activation of CD4 T cells (Stephen et al., 2010).

ZPS-specific T cells are in constant contact with ZPS presented by antigen presenting cells (APCs) of the mucosal immune system. Accordingly, the steady-state presentation of this unique immunomodulatory microbial antigen is beneficial to our immune system as it can play pivotal role in shaping a functionally competent, immune system which is a must element in any successful immunotherapy. Interestingly, upon subcutaneous inoculation, ZPSs induce, in a unique manner, both anti-inflammatory and immunosuppressive T cells at the same tine. The stimulated population of cells includes both regulatory CD4 and CD8 T cells, which secrete the immunosuppressive cytokine IL-10. Thus, the same immunogen can elicit both proinflammatory and anti-inflammatory responses dependent upon the route and mode of administration; this can be regarded as one of the reasons that ZPSs are able to play essential role in modulating/regulating immune system of humans.

3. Mechanisms of immune induction and regulation by ZPSs

ZPSs were found to possess immunostimulatory functions. The in vitro stimulation of human and murine CD4 T cells with ZPSs induces cellular proliferation and inhibits apoptosis of immune cells (Stephen et al., 2005; Groneck et al., 2009). And this activity of ZPSs was found to be conducted mainly via T cell receptor (TCR). In addition, co-stimulatory signals were also found necessary to induce remarkable T-cell responses to ZPSs; the activation of CD4 T cells by ZPS is found to be dependent on a several costimulatory factors. It was found that ZPSs can interact with lymphocytes and antigen presenting cells by particular mechanism(s). ZPSs possess specific immunostimulatory activity, leading to direct activation of antigen-presenting cells (APCs) through Toll-like receptor 2 (TLR2) and T-cell receptors (TCR) on the surface of T cells in co-culture systems. ZPS are therefore, considered TLR2 and TCR agonists, able to activate human and mouse APCs. Since T-regulatory cells and other T-cell subsets express TLR2, and TLR2 engagement modifies functionality and activation state of these cells, it is speculated that most effects induced by natural and chemically derived ZPS may be explained by their TLR2 and TCR agonist properties. Moreover, the presentation of fragmented ZPSs by MHC-class II molecules shows that ZPS-mediated T-cell activation is mediated by non-specific, generalized TCR recognition. Vβ chain repertoire analyses of ZPS-stimulated T-cell populations showed that a broad repertoire of subfamilies, including all of the Vβ subfamilies, was used more than specific Vβ genes (Stingele et al., 2004; Groneck et al., 2009). Therefore, the oligoclonal activation of T cells by ZPS seemed highly probable. Clonotype mapping of T cells that were stimulated in vitro with ZPSs showed oligoclonal T cell expansion. This nonrestricted Vβ usage indicates possible ZPS recognition by the CDR3 antigen-binding domain of the TCR. After TCR stimulation, CD69 is rapidly upregulated by the Ras-MAP kinase signaling pathway (D'Ambrosio et al., 1994); this implies to a notion that this pathway may be involved in ZPS-mediated T-cell activation (Stephen et al., 2010). However, no solid clues suggest the ability of ZPSs to stimulate gamma-delta T lymphocytes, NK or NKT cells.

4. The immunological role of bacterial ZPSs

Pathogenic strains of bacteria, such as *B. fragilis*, *S. pneumoniae*, and *S. aureus*, produce one of the most potent ZPSs in nature (Kolka-Moll et al., 2002); for this reason, bacterial ZPSs offer unique opportunity to exploit their extraordinary potential in stimulating or modulating immune system of humans. The capsular polysaccharide antigens PSA of B. fragilis (NCTC 9343 and 638R) (Kolka-Moll et al., 2001) and Sp1 of S. pneumoniae serotype 1 (Kolka-Moll et al., 2002) are the most widely studied ZPSs. Intra-abdominal abscess formation, which commonly occurs during secondary peritonitis and abdominal surgeries, is actually a ZPS-based protective mechanism used by the body to limit the spread of microbial pathogens. Initially, bacterial ZPS-induced pathologies were shown to be T-cell dependent. In those experiments, T-cell-deficient mice were unable to form abscesses after inoculations with bacterial ZPSs (Shapiro et al., 1986). Further experiments with α/βTCR-knockout mice revealed that immune response towards bacterial ZPSs were dependent on α/β TCR+ T cells (Chung et al., 2003). The activation of CD4 T cells is required for ZPS-mediated intra-abdominal abscess induction because mice lacking CD4 T cells failed to develop abscesses (Chung et al., 2003). As abscess formation was inhibited by the transfer of T cells from animals that were immunized with ZPS, these results suggest that abscess inductions and protection in the presence of ZPS are likely mediated by T-cell components of the adaptive immune system. The immunomodulatory effects of ZPSs require both positive and negative charge motifs as neutralization of a single charge motif abrogates the biological activities of ZPSs in triggering elaborative immune response and in stimulating immune cells altogether (Stephen et al., 2010). In this regard, it was found that the conversion of a nonzwitterionic bacterial molecule into a zwitterion makes the molecule biologically active just like the natural zwitterionic molecules (Gallorini et al., 2009; Stephen et al., 2010). However, bacterial ZPSs exert both wanted and unwanted actions, namely immunostimulatory/ immunomodulatory action and vigorous antigen-based immune response, respectively. This provided evidence for the justification of creating novel approaches for converting bacterial non-ZPSs into ZPSs molecules using chemical in-laboratory methods in a way strengthening their immunostimulatory effect and at the same time lowering their antigen-based immune reaction induction.

5. Model study for the experimentally zwitterionized bacterial polysaccharides to induce immunostimulatory effect in immunosuppressed cancer patients

The unique effect of zwitterionized bacterial polysaccharides as a potent in vitro immunostimulatory agent for immunosuppressed cancer patients was investigated in a novel study. The introduction of zwitterionic motifs into some of bacterial capsular polysaccharides turn these modified polysaccharides into moderately immunogenic and highly immunostimulatory agents. This study was conducted to assess the in vitro immunogenic and immunostimulatory effect of novel zwitterionized polysaccharides of the commercial pneumo-23 vaccine. In vitro proliferation, ELISA-based in vitro cytokine synthesis (IL-2, IFN-γ, and IL-10), and immunofluorescence microscopy-based immune profiling (CD4+, CD8+, and CD21+ cells) assays were used to evaluate the immunostimulatory effect of 48h of zwitterionized pneumo-23 encounter with peripheral blood mononuclear cells (PBMC) of immunosuppressed cancer (CA) patients and healthy control subjects (HC) in comparison with PBMC exposed to Concanavalin A (Con A), the positive control, and to phosphate buffered saline (PBS), the negative control. Zwitterionized pneumo-23, induced remarkable proliferation of PBMC in both CA and HC groups, induced in vitro synthesis of IL-2 and IFN-γ but not IL-10 in CA and borderline increase in IFN-γ and IL-10 in HC group, and expanded CD4+, CD8+, and CD21+ lymphocytes in CA rather than HC group. On contrary, Con A induced proliferation in HC more than CA group, induced only IL-2 synthesis and expanded only CD4+ cells in HC rather than CA group. Therefore, in this regard, it was concluded that a unique in vitro immunostimulatory potential of zwitterionized pneumo-23 vaccine was observed on PBMC of immunosuppressed more than immunocompetent subjects, stimulating the synthesis of core cytokines of T-helper 1, and inducing the CD8+ T cells, which are most probably CD8+ cytotoxic T-cells rather than suppressor cells. Accordingly, introducing zwitterionic motifs into polysaccharides of the commercial penumo-23 vaccine turned it into a unique and potent immunostimulator reverting suppressed immune cells back into normal levels.

Pneumo-23 is a polyvalent pneumococcal polysaccharide vaccine (Pasteur Merieux Connaught, 2004). This vaccine was designed mainly to confer immunity against severe pneumococcal infections in elderly patients and those who underwent splenectomy as part of a management of various hematological disorders, renders the patients unsusceptible to the development of overwhelming sepsis by Streptococcus pneumoniae (Pasteur Merieux Connaught, 2004; Rybachenko et al., 2009; vad der Harst, 2007; Kazancioglu et al., 2000). Pneumo-23 is a clear, colorless liquid prepared from purified pneumococcal capsular antigens. Each dose of 0.5 mL contains purified *S. pneumoniae* polysaccharides (PS), 25 µg of each of the included 23 serotypes (Rybachenko et al., 2009). Although pneumo-23 is composed of non- T cell-dependent polysaccharides, it was observed that pneumo-23 vaccine when is given to elderly people, or immunosuppressed patients, their immune response, in unexplained manner, was moderately enhanced non-specifically in addition to the immune protection achieved against pneumococcal infection(Rybachenko et al., 2009; vad der Harst, 2007; Kazancioglu et al., 2000). In addition, a recent study revealed another immune enhancing feature of pneumo-23 vaccine stating that pneumo-23 vaccine enhanced the opsonization and sustained normal compliment components of C3 and C4 in elderly cancer patients after splenectomy Uslu et al., 2006). This might be attributed to the fact that some of pneumo-23 PS is zwitterionic substances such as polysaccharides of type 1 pneumococci (Gallorini et al., 2007).

Although many studies discussed the specific immunogenicity of pmeumo-23 vaccine against pneumococcal bacterial serotypes in elderly or in HIV-infected patients (de Greef et al., 2007; Peetermans et al., 2005; Sumitani et al., 2008; Valenzuela et al., 2007), very few reports gave remarks on the unexplained potential of pneumo-23 to exert non-specific, generalized, immunostimulating effect and non-specific protection against microbes rather than pneumococci. A study revealed that the protection of pneumo-23 vaccine after splenectomy was perfect against the sepsis of many bacteria other than pneumococci which indicated a dubious role of the non-specific immunostimulatory effect of pneumo-23 vaccine in protecting subjects against bacterial infection in addition to its specific anti-pneumococcal infection (Uslu et al., 2005). Nevertheless, our team examined the possible in vitro immunostimulatory effect of the commercial pneumo-23 vaccine on human peripheral blood mononuclear cells (PBMC); the results showed some immunostimulatory potential of penumo-23 but it did not reach significant levels [data not shown]. This was predicted as the majority of pneumo-23 polysaccharides are T cell-independent substances except for small portion, serotype 1, which possess T cell-dependent zwitterionic motifs (Gallorini et al., 2007; Cobb & Kasper, 2005). Since the commercial pneumo-23 is a pure polysaccharides mixture and unlikely to possess TLR ligands, accordingly, it was believed that the observed slight immunostimulatory effect of the commercial pneumo-23 in the preliminary study of our team and in other studies might belong to the presence of low level of zwitterionic motifs in pneumo-23 vaccine which provide evidence that if polysaccharides of pneumo-23 vaccine were zwitterionized, then this might issue in a very potent and unique bacterial ZPSs that is able to modulate and stimulate immune system of immunosuppressed and debilitated human patients. Therefore, it was hypothesized that introducing zwitterionic motifs into polysaccharides of pneumo-23 vaccine might render it a potent and effective immunostimulatory agent. In the current research, polysaccharides of the commercial pneumo-23 vaccine were modified chemically by adding zwitterionic motifs. The ability of zwitterionized pneumo-23 vaccine to trigger T cell-dependent immunostimulatory effect on PBMC of immunosuppressed cancer patients in comparison with healthy control subjects was scrutinized.

5.1 Patients and methods

5.1.1 The research population

Since, cancer (CA) itself and the related chemotherapy are considered as a well-known condition of immunosuppression (Whiteside, 2006), three kinds of common CA were involved in this study, namely, lung, head and neck, and colorectal cancers. Sixty five immunosuppressed cancer patients of age ranged 42 to 62 years were involved in this study including 42 men with lung (22), head and neck (11), and colorectal (9) cancers and 23 women with lung (13), colorectal (7), and head and neck (3) cancers. They were selected out of 94 cancer patients after excluding the non-confirmed cases of immunosuppression. The selection criteria of the involved cancer patients were: confirmed diagnosis of advanced cancer (stages III and IV), pre-operative, immunosuppressed, engaged regularly in chemotherapy, 6 weeks interval from the last chemotherapy. The selection was done without any bias to certain type of the involved cancer types. This study was conducted in the period from November 2006 to February 2009. Cancer patients were retrieved from a number of central hospitals in Malaysia, Kuala Lumpur. The immunosuppression status of cancer patients was checked twice. First, the clinical presentation of patients which revealed patients' high susceptibility to frequent infections, patients' lymphopenia in complete blood count, and state of hypo-γ-globulinemia where serum IgG < 250 mg/dL, and serum IgA <5 mg/dL. Second, the immunosuppression status was confirmed by the conducted assays of the current study.

On the other hand, 100 age- and sex- matched healthy control (HC) were selected who attended hospitals for minor traumatic therapy. Medical examination was done for HC as well as their medical records were retrieved. They showed no current or previous major illness, no cancer, and normal blood and biochemical laboratory tests, namely erythrocyte sedimentation rate, complete blood count, liver function test, kidney function tests, and total serum proteins. Blood samples were taken from CA and HC groups after obtaining full written consent. Withdrawn blood was held in heparinized tubes for later isolation of PBMC. Permission was granted from the regional committee of ethics for biomedical research.

5.1.2 Zwitterionisation of pneumo-23 polysaccharides

Chemical modification of PSs of the commercial form of pneumo-23 (Sanofi Pasteur, France) was done by adding positive charge motifs in order to convert PS to zwitterionic PSs. The procedure of zwitterionisation was done according to a recent standardized method (Gallorini et al, 2007). Briefly, a chemical oxidation of the aliphatic chain from the terminal

NeuNAc residue using 0.01 M NaIO4, sodium metaperiodate, (Sigma, USA) for 90 min at room temperature was conducted leaving an aldehyde group. NaIO4 was used as limiting (30%) or stoechiometric (100%) reagent of the reaction. The periodate oxidation selectively cleaves the C8-C9 bond between vicinal hydroxyl groups (-CHOH-CH_2OH) of NeuNAc residues, leaving an aldehyde group (-CHO) at C8. This group was converted to a cationic -$NH3^+$ group by reductive amination using 300 mg/ml NH_4Ac, ammonium acetate, (Sigma, USA) and 49 mg/ml $NaBH_3CN$, sodium cyanoborohydride, (Sigma, USA) at pH 6.5 for 5 days at 37°C. PS obtained, R-CH_2NH_2, were treated with 37% formaldehyde (Merck, Germany) in the presence of sodium cyanoborohydride to convert the generated free amino group to a tertiary dimethylamine, R-$CH_2NH(CH_3)_2^+$ such that it retained a positive charge. This conversion was confirmed by the routine application of NMR spectroscopy Avance 600 MHz (Bruker, Germany) using 5-mm triple-resonance NMR probe as evidenced by the resonance at 2.9 ppm. The NMRShiftDB was used for processing data obtained (Fig. 1).

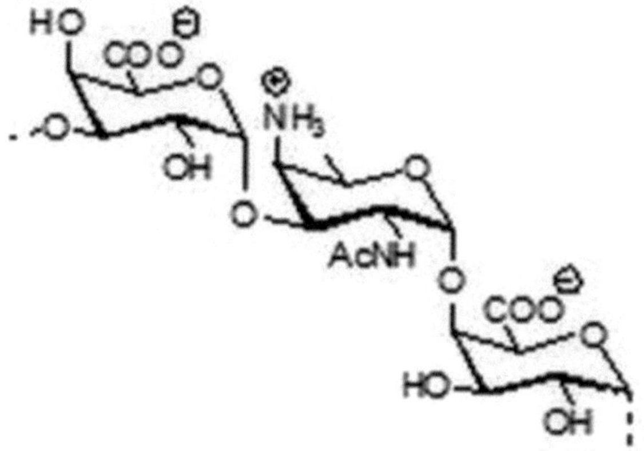

Fig. 1. The chemical structure of the zwitterionized polysaccharide (ZPS) of Streptococcus pneumoniae.

5.1.3 The strategy of conducting in vitro assays

The in vitro PBMC challenge with modified pneumo-23, the in vitro proliferation assay, the in vitro PBMC cytokine synthesis assay and the in vitro peripheral blood lymphocytes (PBL), part of PBMC, subsets markering assay were all conducted double blindly by two immunologists, the first from inside and the second from outside the research team. After finding that the results were minimally different between double blind runs of each assay, the final results were averaged. This strategy was necessary to keep the fidelity of the findings of the current study as this study is a pilot research on zwitterionized pneumo-23 vaccine and because some of the novel findings in this study need to be verified prudently in order to avoid causal or biased results.

5.1.4 Isolation of peripheral blood mononuclear cells

Isolation of PBMC from the heparinized whole blood of 65 CA and 100 HC subjects was conducted to prepare a population of cells containing T and B lymphocytes for the subsequent in vitro assays. PBMC separation was carried out in ultraviolet hood. The procedure was based on the gradient density sedimentation technique by using Ficoll hypaque (Sigma) (Wahlstorm et al., 2005). Cell viability was done; >99% of cells were found viable. Final concentration of the isolated PBMC suspension was adjusted to $1x10^6$ cells/mL.

5.1.5 PBMC challenge with modified pneumo-23 and concanavalin A

One hundred µl of $1x10^6$ cells/mL of PBMC suspension in complete RPMI–1640 medium (Merck, Germany) with 200 U/mL penicillin G (Sigma, USA), 200 µg/mL streptomycin (Merck, Germany), and 10% human AB serum (BDH, UK) were added to 96 wells microtiter plate in duplicates. Initially, cells were cultured for 1 day in a humid sterile incubator; then, 10 µl of 40ug/mL Concanavalin A (Con A) mitogen were added as positive control, 10 µl of 5 µg/mL diluted in PBS of modified pneumo-23 vaccine were added as test sample, and 10 µl of PBS alone were added as negative control. The used concentration of modified pneumo-23 vaccine, 5 µg/mL, was adjusted repeatedly after many standardization trials. PBMC in complete RPMI-1640 medium were incubated with modified pneumo-23, Con A, and PBS for 48 hours at 37 °C. Afterwards, PBMC were subjected to three in vitro assays; MTT assay to measure the proliferative potential of PBL, ELISA for in vitro synthesis of PBMC cytokines, IL-2, IFN-γ, and IL10, and PBL subset profiling namely, CD4, CD8, and CD21.

5.1.6 In vitro prolifertative assay

After 48 hours of PBMC incubation with Con A, modified penumo-23, and PBS, 40 µl of 3-[4,5,dimethylthiazol-2-yl]-2,5diphenyl tetrazolium bromide microculture, MTT, reagent (Sigma, USA) at 5 mg/mL were added to the microtiter plate and incubated for 4 hours at 37 °C. Finally, the supernatant was removed by Pasteur pipette and 100 µl of isopropanol was added. ELISA reader was used to measure the optical density (OD) at 540 nm Wigzell & Andersson, 1971). By using MTT assay, the proliferative activity of living PBMC exposed to mitogenic substances was measured (Shimoyama et al., 1989). The proliferative percentage of the challenged PBMC with Con A and zwitterionized penumo-23 was calculated in relation to the negative control, PBS, according to the below-mentioned equation (Kane e al., 1999):

Proliferative % of modified pneumo-23 = [absorbency of experimental wells "PBMC exposed to modified pneumo-23" / absorbency of negative control wells "PBMC exposed to PBS"] - 1 x 100

Proliferative % of the positive control (Con A) = [absorbency of positive control wells "PBMC exposed to Con A" / absorbency of negative control wells "PBMC exposed to PBS"] - 1 x 100.

5.1.7 ELISA for in vitro synthesis of PBMC cytokines

After 48 hours of PBMC incubation with modified penumo-23, Con A, and PBS, PBMC were centrifuged at 3000 g for 5 minutes and the supernatant was withdrawn separately. After a series of standardization steps, mouse monoclonal anti-human IL-2, IFN-γ, and IL-10 capturing antibodies (Dako, Denmark) were diluted 1:10 in carbonate-bicarbonate coating buffer (1.59g/L carbonate & 2.93 g/L bicarbonate) (Sigma, USA) at final concentration 0.1 mg/mL. Fifty µl/well of the diluted capturing antibodies in coating buffer were added and incubated overnight at 4 °C. Next day after washing step, 50 µl/well of the supernatant diluted 1:4 in blocking buffer, bovine serum albumin (Sigma, USA), were added in duplicates and the microtiter plate was incubated for 1 hour at 37 °C. Horseradish-peroxidase-labeled rabbit monoclonal anti-human IL-2, IFN-γ, and IL-10 antibodies (ICN immunologicals, UK) were diluted 1:100 in the antibody dilution buffer (ICN immunologicals, UK) at final concentration, 0.01, 0.005, and 0.0.005 mg/mL respectively. After a washing step, 50 µl/well of the diluted horseradish-peroxidase-labeled rabbit monoclonal anti-human IL-2, IFN-γ, and IL-10 antibodies were added and incubated for 1 hour at 37°C. The conjugated antibodies recognize different epitopes in IL-2, IFN-γ, and IL-10 from these recognized by the capturing antibodies. After washing step, 50 µl/well of OPD-H2O2 as chromogen-substrate (Sanofi diagnostics, France) were added for 20 minutes at 37 °C. For each run, duplicate wells of the negative control of the run were used by adding antibody dilution buffer alone instead of monoclonal antibodies. ELISA readings in terms of OD were measured at wavelength 492 nm (Schuurs & Weeman, 1977). A series of standards for IL-2, IFN-γ, and IL-10 (Sigma, USA) were used to obtain the linear regression analysis of the resulted standard curve. Moreover, the median value of the standard curve was considered as the positive control of the ELISA run. The achieved correlation coefficient of the standard curve was 0.81 which indicated a high linear behavior of the customized ELISA. The minimal detection limits for IL-2, IFN-γ, and IL-10 were 0.1, 0.08, and 0.1 ng/mL, respectively.

5.1.8 Immune phenotyping via direct immune fluorescence microscopy

For the Fixation of PBMC cells, after 48 hours of PBMC incubation with modified penumo-23, Con A, and PBS, PBMC were centrifuged at 3000 g for 5 minutes and the pellet was resuspended in PBS. Fifteen µl of $1x10^6$ cells/mL of PBMC suspension were added onto circular depressions of the immunofluorescence slides. Slides were allowed to dry up for about 1 to 2 hours. Fifteen µl of fixative solution, which is buffered formal acetone (BFA) composed of 5.7% v/v PBS, 24% v/v 40 % formalin, and 43% v/v acetone from (Merck, Germany), were added per depression to cover all the dried lymphocytes and stored at -20 0C for later use Taylor et al., 1970).

For the Fluorescent microscopy, 15 µl of immunofluorescence-labeled monoclonal antibodies, namely anti-CD4, anti-CD8 and anti-CD21 (Dako, Denmark) diluted 1:5 in antibody dilution buffer (Dako, Denmark) at final concentrations 0.1, 0.1, and 0.05 mg/mL respectively. These antibodies were added onto slide depressions in duplicates for 1 hour at 37 °C with mild shaking. After dipping and stirring slides in PBS-filled jar for 10 minutes, 1-2 drops of mounting fluid were added. After adding cover slips, examination of slides was conducted under immunofluorescent microscope at 40X and 100X. At light microscopy phase, a suitable countable field was chosen to count the total number of lymphocytes. At UV light phase, the fluorescently stained cells were only counted. The average percentage of the fluorescently stained cells was calculated from the total PBL cells in 5 high power fields multiplied by 100 (Ben Trividi et al., 1990).

5.1.9 Statistical analysis

The statistical analysis was preformed using software SPSS version 10 and MS Excel 2000. Kolmogorov-Semirnov tests were used for confirming the normal distribution pattern of MTT, ELISA, and immunofluorescent CD marketing values. Therefore, mean ±SEM of the averaged values as well as parametric multivariate student t-tests were used to evaluate the significance of differences. P value <0.05 was considered significant.

5.2 Results

5.2.1 The confirmation of the immunosuppression status of cancer patients

As part of the research plan, the immunosuppression status of the involved CA patients, who were already shown as immunosuppressed at the clinical and laboratory hospital tests, was confirmed. All of the selected immunosuppressed CA patients showed significantly lower prolifertative rates of PBMC, lower IL-2 and IFN-γ concentrations, and lower CD4+, CD8+, and CD21+ cells percentages than in HC ($P<0.05$). These comparisons are clarified as dashed lines between the negative control group of HC to that of CA (Fig. 2- A&B, Fig. 4-A&B, and Fig. 5-A&B).

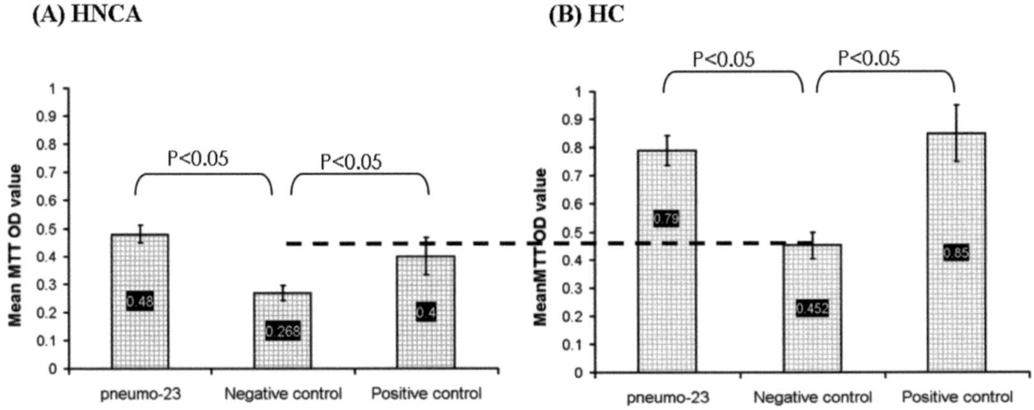

Fig. 2. Mean MTT OD values for negative control (PBS), zwitterionized pneumo-23 vaccine, and positive control (Con A) groups in both (A) CA patients and (B) healthy control subjects (HC). This histogram shows that pneumo-23 induces remarkable PBMC proliferation in immunosuppressed CA and immunocompetent HC subjects. The dashed line depicts the confirmed status of immune suppression represented by the significantly lower proliferation of un-stimulated PBMC, negative control, of CA patients than that of HC.

5.2.2 The in vitro proliferative assay

In this study, two groups were involved, CA and HC group. Each group was subdivided into three categories; test group where PBMC exposed to modified pneumo-23 vaccine, negative control group where PBMC cells exposed to PBS, and positive control group where PBMC exposed to Con A. It was found that the modified, zwitterionized, pneumo-23 vaccine exerted remarkable stimulatory effect on PBMC proliferation of immunosuppressed CA patients in that the mean MTT OD value of modified pneumo-23 group in CA, 0.48±0.033, and in HC, 0.79±0.053, were higher than in the negative control of CA, 0.268±0.027, and of HC, 0.452±0.048 respectively ($P<0.05$) (Fig. 2-A and 2-B). Moreover, the mean MTT readings for PBMC exposed to modified pneumo-23 vaccine were close to that of Con A in HC, 0.85±0.1, and borderline higher than Con A in CA, 0.4±0.068 ($P>0.05$) (Fig. 2-A and B). Nevertheless, by using the calculated proliferative percentage of MTT, a significant difference was clear and evident between the proliferative percentage of modified pneumo-23 and that of Con A in immunosuppressed CA patients. The mean proliferative percentage of PBMC of CA patients exposed to modified pneumo-23, 81%,±7.6, was significantly higher than that exposed to Con A, 51%±8.9, (P<0.05) while in HC group, both con A, 89%±9.6, and penum-23, 75%±8.4, were close to each other (P>0.05) (Fig. 3). In other words, the zwitterionized pneumo-23, unlike the unmodified penumo-23 [data not shown], induced efficiently a remarkable proliferation in both immunosuppressed and immunocompetent groups while Con A induced proliferation efficiently only in immunocompetent group rather than the immunosuppressed group (Figure 2). Moreover, there was no differences in the modified pneumo-23 or Con A -driven proliferation in PBMC of CA patients in respect cancer type, age, or sex of patients (P>0.05).

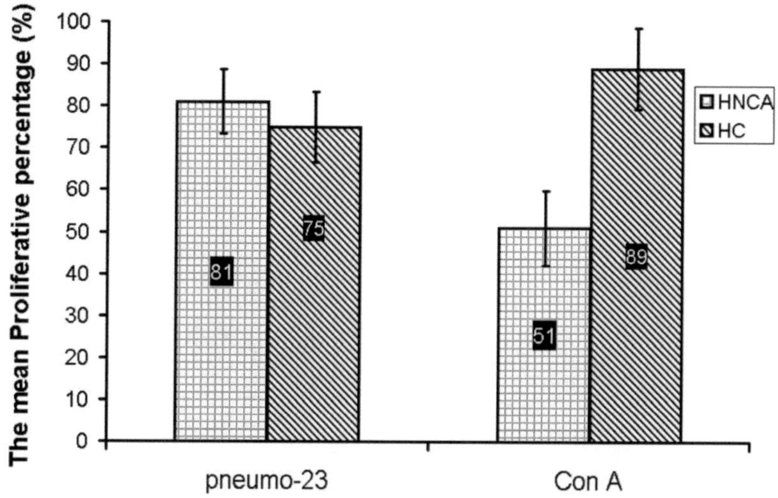

Fig. 3. The calculated proliferative percentage of PBMC in immunosuppressed CA and immunocompetent HC groups in response to zwitterionized pneumo-23 vaccine and Con A measured by MTT assay. The proliferative percentage of PBMC exposed to zwitterionized penumo-23 was closely high in both CA and HC groups (P>0.05) while Con A induced much higher PBMC proliferation in HC than in CA group (P<0.05).

5.2.3 The in vitro synthesis of cytokines

ELISA for in vitro synthesis of cytokines was conducted on PBMC of both CA and HC groups that each was subdivided into three groups; test group, negative control, and positive control where PBMC were exposed to modified pneumo-23, PBS, and Con A respectively, for 48 hours. In CA group, it was found that the mean synthesis of soluble IL-2, 0.61±0.063 ng/mL, and IFN-γ, 0.45±0.052 ng/mL, in PBMC exposed to modified pneumo-23 was much higher than that exposed to PBS, 0.41±0.03 and 0.29±0.051 ng/mL respectively and that exposed to Con A, 0.45±0.028 and 0.42±0.03 ng/mL respectively (P<0.05) (Fig. 4-A) while the mean synthesis of soluble IL-10, 0.36±0.042 ng/mL exposed to modified pneumo-23 was not different from that exposed to PBS and Con A, 0.4±0.041 and 0.42±0.027 ng/mL respectively (P>0.05) (Fig. 4-A).

On the other hand, in HC group, no similar upsurge was found in the mean synthesis of IL-2, 0.67±0.061 ng/mL in PBMC exposed to modified neumo-23 when compared to the negative control, 0.62±0.034 ng/mL (P>0.05) and, on contrary to CA, it was lower than in PBMC exposed to Con A, 0.82±0.042 ng/mL (P<0.05) (Fig. 4-B). Regarding IFN-γ and IL-10, they were close to each other with borderline higher levels of IFN-γ and IL-10 in PBMC exposed to modified pneumo-23, 0.52±0.031 and 0.41±0.03 ng/mL respectively than in PBMC exposed to PBS, 0.45±0.034 and0.37±0.052 ng/mL respectively and PBMC exposed to Con A, 0.47±0.042 and 0.36±0.017 ng/mL respectively (P ranged 0.051 to 0.048). (Fig. 4-B). In addition, there was no significant differences in the pneomo-23 and Con A -driven synthesis of IL-2, IFN-γ, and IL-10 in PBMC of the CA patients in respect to cancer type, age, and sex (P>0.05). These results collectively indicated that zwitterionized pneumo-23 exerted a unique potent cytokine stimulatory effect, IL-2 and IFN-γ, on PBMC of immunosuppressed cancer patients while a powerful mitogenic substance, Con A, exerted a mild cytokine stimulatory effect, IL-2, on immunocompetent healthy group only.

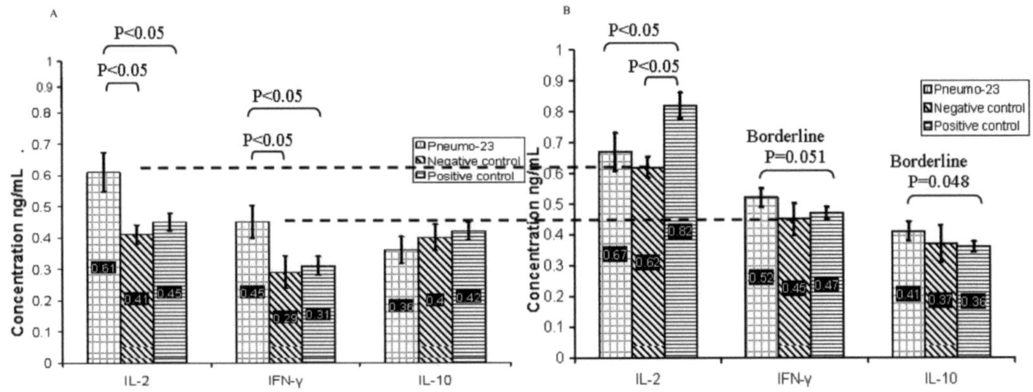

Fig. 4. (A) the concentrations of in vitro synthesis of IL-2 and IFN-γ but not IL-10 in CA PBMC exposed to zwitterionized pneumo-23 was higher than in PBMC of the negative control, PBS, and the positive control, Con A. (B) The concentration of IL-2 in HC PBMC exposed to Con A was higher than in PBMC exposed to zwitterionized penumo-23 whereas borderline higher IFN-γ and IL-10 synthesis is seen by HC PBMC exposed to zwitterionized penumo-23 than by PBMC exposed to Con A. The dashed line depicts the confirmed status of immune suppression represented by the significantly lower synthesis of IL-2 and IFN-γ by PBMC of the CA patients than that of negative control group of HC.

5.2.4 The immune phenotyping of lymphocytes subsets

The immune phenotyping of PBL exposed to modified pneumo-23, PBS, and Con A was investigated. Although the percentages of CD4+, CD8+, and CD21+ cells in CA group were lower than in HC group, these percentages were within the lowest tier of normal ranges, 30-60% for CD4+, 20-50% for CD8+ cells, and 4-14% for CD21 [14]. IN CA, the mean percentage of CD8+, CD4+, and CD21+ cells in modified pneumo-23 group, 39.3±4.7, 42.7±3.2, and 8.1±2.1% respectively, was higher than in PBS group, 25.6±3.1, 31.9±4.1, and 4.2±1.7% respectively, (P<0.05) and in Con A group, 27.2±2.8, 35.8±3.6, and 4.1±0.8 respectively (P<0.05) (Fig. 5-A) while no significant difference found between con A and PBS groups regarding the mean percentage of CD8+, CD4+, and CD21+ cells (P>0.05).

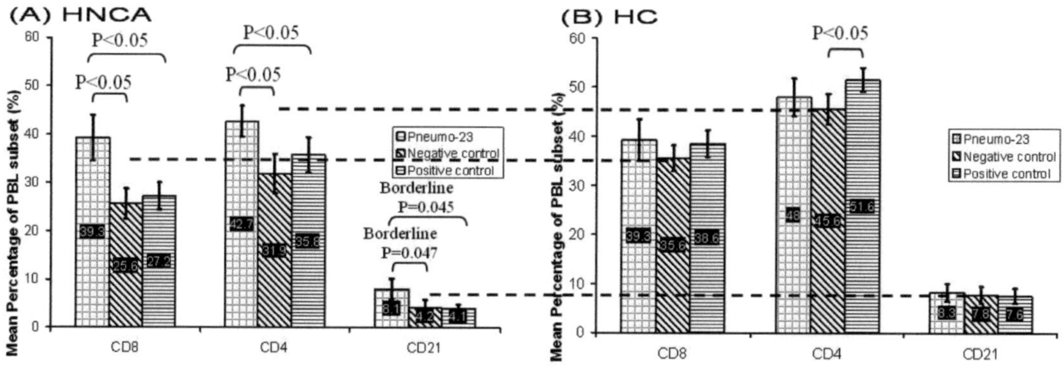

Fig. 5. (A) The mean percentage of CD8+, CD4+ and CD21+ cells was higher in CA PBMC exposed to zwitterionized penumo-23 than both these exposed to PBS or Con A. (B) CD4+ cells was higher in HC PBMC exposed to Con A than these exposed to PBS but not zwitterionized pneumo-23. The dashed lines depicts the confirmed status of immune suppression represented by the significantly higher percentages of CD8+, CD4+, and CD21+ cells in PBMC of the negative control group of HC than that of CA patients.

On the other hand, there was no significant difference in the percentage of CD8+, CD4+, and CD21+ cells in HC PBL exposed to modified pneumo-23, 39.3±4.2, 48±5.8 and 8.3±2.2% respectively, when compared to cells exposed to PBS, 35.6±2.6, 45.6±3.8, and 7.8±2.4% respectively (P>0.05) (Fig. 5-B). However, Con A was shown to increase the percentage of CD4+ cells, 51.6±2.4 more than PBS group (P<0.05) and pneumo-23 (P>0.05) (Fig. 5-B). In addition, there was no significant differences in the percentage of CD4+, CD8+, and CD21+ cells in PBMC exposed to modified pneumo-23 or Con A in respect to cancer type, age, or sex of CA patients (P>0.05).

5.3 Discussion

The immunostimulatory effect of the zwitterionized pneumo-23 was tested on PBMC of immunosuppressed CA patients in comparison with HC group regarding the in vitro proliferative potential, the in vitro cytokine synthesis, IL2, IFN-γ, and IL-10, and immune phenotyping, CD4+ as T helper cells, CD8+ as T cytotoxic/suppressor cells (Kalinski et al., 2006; Knustion & Disis, 2005), and CD21+ as B cells (Knustion & Disis, 2005) by using the accurate and simple microculture tetrazolium (MTT) assay for the in vitro prolifertative assay (Ben Trivdei et al., 1990; Iwatsuki et al., 2004), ELISA for in vitro cytokines synthesis, and direct immunofluoresecence microcopy for immune phenotyping assays.

Unlike the commercial pneumo-23 vaccine [data not shown], the chemically modified pneumo-23 vaccine, in a unique manner, augmented the proliferative potential of PBMC in both immunosuppressed, CA, and immunocompetent, HC, groups, inducing remarkable in vitro synthesis of PBMC soluble IL-2 and IFN-γ but not IL-10 in CA versus just borderline increase in IFN-γ and IL-10 in HC group, and augmented the proliferation of CD8+, CD4+, and CD21+ PBL selectively in CA rather than HC group. On contrary, the positive control, Con A, induced PBMC proliferation, increased in vitro synthesis of IL-2, but not IL-10 or

IFN-γ, and increased CD4+, but not CD8+ or CD21+ cells, in immunocompetent, HC, rather than immunosuppressed, CA group.

Unfortunately, no previous report was found utilizing zwitterionized pneumococcal PSs as enhanced immunogenic vaccine or as immunostimulatory agent to compare with. Nevertheless, the findings of the current research showed that the zwitterionized pneumo 23 exerted a highly remarkable in vitro T cell dependent and/or mitogenic triggering of a robust immune response in just 48 hours of exposure. Moreover, in unexplained manner, the immunosuppression status, interestingly, did not hinder the zwitterionized pneumo-23, unlike Con A, to stimulate immune cells proliferation, cytokines synthesis, and PBL subsets proliferation and expansion. Con A, a powerful mitogenic substance, failed in triggering an efficient immune stimulation in immunosuppressed PBMC like that seen in immunocompetent PBMC. Therefore, the immune triggering pathway of the zwitterionized pneumo-23 might be unique.

Collectively, the zwitterionized pneumo-23 vaccine was shown to act as a normalizing immunostimulatory agent for the immunosuppressed cells. In other words, it served to revert the suppressed 'lazy' immune cells back to normal 'alert' status while it did not stimulate much the already competent 'alert' immune cells. The findings of the current study might explain how the commercial pneumo-23 showed some signs of immune stimulation, which is most likely due to the presence of small fraction of natural zwitterionic type 1 PSs (Gallorini et al., 2007). Beside the report of the manufacturing company on the immunostimulatory effect of pneumo-23, there was a report supports the findings of the current research which showed that the protection of pneumo-23 vaccine after splenectomy was perfect against the sepsis of many bacteria other than pneumococci (Uslu et a., 2006). This suggests strongly the presence of non-specific immune stimulation, which was augmented and shown in the current study after the zwitterionisation of the commercial pneumo-23 vaccine

The modified pneumo-23 vaccine was shown to stimulate the cell-mediated immunity (CMI) more than the humeral arm of immune response as it induced CD8+ and CD4+ cells far higher than CD21+ cells. These findings might render zwitterionized pneumo-23 vaccine as a practicable choice for stimulating the suppressed CMI in attempts to augment immunity against diseases. The current study also showed that the immune stimulation of zwitterionized pneumo-23 vaccine in CA patients was attributed partially to the synthesis of IL-2 and IFN- γ, T helper 1 cytokines, rather than IL-10, T helper 2 cytokine, as well as stimulating vigorously CD8+ T cells. Collectively, this provided evidence that the zwitterionized pneumo-23 stimulate T-helper 1 profile of CMI. This might be supported indirectly by other studies which stated that the atopic bronchial asthma children, from a past case of outhospital pneumonia, which were given pneumo-23 vaccine showed tendency towards decreased level of serum IgE (Markelova et al., 2005; Ryzhov et al., 2005). This was either due to complete eradication of the chronic infection of pneumococcal bacteria and/or the deviation of the immune system towards T-helper one which counteracts the T-helper two atopic arm of immunity (Markelova et al., 2005; Ryzhov et al., 2005). Moreover, the nature of the remarkably increased CD8+ cells in response to the modified pneumo-23 was more likely cytotoxic rather than suppressive CD8+ cells because the enhanced prolifertative rate of PBMC, the in vitro high level of synthesis of IL-2 and IFN-γ, and the high rates of CD4+ and CD21+ cells in PBMC exposed to modified penumo-23 contradict strongly the possibility of the suppressive nature of CD8+ cells. Accordingly, zwitterionized pneumo-23 more likely augments the cytotoxic arm of CMI which is essential against most of viral infections and tumor diseases.

A question might be presented, whether the zwitterionized penumo-23 is an immunostimulatory agent or it is just an antigen that induced immune reaction. The findings of the current study showed that pneumo-23 mostly acts as potent immunostimulator as well as an effective T cell-dependent antigen rather than just an antigen. The findings supporting the immunostimulatory action of pneumo-23 are: first, peumo-23 induced consistent upsurge in PBMC proliferation, IL-2 and IFN-γ synthesis, and CD 4+, CD8+, and CD21+ cells in immunosuppressed CA patients more than immune competent HC group which is exactly the contrary to what should happen in the antigenic stimulation. Second, the magnitude of increase in PBMC proliferation, cytokines synthesis and expansion percentage of PBL subsets in just 48 hours favors the immunostimulatory effect in addition to antigenic effect.

The mechanism of the observed immunostimulatory action of zwitterionized pneumo-23 vaccine has not yet been understood. It could be a combination of T cell-dependent antigen triggering pathway via T cell receptor (TCR), a non-specific mitogenic signal through bridging of multiple costimulatory receptors, or acting as a ligand on Toll-like receptors (TLR). A recent study revealed that TLR2 engagement in T-regulatory cells and other T-cell subsets with zwitterionic motifs of PS modifies functionality and activation state of these cells and the most effects induced by natural and chemically derived zwitterionized PS may be explained by their TLR2 agonist properties on T cells Wack & Gallorini, 2008). Regardless the previous study conclusions, the immunostimulatory effect of zwitterionized pneumo-23 vaccine needs further studies designed specifically for investigating the mechanism and pathways of its immunostimulatory effect in vivo using experimental animals to explore why it is more evident in immunosuppressed rather than immunocompetent subjects. And to explore its effects on natural killer cells, antigen presenting cells, TLR, other cytokines, and other CD markers. Moreover, a long-term prospective study might be needed to evaluate the in vivo immunostimulatory effect of pneumo-23 vaccine on laboratory animals and later, after proving its safety, on human beings.

Taken together, the zwitterionized, but not the commercial, pneumo-23 vaccine appeared to exert a remarkable in vitro immunostimulatory effect on the isolated PBMC of immunosuppressed cancer patients more than the immune competent individuals. In addition, it drives the immunity towards T-helper one profile and triggers largely CD8+ cells. Basing on the findings of the current study, it seems that the zwitterionized PSs exert a unique immunostimulatory pathway that tends to correct the immune suppression status of CA patients' immune cells to normal levels while such normalizing effect was not observed in the immunocompetent healthy subjects. Therefore, zwitterionized PSs, such as pneumo-23, can be developed, after securing its safety in humans, as a potent immunostimulatory drug for cancer immunosuppressed patients.

6. Conclusion

Zwitterionization can be one of the most recent approaches for immuno- stimulating /modulating the immune system of cancer patients. The process of zwitterionization is a cheap, simple, and fast; it is a chemical procedure by which natural, non-immunostimulating and non-immunomodulating polysaccharides are converted to universal TCR-based immunostimulator and immunomodulators. ZPSs are found to be useful in correcting the immune suppression and immune deviation in incompetent immune systems in cancer patients. Patients with cancer might be immunosuppressed due to disease itself or due to cancer chemotherapy. In both cases, correction of the immune system of cancer patients is necessary taken into account that fatality in cancer patients due to infections is very high. In addition, immune suppression itself can be considered one of the serious causes for the development of some tumors because of the loss of immune surveillance exerted by immune system which daily scavenges any cancerous neoplastic cells. In addition, ZPSs can be used as adjuvant elements along with other modalities of cancer immunotherapy to overcome the long achieved failures in this field. It is well known that most cases of failures in cancer immunotherapy are attributed to the ability of cancerous cells to escape immune defense mechanisms as well as immunotherapy approaches used. In this instance, ZPSs can change the fate of cancer immunotherapy to a more optimistic modality of therapy. One of the essential conclusions incurred from the use of ZPSs in cancer patients is that ZPSs exert immunostimulatory action on cancerous cells much more remarkably than on non-cancerous cells. The mechanism underlying this is still unknown; however, this implies to a very important phenomenon which might be highly useful in combating immune evasive nature of cancerous cells without affecting other normal cells.

7. Acknowledgments

Appreciation goes to UPM for supporting this chapter and financing the model study of zwitterionization process. In addition, we would like to acknowledge the important role played by oncology specialists and patients for achieving this research.

8. References

Baumann, H., Tzianabos, A. O., Brisson, J.-R., Kasper, D. L., Jennings, H. J. (1992). Structural elucidation of two capsular polysaccharides from one strain of Bacteroides fragilis using high-resolution NMR spectroscopy, *Biochemistry*, vol. 31, No.16, pp. 4081–4089.

Ben Trivedi, A., Kitabatake, N., Doi, E. (1990). Toxicity of dimethyl sulfoxide as a solvent in bioassay system with HeLa cells evaluated colorimetrically with 3-(4,5-dimethylthiazol-2-yl)-2,5-diphenyl-tetrazolium bromide. *Agricultural Biology & Chemistry*, Vol. 54, No. 3, pp. 2961-2966.

Chung, D.R., Kasper, D.L., Panzo, R.J., Chitnis, T., Grusby, M.J., Sayegh, M.H., Tzianabos, A.O., (2003). CD4+ T cells mediate abscess formation in intra-abdominal sepsis by an IL-17-dependent mechanism. J Immunol, Vol. 170, No. 4, pp. 1958-1963.

Cobb, B. A., Kasper, D. L. (2005). Zwitterionic capsular polysaccharides: the new MHCII-dependent antigens. *Cell Microbiology*, Vol. 7, N0.5, pp. 1398-1403.

Coyne, M. J., Kalka-Moll, W., Tzianabos, A. O., Kasper, D. L., Comstock, L. E. (2000). Bacteroides fragilis NCTC9343 produces at least three distinct capsular polysaccharides: cloning, characterization, and reassignment of polysaccharide B and C biosynthesis loci, *Infection and Immunity*, Vol. 68, No. 11, pp. 6176–6181.

D'Ambrosio, D., Cantrell, D. A., Frat, L., Santoni, A., Testi, R. (1994). Involvement of p21(ras) activation in T cell CD69 expression, *European Journal of Immunology*, Vol. 24, No. 3, pp. 616–620.

de Greeff, S. C., Sanders, E. A., de Melker, H. E., van der Ende, A., Vermeer, P. E., Schouls, L. M. (2007). Two pneumococcal vaccines: the 7-valent conjugate vaccine (Prevenar) for children up to the age of 5 years and the 23-valent polysaccharide vaccine (Pneumo 23) for the elderly and specific groups at risk. *Ned Tijdschr Geneeskd*, Vol. 151, No. 9, pp. 1454-1457.

Gallorini, S., Berti, F., Mancuso, G., Cozzi, R., Tortoli, M., Volpini, G., Telford, J.L., Beninati, C., Maione, D., Wack, A., (2009). Toll-like receptor 2 dependent immunogenicity of glycoconjugate vaccines containing chemically derived zwitterionic polysaccharides. Proc Natl Acad Sci U S A, Vol. 106, No. 41, pp. 17481-17486, 1091-6490.

Gallorini, S., Berti, F., Parente, P., Baronio, R., Aprea, S., D'Oro, U., Pizza, M., Telford, J. L., Wack, A. (2007). Introduction of zwitterionic motifs into bacterial polysaccharides generates TLR2 agonists able to activate APCs. *Journal of Immunology*, Vol. 179, No. 8, pp. 8208-8215.

Groneck, L., Schrama, D., Fabri, M., Stephen, T.L., Harms, F., Meemboor, S., Hafke, H., Bessler, M., Becker, J.C., Kalka-Moll, W.M., (2009). Oligoclonal CD4+ T cells promote host memory immune responses to Zwitterionic polysaccharide of Streptococcus pneumoniae. Infect Immun, Vol. 77, No. 9, pp. 3705-3712.

Iwatsuki, K., Yamamoto, T., Tsuji, K., Suzuki, D., Fuji, K., Matsuura, H., Oono, T. A. (2004). Spectrum of clinical manifestations caused by host immune responses against Epstein-Barr virus infections. *Acta Medical Okayama*. Vol. 58, pp. 169-180.

Kalinski, P., Nakamura, Y., Watchmaker, P., Giermasz, A., Muthuswamy, R., Mailliard, R. B. (2006). Helper roles of NK and CD8+ T cells in the induction of tumor immunity. Polarized dendritic cells as cancer vaccines. *Immunological Research*, Vol. 36, No. 8, pp. 137-146.

Kalka-Moll, W. M., Wang, Y., Comstock, L. E., Gonzalez, S. E., Tzianabos, A. O., Kasper, D. L. (2001). Immunochemical and biological characterization of three capsular polysaccharides from a single Bacteroides fragilis strain, *Infection and Immunity*, Vol. 69, No. 4, pp. 2339–2344.

Kalka-Moll, W.M., Tzianabos, A.O., Bryant, P.W., Niemeyer, M., Ploegh, H.L., Kasper, D.L., (2002). Zwitterionic polysaccharides stimulate T cells by MHC class II-dependent interactions. J Immunol, Vol. 169, No. 11, pp. 6149-6153.

Kane, M. D., Schwarz, R. D., St Pierre, L., Watson, M. D., Emmerling, M. R., Boxer, P. A., Walker, G. K. (1999). Inhibitors of V-type ATPases, bafilomycin A1 and concanamycin A, protect against beta-amyloid-mediated effects on 3-(4,5-dimethylthiazol-2-yl)-2,5-diphenyltetrazolium bromide (MTT) reduction. *Journal of Neurochemistry*, Vol. 72, No. 5, pp. 1939-1947.

Kazancioglu, R., Sever, M. S., Yuksel-Onel, D., Eraksoy, H., Yildiz, A., Celik, A. V., Kayacan, S. M., Badur, S. (2000). Immunization of renal transplant recipients with pneumococcal polysaccharide vaccine. *Clinical Transplantation,* Vol. 14, N0.10, pp. 61-5.

Knutson, K. L., Disis, M. L. (2005). Tumor antigen-specific T helper cells in cancer immunity and immunotherapy. *Cancer Immunology & Immunotherapy.* Vol. 54, No. 6, pp. 721-728.

Markelova, E. V., Gushchina, S., Kostinov, M. P., Zhuravleva, N. V. (2005). [Clinical and immunological effect produced by vaccination with "Pneumo 23" of children with atopic bronchial asthma]. *Zh Mikrobiology Epidemiology & Immunobiology,* Vol. 4, No. 2, pp. 83-85.

Mazmanian, S. K., Cui, H. L., Tzianabos, A. O., Kasper, D. L. (2005). An immunomodulatory molecule of symbiotic bacteria directs maturation of the host immune system, *Cell,* Vol. 122, No. 1, pp. 107–118.

Pasteur Merieux Connaught. (2004). Immunodefficiency In:.*Vaccine against pneumococcal infection,* pp. 12-14.

Peetermans, W. E., Van de Vyver, N., Van Laethem, Y., Van Damme, P., Thiry, N., Trefois, P., Geerts, P., Schetgen, M., Peleman, R., Swennen, B., Verhaegen, J. (2005). Recommendations for the use of the 23-valent polysaccharide pneumococcal vaccine in adults: a Belgian consensus report. *Acta Clinica Belgica,* Vol. 60, No.11, pp. 329-337.

Richard, J. P., Amyes, T. L. (2004). On the importance of being zwitterionic: enzymatic catalysis of decarboxylation and deprotonation of cationic carbon. *Bioorganic Chemistry,* Vol. 32, No. 3, pp. 354-66.

Rybachenko, V. V., Sementsov, V. K., Manuilov, V. M., Zabolotnyi, S. P. (2009). [About the results of using vaccine "Pneumo-23" in Northern fleet]. *Voen Med Zh,* Vol. 330, No. 2, pp. 11-3.

Ryzhov, A. A., Katosova, L. K., Kostinov, M. P., Volkov, I. K., Magarshak, O. O. (2005). [Evaluation of the influence of the bacterial vaccines Pneumo-23 and Act-HIB on the course of the chronic inflammatory process of the respiratory organs in children]. *Zh. Mikrobiology Epidemiology & Immunobiology,* Vol. 3, No. 4, pp. 84-87.

Schuurs, A., Weeman, V. (1977). Enzyme innunoassay. *Clinica Chimica Acta,* Vol. 31, pp. 1-12.

Shapiro, M.E., Kasper, D.L., Zaleznik, D.F., Spriggs, S., Onderdonk, A.B., Finberg, R.W., (1986). Cellular control of abscess formation: role of T cells in the regulation of abscesses formed in response to Bacteroides fragilis. J Immunol, Vol. 137, No. 1, pp. 341-346.

Shimoyama, Y., Kubota, T., Watanabe, M., Ishibiki, K., Abe, O. (1989). Predictability of in vivo chemosensitivity by in vitro MTT assay with reference to the clonogenic assay. *Journal of Surgical Oncology,* Vol. 41, No. 7, pp. 12-18.

Stephen, T.L., Groneck, L., Kalka-Moll, W.M., (2010). The modulation of adaptive immune responses by bacterial zwitterionic polysaccharides. Int J Microbiol, Vol. 2010, No. pp. 917075, 1687-9198.

Stephen, T.L., Niemeyer, M., Tzianabos, A.O., Kroenke, M., Kasper, D.L., Kalka-Moll, W.M., (2005). Effect of B7-2 and CD40 signals from activated antigen-presenting cells on the ability of zwitterionic polysaccharides to induce T-Cell stimulation. Infect Immun, Vol. 73, No. 4, pp. 2184-2189.

Stingele, F., Corthesy, B., Kusy, N., Porcelli, S.A., Kasper, D.L., Tzianabos, A.O., (2004). Zwitterionic polysaccharides stimulate T cells with no preferential V beta usage and promote anergy, resulting in protection against experimental abscess formation. J Immunol, Vol. 172, No. 3, pp. 1483-1490.

Sumitani, M., Tochino, Y., Kamimori, T., Fujiwara, H., Fujikawa, T. (2008). Additive inoculation of influenza vaccine and 23-valent pneumococcal polysaccharide vaccine to prevent lower respiratory tract infections in chronic respiratory disease patients. *Internal Medicine,* Vol. 47, No.5, pp. 1189-1197.

Taylor, R. B., Duffusm P. H., Raffm M. C., De petrism S. (1970). Redistribution and pinocytosis of lymphocyte surface immunoglobulin molecules induced by anti-immunoglobulin. *iNa New Biol.* Vol. 12, No. 12, pp. 225-29.

Tzianabos, A. O., Finberg, R. W., Wang, Y. (2000). T cells activated by zwitterionic molecules prevent abscesses induced by pathogenic bacteria, *Journal of Biological Chemistry,* Vol. 275, No. 10, pp. 6733–6740.

Tzianabos, A. O., Pantosti, A., Baumann, H., Brisson, J.-R., Jennings, H. J., Kasper, D. L. (1992). The capsular polysaccharide of Bacteroides fragilis comprises two ionically linked polysaccharides, *Journal of Biological Chemistry,* Vol. 267, No. 25, pp.18230–18235.

Uslu, A., Yetis, H., Aykas, A., Karagoz, A., Dogan, M., Simsek, C., Nart, A., Yuzbasioglu, M. F. (2006). The efficacy and immunogenicity of Pneumo-23 and ACT-HIB in patients undergoing splenectomy. *Ulus Travma Acil Cerrahi Derg.* Vol. 12, No. 3, pp. 277-281.

Valenzuela, M. T., Altuzarra, R. H., Trucco, O. A., Villegas, R. R., Inostroza, J. S., Granata, P. S., Fleiderman, J. V., Maggi, L. C. (2007). Immunogenicity of a 23-valent pneumococcal polysaccharide vaccine in elderly residents of a long-term care facility. *Brazilian Journal of Infectious Diseases,* Vol. 11, No.5, pp. 322-326.

van der Harst S. (2007). [Two pneumococcal vaccines: the 7-valent conjugate vaccine (Prevenar) for children up to the age of 5 years and the 23-valent polysaccharide vaccine (Pneumo 23) for the elderly and specific groups at risk]. *Ned Tijdschr Geneeskd,* Vol. 151, No. 6, pp. 1853-1854.

Wack, A., Gallorini, S. (2008). Bacterial polysaccharides with zwitterionic charge motifs: toll-like receptor 2 agonists,t cell antigens, or both? *Immunopharmacology & Immunotoxicology.* Vol. 30, No. 10, pp. 761-770.

Wahlstrom, J., Berlin, M., Skold, C. M., Wigzell, H., Eklund, A., Grunewald, J. (1999). Phenotypic analysis of lymphocytes and monocytes/macrophages in peripheral blood and bronchoalveolar lavage fluid from patients with pulmonary sarcoidosis. *Thorax,* Vol. 54, No. 12, pp. 339-346.

Wang, Y., Kalka-Moll, W. M., Roehrl, M. H., Kasper, D. L. (2000). Structural basis of the abscess-modulating polysaccharide A2 from Bacteroides fragilis, *Proceedings of the National Academy of Sciences of the United States of America,* Vol. 97, No. 25, pp. 13478–13483.

Whiteside, T. L. (2006). Immune suppression in cancer: effects on immune cells, mechanisms and future therapeutic intervention. *Seminars in Cancer Biology,* Vol. 16, pp. 3-15.

Wigzell, H. (1971). Andersson, B. Isolation of lymphoid cells with active surface receptor sites. *Annual Reviews in Microbiology,* Vol. 25, No.10, pp. 291-308.

9

Type III Interferons IL-28 and IL-29: Novel Interferon Family Members with Therapeutic Potential in Cancer Therapy

Hitomi Fujie and Muneo Numasaki
Department of Nutrition Physiology, Pharmaceutical Sciences, Josai University, Sakado, Saitama, Japan

1. Introduction

Type I interferons (IFNs), namely IFN-α/ß, were originally discovered due to its powerful antiviral activity [1, 2]. Type I IFNs were later shown to have pleiotropic biological activities, including modulation of innate and acquired immune responses, cell growth and apoptosis, in addition to their well-known ability to inhibit virus replication [3]. Type I IFN forms a vast multigenic family [4]. The human genome carries the intronless genes encoding 13 functionally and structurally related IFN-α subtypes and a single IFN-ß molecule [5]. In addition, it contains genes encoding for IFN-κ [6], IFN-ε/τ [7], and IFN-ω [8]. In spite of this remarkable variability, all type I IFN subtypes appear to bind the same heterodimeric receptor [4].

Type I IFNs have been used for the clinical treatment of several malignancies including renal cell carcinoma, melanoma, Kaposi's sarcoma, hairy cell leukemia and chronic myeloid leukemia. For a long time, it was thought that the direct actions on tumor cells were the major mechanisms involved in the antitumor responses observed in type I IFN-treated patients [9]. Actually, type I IFNs are able to directly inhibit the proliferation of tumor cells *in vitro* and *in vivo*, and exert other direct effects on tumor cells including induction of apoptosis and enhancement of major histocompatibility complex (MHC) class I expression, which can enhance immune recognition [10]. In addition to the direct effects on tumor cells, type I IFNs exert multiple biological effects on host immune cells, especially T cells and dendritic cells, that can play a central role in the overall antitumor responses [11].

Type III IFNs, also termed IFN-λs, were discovered independently by 2 different research groups in 2003 [12, 13]. The type III IFN family consists of IFN-λ1, IFN-λ2 and IFN-λ3, also referred to as interleukin (IL)-29, IL-28A and IL-28B, respectively. On the basis of sequence and protein structure, type III IFNs are more similar to the IL-10 family of cytokines, but the deciding factor that led to the classification of IL-29, IL-28A and IL-28B as IFNs was their antiviral function and induction of IFN-stimulated genes (ISGs) [12, 13]. In humans, among these molecules, only IL-29 is glycosylated [12, 13]. In the mouse system, the IL-29 gene is a pseudogene. The IL-28A and IL-28B genes encode glycosylated protein [14].

Type III IFN expression has been shown to depend on the same triggers (viral infection or Toll-like receptor (TLR) ligands) [12, 13, 15, 16, 17, 18, 19, 20] and signal transduction pathway as those inducing type I IFN expression. Type I IFNs and type III IFNs bind distinct heterodimeric receptors [12, 13]. The type I IFN receptor is made of the ubiquitously expressed IFN-αRα and IFN-αRß subunits [21]. The type III IFN receptor is comprised of the IL-10Rß subunit which is widely expressed and shared by other IL-10-related cytokines, and of the IL-28R subunit, which is specific to type III IFN and responsible for signal transduction [12, 13, 21]. While the receptor subunits of type III IFNs display no detectable homology to those of type I IFNs, they elicit strikingly similar intracellular responses, mostly through the activation of several latent transcriptional factors of the signal transducer and activator of transcription (STAT) family including STAT1, STAT2, STAT3, STAT4 and STAT5 [12, 22, 23]. In particular, type III IFN receptor engagement leads to the phosphorylation of STAT1 and STAT2 and the formation of the interferon-stimulated gene factor 3 (ISGF3) transcription complex, which is composed of STAT1, STAT2 and IFN regulatory factor (IRF) 9/p48 [12], and to the induction of myxovirus resistance A (MxA) and oligoadenylate synthetase (OAS)1, which mediate the antiviral effects of type I IFN [12, 24]. Initially, type I IFNs and type III IFNs were also considered to lead to activation of the mitogen-activated protein (MAP) kinases c-Jun N-terminal kinase (JNK) and p38, but not extracellular signal-regulated kinase (ERK) [24]. Accordingly, type III IFNs have been shown to elicit biological activities including antiviral, antiproliferative and immunomodulatory properties, similar to those of type I IFNs. Therefore, despite the structural difference and the utilization of a distinct receptor system, type III IFN seems to be functionally related to type I IFN.

In the first half of this chapter, we will summarize the current knowledge on the novel IFN family member type III IFN and, in the latter half, we will review studies from several laboratories, including our group, displaying direct and indirect antitumor activities of type III IFNs with the usage of various histological types of human tumor cell lines and xenogeneic models of human esophageal carcinoma and non-small cell lung cancer (NSCLC), and genetically modified tumor cells in murine tumor models.

2. Type III IFN-encoding genes and regulation of production

In 2003, two research groups independently reported the identification of a small family of interferon like cytokines through computational analysis of the human genome sequence database [12, 13]. This novel family of interferon consists of three family members, which were referred to alternatively as IFN-λ1, IFN-λ2 and IFN-λ3, or IL-29, IL-28A, and IL-28B, respectively. The genes encoding human IL-28A, IL-28B and IL-29 are located on the same genomic contig, which is from chromosomal region 19q13.13 [12, 13]. This chromosomal location differs from the type I and type II interferon families clustered on chromosome 9 and chromosome 12, respectively. The genes encoding type III IFNs are composed of multiple exons, 5 for IL-29, and 6 for IL-28A and IL-28B, resembling the structural organization of genes encoding IL-10-related cytokines [12, 13]. This is in clear contrast to type I IFNs, which are encoded within a single exon. At amino acid level, IL-28A has an 81-96% identity to IL-28B and IL-29, 11-13% identity to IL-10 and 15-19% identity to IFN-γ and IL-22 [12, 13].

Mouse type III interferon-encoding genes were mapped to chromosome 7A3. This region has a similar organization as the human type III interferon locus [14]. Two genes colinear with the human IL-28A and IL-28B genes are intact and are predicted to encode functional proteins, which are designated mouse IL-28A and IL-28B in accordance with the corresponding human genes [14]. Mouse IL-28A and IL-28B have higher sequence identity to human IL-28A and IL-28B than to IL-29 [14]. In contrast to the IL-28A and IL-28B genes, the mouse IL-29 gene has lost the entire exon 2 and acquired the stop codon within exon 1, resulting in a pseudogene in all murine strains studied [14]. Both mouse IL-28A and IL-28B possess a site for N-linked glycosylation (Asn^{105}-Met-Thr in IL-28A and Asn^{107}-Asp-Ser in IL-28B) [14].

Like type I IFNs, type III IFN mRNAs expression was detected at low levels in human blood, brain, lung, ovary, pancreas, pituitary, placenta, prostate, and testis by RT-PCR analysis [25]. Furthermore, there have been many reports that infection of encephalomyocarditis virus (EMCV) [13], Sindbis virus [25], Dengue virus [12], vesicular stomatitis virus (VSV) [10], mengo virus [23], cytomegalo virus (CMV) [24], and Sendai virus [27, 28, 29] leads to transcriptional activation of IL-28A, IL-28B, and IL-29 variously in human peripheral mononuclear cells (PBMC), monocyte-derived dendritic cells (MD-DCs), bronchial epithelial cells and a number of human cell lines. Respiratory syncytial virus induces expression of type III IFNs in monocyte-derived macrophages [30]. Type III IFN mRNAs are co-expressed with IFN-α and IFN-ß in virally infected cells [10, 11]. Sendai virus infection readily activates the expression of IFN-α, IFN-ß, and IFN-λ genes, whereas influenza A virus (IAV)-induced activation of these genes is mainly dependent on pretreatment of A549 lung alveolar cell carcinoma with IFN-α or tumor necrosis factor (TNF)-α [31]. Although virtually any cell type following viral infection can express type III IFNs, PBMC, MD-DCs and plasmacytoid DCs appear to be the major cellular sources [10, 11, 32]. The antigen presenting cells (APCs) such as DCs and macrophages have been shown to produce and secrete type III IFNs following stimulation with TLR agonists [25, 33]. MD-DCs express low levels of type III IFNs when stimulated with TLR agonists such as lipopolysaccharide (LPS) or polyinosinic:polycytidylic acid [poly(I:C)]. In addition, type III IFNs also have a positive regulatory effect on the expression of type III IFNs. Siren *et al.* [27] demonstrated this clearly, whereas pretreatment with type III IFNs was shown to enhance the production of type III IFNs by macrophages stimulated with TLR3 and TLR4 agonists. TLR3 ligand poly(I:C) up-regulated IFN-ß, IFN-λ, and TLR3 expression in HUVECs but not in A549 cells. Similarly, IFN-α pretreatment also strongly enhanced poly(I:C)-induced activation of IFN-β and IFN–λ genes in HUVECs [33]. Although type III IFNs differ genetically and structurally from type I IFNs and use their own specific receptor, the expression of type III IFNs and type I IFNs is regulated in a similar fashion in virus-infected cells exhibiting both early and late phases of interferon induction [15]. However, type III interferon genes are under a more complex regulation than type I interferon genes, since type III interferon genes have a higher number of regulatory elements on their promoters [15]. Type III interferon gene promoters have several putative IFN-stimulated response elements (ISRE) and NF-κB binding sites [30]. The promoter sequences of IL-28A and IL-28B genes are almost identical, whereas the promoter of IL-29 is somewhat different from the IL-28A/B promoters [25]. Namely, NF-κB and multiple IRF family members induce the expression of IL-29 gene [25]. In contrast to IL-29, the IL-28A/B genes are predominantly regulated by an IFN regulatory factor (IRF) family member IRF7 [25]. Therefore, the IL-29 gene is mainly regulated by virus-activated IRF3 and IRF7, resembling that of the IFN-ß gene, whereas IL-28A/B gene expression is mainly controlled by IRF7, resembling those of IFN-α genes [25]. Viral infection serves to activate IRF3, which is expressed broadly and constitutively at high levels in cells, via specific serine phosphorylation events, leading to the synthesis and release of IFNs, predominantly IL-29 and IFN-ß. In paracrine fashion, these newly released IFNs are free to act on neighboring cells. The binding of IFNs to the respective specific receptor induces expression of another transcriptional activator, IRF7, in a STAT1-dependent manner. When cells expressing other IRF7 are in turn infected with viruses, IRF7 is phosphorylated, and the cells respond by expressing other type III IFN and type I IFN genes, such as IL-29, IL-28A/B, IFN-α and INF-ß.

3. Type III IFN receptor subunit IL-28R

Type III IFNs act through a cell surface receptor which is composed of the newly identified IL-28R and IL-10Rß with both chains apparently required for full binding affinity [12, 13]. At the time of its discovery, IL-10Rß has been already known as the second chain of the IL-10 [34], IL-22 [35, 36], or IL-26 receptor [37], formerly known as the class II cytokine receptor (CRF2)-9. IL-28R belongs to members of the class II cytokine receptor family, which are tripartite single-pass transmembrane proteins defined by structural similarities in the extracellular domain including the ligand binding residues [37, 38]. In accordance with the CRF2 characteristics, both transmembrane chains have an extracellular moiety containing two tandem fibronectin III domains, a structural motif in the immunoglobulin fold superfamily, with several amino acid (aa) positions conserved within this receptor family [38, 39]. Like IL-10, IL-22 and IL-26, the binding of type III IFN to IL-28R induces a conformational change that enables IL-10Rß to interact with the newly formed ligand-receptor complex [40].

The human IL-28R-encoding gene is located on chromosomoe 1p36.11, near the *IL22RA1* locus, while the IL-10R-encoding gene is located on 21q22.11, near the *IFNAR1*, *IFNAR2*, and *IFNGR2* loci [12, 13, 41]. The first exon of the human IL-28R-encoding gene contains 5-UTR and the signal peptide [12, 13]. The transmembrane moieties are predicted to be encoded by sequences derived from exon 6 of the corresponding genes [12, 13]. The longer intracellular moiety of IL-28R (predicted 271 aa versus 79 aa in the IL-10Rß) contains three tyrosine residues, which are potential targets for phosphorylation [12, 13]. Dumoutier *et al.* indicated two tyrosines Tyr^{343} and Tyr^{517} of human IL-28R can independently mediate STAT2 activation by type III IFNs [23]. This work also showed that when both $tyrosines^{343 \text{ and } 517}$ were mutated to phenylalanine, antiviral and antiproliferative activities of type III IFNs were completely abolished [23]. The extracellular domains of IL-28R and IL-10Rß contain four putative N-linked glycosylation sites [12, 13].

The murine genes encoding IL-28R and IL-10Rß are located on chromosome 4D3 and 16C4, respectively [14]. The mouse IL-28R chain is ~67% similar to its human counterpart [14]. Although the mouse and human IL-28R sequences are similar, only two of three tyrosine residues of the human receptor intracellular domain are conserved in the mouse orthologue [14]. The mouse receptor contains three additional tyrosine residues [14]. The Try^{341}-based motif of mouse IL-28R (YLERP) shows similarities with that surrounding Tyr^{343} of human

IL-28R (YLERP). In addition, the COOH-terminal amino acid sequence of mouse IL-28R containing Tyr533 (YLVRstop) is similar to the COOH-terminal amino acid sequence of human IL-28R containing Tyr517 (YMARstop). Therefore, both the mouse and human IL-28R chains contain similar docking sites for STAT2 recruitment and activation. Human IL-28R has a stretch of negatively charged residues close to the end of the intracellular domain. This region in the mouse IL-28R is significantly altered by a short insertion and substitution of several amino acid residues, resulting in a longer and more negatively charged region in the mouse receptor [14].

Several research groups including our own have examined the expression of IL-28 receptor complex components. The IL-10Rß chain is ubiquitously expressed, which can be explained by its function as part of several cytokine receptors. The one notable exception is the brain, where the IL-10Rß chain seems to be expressed at very low levels [42]. Therefore, the expression of the IL-28R chain should determine whether a cell is responsible to the type III IFNs or not [12, 13]. The near relation of type III IFNs to type I IFNs and IL-10 initially suggested extensive effects of type III IFNs on various cell populations. Actually, Sheppard *et al.* observed at first that, using northern blot analysis, various organs variably expressed the major IL-28R transcript and therefore contain putative target cells in humans [13]. These organs include the adrenal gland and kidney, and those from the digestive (stomach, small intestine, colon and liver), respiratory (lung) and immune (spleen and thymus) systems, with the highest expression found in the pancreas, thyroid, skeletal muscle, heart, prostate, and testis [13]. Interestingly, most IL-28R mRNA-expressing tissues form outer body barriers and contain epithelial cells [43]. These quantitative results are in line with the data published by Kotenko *et al.* [9]. A pattern similar to that obtained in tissues using northern blot analysis was found in corresponding hematopoietic (HL-60 promyelocytic leukemia, K-562 erythroleukemia, MOLT-4 T-cell leukemia and Raji B-cell leukemia) and non-hematopoietic (HeLa S3 cervical adenocarcinoma, Caco-2, SW480, HCT116, SW480 and DLD-1 colorectal adenocarcinoma, A549 lung alveolar cell carcinoma, LK-1 lung adenocarcinoma and G-361 melanoma) cell lines [12, 44, 45].

At present, it has been thought that the surface expression of IL-28R is more restricted relative to the type I IFN receptor although detailed information regarding with the expression level and cell distribution of the type III IFN specific receptor IL-28R is relatively limited. Therefore, whereas type I IFN signaling is observed for a broad spectrum of cell types, type III IFN signaling is generally weaker and more restrictive, which is correlated with a low expression of the IL-28R subunit of the type III IFN receptor. Actually, at the cellular level, B cell lymphoma Raji and hepatoma HepG2 cells respond well to type III IFNs. On the contrary, in HT1080 fibrosarcoma, Sw13 adrenal carcinoma cells and MCF-7 breast cancer cells, all of which respond to type I IFNs, no significant response to type III IFNs was observed [26]. Furthermore, in humans, primary bronchial epithelial cells and primary gastric epithelial cells are responsive to type III IFNs, whereas primary fibroblasts and umbilical vein endothelial cells do not express IL-28R and therefore are not responsive to type III IFNs (14 and our unpublished observation).

In mouse, IL-28R mRNA expression has been found in keratinocyte and lung fibroblast [14, 46]. In immune systems, our studies using RT-PCR did not detect any expression of IL-28R mRNA in primary spleen cells from C57BL/6 mice [43, 46]. Moreover, we could not detect any IL-28R expression in resting primary immune cells such as B cells and T cells [46]. Lasfar *et al.* also observed that primary lymphocytes and macrophages, the major players in specific antitumor immunity, are found to be unresponsive to type III IFN [14]. In accordance with the results obtained with primary immune cell subpopulations, corresponding cell lines (EL4 and P815) expressed IL-10Rß but not IL-28R [44]. On the contrary, Siebler *et al.* reported the opposite finding that the IL-28R mRNA is expressed in primary murine CD4 T cells [48]. In the case of NK cells, Murakami's group demonstrated the mRNA expression of IL-28R [47]. Further analyses are needed to determine the precise expression profile among immune cells. In general, tissues which are mainly composed of epithelia such as intestine, skin, or lung are the most responsive to type III IFNs. These data indicate that a key difference between the type I IFN and type III IFN systems could be the cell specificity of their respective receptor expression.

4. Signal transduction of type III IFNs

Signaling induced by a cytokine binding to type II cytokine receptor, whose extracellular parts commonly consist of tandem fibronectin type III domains and the cytoplasmic domain is associated with a tyrosine kinase of the Janus kinase (Jak) family, is known to occur primarily via the Jak/STAT pathway. Both IL-28R and IL-10Rß subunits are necessary to form a functional type III IFN receptor. The formation of the IL-28R-IL-10Rß ternary complex initiates signaling events by activating the transduction elements bound to the intracytoplasmic part of the two chains composed of functional type III IFN receptor. Type III IFNs induce the activation of a Jak/STAT signaling pathway leading to tyrosine phosphorylation of STAT1, STAT2, STAT3, STAT4 and STAT5 [12, 13, 22, 23, 49]. In structure, IL-28R is most closely related at the sequence level with the soluble class II cytokine receptor IL-22Rα2, whereas a second type III IFN receptor chain IL-10Rß is commonly utilized by IL-10, IL-22 and IL-26 [38]. IL-10, IL-22 and IL-26 can stimulate STAT3 phosphorylation, and IL-22 and IL-26 have been shown to phosphorylate STAT1. On the other hand, only the type III IFN family induces tyrosine phosphorylation of STAT2. The characteristics to be able to phosphorylate STAT1, STAT2 and STAT3 are common to the type III IFN family and the type I IFNs. Thus, STAT2 activation has been, at present, restricted to type I IFNs and type III IFNs. From studies of IL-10 and IL-22 signal transduction, it is known that its short (82 amino acids) intracytoplasmic part binds tyrosine kinase Tyk2 but does not provide STAT recruitment sites [50]. Jak1 was shown to be critical in mediating IFN-induced STAT phosphorylation [22]. Thus, it is likely that, as for the type I IFN receptor system, Jak1 and Tyk2 are the two tyrosine kinases associated with the type III IFN receptor subunit and mediating STAT activation. STAT2 is specifically recruited in the ISGF3 transcription factor that translocates to the nucleus and drives the expression of the gene family carrying an ISRE sequence in their promoter. ISGF3 is formed by dimerization of STAT1 and STAT2 via SH2 phosphotyrosine interactions and association of the heterodimer with IRF9. Type III IFNs induce the formation of both ISGF3 and STAT1 homodimers, which are able to recognize ISRE and GAS sequences [12, 14, 23]. Among the IFN-induced genes, suppressor of cytokine signaling (SOCS)1 and SOCS3 are involved in the negative regulation of type III IFN signaling [51, 52]. Overexpression of SOCS1 in hepatic cell lines inhibits type III IFN signaling as well [51]. Additionally, type I IFNs can activate a variety of signaling molecules and cascades, which may operate in concert with or independently of STATs. Similarly, type III IFNs were shown to activate ERK 1/2 and Akt in an intestinal epithelial cell line [44].

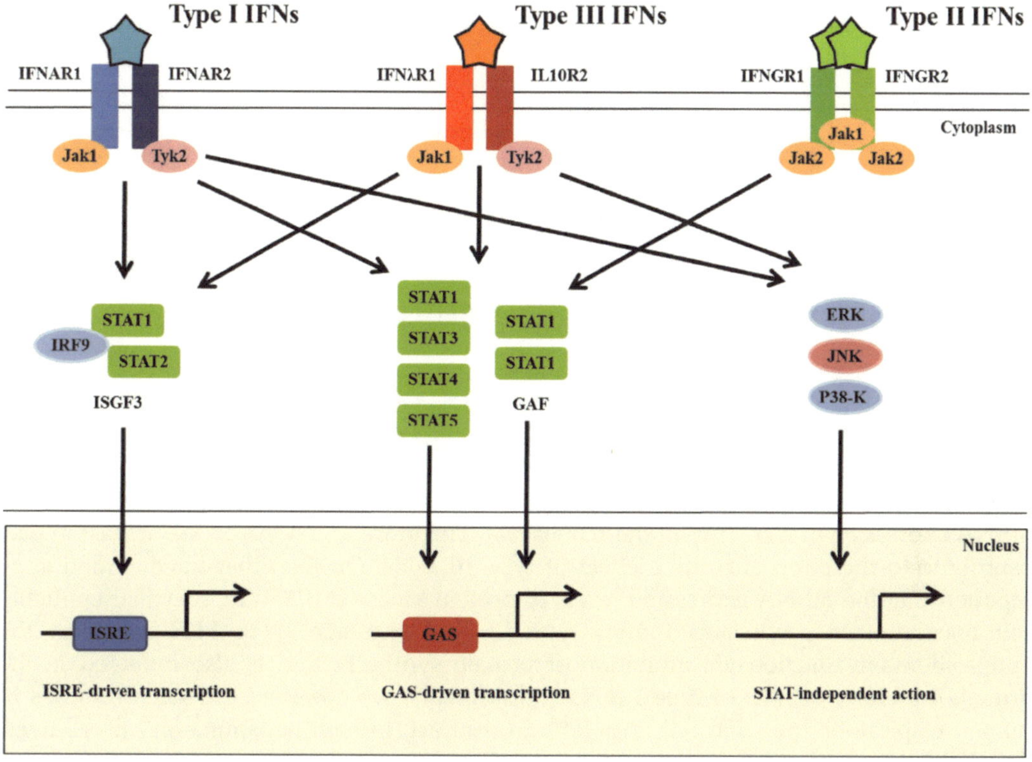

Fig. 1. Signaling pathways of type III IFNs, which activate similar intracellular signaling components and genes to type I IFNs.

5. Direct antitumor activity of type III IFNs

One of the most important properties of type I IFNs is their potential in cancer treatment. Type I IFNs represent the cytokines exhibiting the longest record of use in clinical oncology [53]. Even though today some new anticancer drugs somehow replaced type I IFNs in the treatment of certain hematological malignancies such as hairy cell leukemia and chronic myeloid leukemia, type I IFN therapy continues to be widely used in the adjuvant treatment of certain malignancies such as melanoma and renal cell carcinoma [54, 55]. As mentioned earlier, signaling components are shared between type I IFNs and type III IFNs. Therefore, based on the similar functional profiles with type I IFNs, it would be anticipated that type III IFNs would have redundant antitumor properties.

Several research groups have investigated the antitumor potential of type III IFNs. Until now, growth-inhibitory action of type III IFNs has been documented in certain histological types of human tumors such as neuroendocrine tumors [52], esophageal carcinoma [56], colorectal/intestinal carcinoma [51], hepatocellular carcinoma [16, 57, 58], lung adenocarcinomas [45], Burkitt's lymphoma [26], and melanoma [59]. These are summarized in Table 1.

Experimental system	Possible mechanism	References
Human glioblastoma LN319 cell line	Growth inhibition	Meager et al. (2005)
Human neuroendocrine BON1 tumor cells	Induction of apoptosis	Zitmann et al. (2006)
Murine BW5147 thymoma cell line	Growth inhibition	Dumoutier et al. (2003)
Human keratinocyte cell line HaCaT,	Induced apoptosis, extended STAT activation,	Maher et al. (2008)
Human fibrosarcoma 2fTGH cell line	prolonged ISG expression	Maher et al. (2008)
Murine melanoma	Engaged host mechanisms to exert their antitumor functions	Lasfer et al. (2006)
Murine fibrosarcoma	Induce innate and adaptive immune responses against tumors,	Numasaki et al. (2007)
	including increase of IFN-γ production and	
	polymorphonuclear neutrophils, NK cells, and CD8 T cell activity	
Murine melanoma, colon cancer	Induced tumor apoptosis and innate immune responses	Sato et al. (2006)
Murine hepatoma	including IFN-γ, IL-12, NK cells and dendritic cells	Abushahba et al. (2010)

Table 1. Representative antitumor activity of type III IFNs

In vitro studies using multiple human cell lines including B cell lymphoma, hepatoma, neuroendocrine and colorectal tumor cell lines provide evidence that, in these lines, type III IFNs can induce 2′-5′ oligoadenylate synthetase (2′,5′-OAS), which is involved in type I IFN-induced antiproliferative effects [12, 23, 44]. A study of ours also displayed that type III IFNs significantly suppressed *in vitro* growth of human NSCLC lines and markedly up-regulated mRNA expression of 2′,5′-OAS in these lines [60]. Therefore, 2′,5′-OAS could, at least in part, contribute to the antiproliferative effect of type III IFNs. On the other hand, Brand *et al.* reported that the mRNA expression levels of protein kinase R (PKR) in intestinal epithelial cell lines remained unchanged after type III IFN treatment [44]. PKR mediates the antiproliferative function via inhibition of protein synthesis, and is also involved in the growth-inhibitory actions of type I IFNs. Additionally, we observed the same findings in human respiratory epithelial cell lines [60]. In contrast, in both hepatoma and B cell lines, type IIII IFNs mediated PKR gene induction [57]. Collectively, PKR could be involved in type III IFN-induced antiproliferative effect in a limited range of cell types.

Type I IFNs can exert a more direct negative regulatory effect on the cell cycle by specifically up-regulating expression of a number of cyclin-dependent kinase inhibitors (CKIs). Type I IFNs specifically enhance the expression level of $p21^{Waf1/Cip1}$, which plays a crucial regulatory role in the progression from the G1 to S phase [61]. Type I IFNs also increase expression of another CKI $p15^{Ink4b}$ that can complex specifically with Cdk4 [62]. A third protein $p27^{Kip1}$ preferentially binds to cyclinE/Cdk2 complexes, and dissociation of the retinoblastoma gene product (pRb) and the related pocket proteins (p107 and p130) is concomitantly suppressed [63]. Rb and the related pocket proteins, in their non-phosphorylated forms, interact strongly with the E2F family of transcription factors, thus inhibiting their activity [64]. Phosphorylation of Rb (and p107 or p130) normally releases E2F transcription factors, and permits transition from the G1 to S phase.

Our recent study demonstrated that, in a panel of human esophageal carcinoma cell lines, the T.Tn cell line was susceptible to the apoptotic effects of type III IFNs, whereas type I IFNs elicited neither an antiproliferative nor a pro-apoptotic response [56]. $p21^{Waf1/Cip1}$ was initially expressed at high levels in T.Tn cells, and a large fraction of these cells were in the G0/G1 phase as a possible consequence of high levels of $p21^{Waf1/Cip1}$ expression. In addition, our studies using multiple human NSCLC lines displayed elevated $p21^{Waf1/Cip1}$ mRNA expression and, to a lesser extent, $p27^{Kip1}$, but not $p15^{Ink4b}$, expression with type III IFN treatment, and that knockdown of p21$^{Waf1/Cip1}$ with a p21$^{Waf1/Cip1}$-specific double-stranded small inhibitory RNA (p21-siRNA) oligonucleotide largely attenuated the observed antiproliferative effect, suggesting the major role of p21$^{Waf1/Cip1}$ in the growth-inhibitory function of type III IFNs [60]. Analysis of cell cycle distribution displayed that treatment of NSCLC lines with type III IFNs resulted in an accumulation of cell numbers in the G1 phase in a dose-dependent manner. This increase of the G1 population was accompanied by the reduction of S and G2 populations. Taken collectively, our results demonstrated that type III IFNs could induce cell cycle arrest at the G1 phase. These findings are in line with the result published earlier by Sato *et al.* [47].

Another important mechanism for type III IFNs to exert an antiproliferative effect was reported by Zitzmann's research group [52]. They demonstrated that treatment with type III IFN significantly suppressed the growth of human neuroendocrine BON1 tumor cells, but did not result in a significant accumulation in G1 phase [52]. Moreover, the same research group indicated that incubation with type III IFN significantly increased the amount of cleaved caspase-3- and poly(ADP-ribose)polymerase (PARP)-products in BON1 tumor cells [52]. In this case, treatment with type III IFN resulted in induction of apoptosis rather than in the interference of cell cycle progression. Moreover, Sato *et al.* reported that type III IFNs up-regulated surface expression of FAS, dephosphorylated Rb and activated both caspase-3 and caspase-7 in B16 melanoma cells, suggesting the promotion of apoptosis [47]. Our studies displayed that type III IFNs induced apoptosis in NSCLC cells by measuring DNA fragmentation and surface Annexin V expression when NSCLC cells were treated for relatively long periods [60]. In addition, Brand *et al.* indicated that type III IFNs did not influence FAS ligand-induced apoptosis but decreased cell proliferation in human intestinal epithelial cells [24].

Maher *et al.* demonstrated that type III IFN treatment induced a prolonged but overall stronger activation of STAT1 and STAT2 in the immortalized keratinocyte line HaCaT compared with IFN-α treatment [65]. Another distinctive difference was the induction of ISGs by IFN-α, which peaked early and declined thereafter, whereas IFN-λ-induced ISGs levels peaked later but were sustained longer. A substantial growth inhibitory response, activation of caspase-3 and caspase-7, and ultimately apoptosis ensued. Although IFN-α induced a modest antiproliferative effect, it did not promote apoptosis, suggesting that the prolonged STAT activity and subsequent induction and sustained expression of ISGs are what may have favored the activation of programmed cell death. Pretreatment of HaCaT cells with pan-caspase inhibitor benzyloxycarbonyl-Val-Ala-Asp (OMe) fluoromethylketone (Z-VAD-fmk) inhibited apoptosis, indicating a requirement for caspases in the promotion of type III IFN-induced cell death. The combination of IFN-α and type III IFN had additive an antiproliferative effect, suggesting that the distinct receptor complexes did not compete for available JAKs and STATs or, alternatively, the type I IFN and type III IFN signaled partially through alternative pathways. Li *et al.* [66] have also demonstrated that type III IFN signaling leads to the activation of apoptosis. In their model, a human HT29 colorectal adenocarcinoma cell line with ectopic expression of a chimeric IL-10Rß/IL-28R that binds IL-10, but signals through the intracellular domain of IL-28R, was shown to undergo apoptosis when treated with IL-10. The early response was antiproliferative but later switched to one of apoptosis as a drastic increase in the proportion of sub-G0 cells was observed. Caspase-3, caspase-8 and caspase-9 were cleaved and activated, and pretreatment with Z-VAD-fmk abrogated caspase-3 and caspase-9 activities, but did not block the death-inducing effect of IL-10, indicating the presence of an additional cell death pathways. Surprisingly, Z-VAD-fmk increased the cleavage of pro-caspase-9 into caspase-9. The strength of STAT1 activation by IL-10 through the chimeric receptor was more robust than treatment with type III IFN that signaled through the endogenous IL-28R complex. Of note, HT29 cells express low levels of IL-28R and can respond to type III IFN by up-regulating MHC class I expression, but they are not growth inhibited by type III IFN. This raises an important point as it suggests that a sufficient number of cell surface IL-28R must be expressed and engaged for type III IFN to induce an antiproliferative effect. These studies are in agreement with our findings and strongly suggest that the strength of type III IFN signaling through STAT activation may be the determining factor that favors an apoptotic response.

Antiproliferative and pro-apoptotic effects of type III IFN can be augmented when used in combination with chemotherapy drugs. Lesinski *et al.* reported that co-treatment of F0-melanoma cells with proteasome inhibitor Bortezomib and type III IFN synergistically increased cell death, similar to the combination of IFN-α and Bortezomib [67]. We also observed that the combination of 5-fluorouracil (5-FU) or cisplatin (CDDP) with type III IFN drastically inhibited cell growth of the esophageal carcinoma cell lines [56]. When esophageal carcinoma cell lines TE-11, YES-5 and T.Tn cells, which were sensitive to antiproliferative effect of type III IFN IL-29, were cultured with various doses of 5-FU or CDDP, IL-29 significantly enhanced the cytotoxicity of 5-FU or CDDP. This combinatory effect was additive irrespective of the agents. In contrast, IL-29 scarcely influenced the cytotoxicity of 5-FU or CDDP in normal and Het-1A cells, whereas IFN-α enhanced the sensitivity of normal and Het-1A cells to 5-FU or CDDP.

Our recent study demonstrated that antiproliferative effects of type III IFNs could be also enhanced when combined with type I IFN IFN-α [60]. Treatment with interferon combination of type III IFN and type I IFN increased $p21^{Waf1/Cip1}$ expression, and induced apoptotic cell death more efficiently, and consequently exerted an additive growth-inhibitory effect on NSCLC lines *in vitro*. In addition, interferon combination therapy of IL-29 and IFN-α inhibited *in vivo* growth of xenogeneic NSCLC OBA-LK1 tumors more effectively than individual regent alone [60].

One of the important mechanisms of antitumor activities of type I IFNs is inhibition of tumor-induced angiogenesis [68]. Type I IFNs can inhibit a number of steps in the angiogenic processes, including proliferation and migration of vascular endothelial cells [69, 70, 71, 72]. Type I IFNs can also affect the expression of several angiogenic factors, including vascular endothelial growth factor (VEGF) [73], bFGF [74], IL-8 [75], and collagenase type IV in tumor cells and surrounding stroma cells [76]. Indeed, systemic therapy with the use of recombinant type I IFNs produces antiangiogenic effects in vascular tumors including hemangioma [77], Kaposi's sarcoma [78], melanoma [79], and bladder carcinoma [80].

In contrast to type I IFNs, there have been no reports demonstrating type III IFNs possess antiangiogenic activities. One of the key differences reported between the type I IFN and type III IFN systems is in the expression of their respective receptor subunits. For example, vascular endothelial cells express IFN-αRα, IFN-αRß and IL-10Rß, but not IL-28R, on the cell surface [14]. Therefore, vascular endothelial cells appear to be, in general, unresponsive to type III IFNs. In addition, type III IFN treatment up-regulated, not suppressed, the secretion of proangiogenic cytokine IL-8 from human colon cancer cells [24]. Additionally, exposure of human macrophages to type III IFN IL-29 significantly induces IL-8 production [81]. In contrast, Pekarek *et al.* reported that, using human peripheral blood mononuclear cells, type III IFN member IL-29 elevated mRNA expression levels of three chemokines, monokine induced IFN-γ (MIG), IFN-γ inducible protein 10 (IP-10) and IFN-γ inducible T cell α chemoattractant (I-TAC) in the absence of other stimuli [82]. These factors are members of the ELR- subfamily of CXC chemokines and display potent inhibitory effects on angiogenesis. In our xenogeneic NSCLC tumor models, daily intratumoral administration of IL-29 significantly suppressed *in vivo* tumor growth, but did not affect the tumor microvascular density [78]. Taken collectively, it is still now unknown whether type III IFNs possess antiangiogenic properties like type I IFNs. Further detailed analyses are needed to elucidate the biological role of type III IFN in angiogenesis.

6. Induction of antitumor immunity by type III IFNs

Several laboratories including ours carried out an ensemble of studies where the mouse type III IFN IL-28A gene was transduced into different types of mouse tumor cells and *in vivo* behavior of genetically modified cells constitutively secreting IL-28A was evaluated after injection into immunocompetent syngeneic mice [14, 46, 47]. In these experiments, a gene therapy approach was introduced to investigate whether type III IFNs may possess antitumor actions instead of systemic therapy because cytokine gene therapy has many advantages in comparison with systemic administration of cytokine. Systemic delivery of cytokines at pharmacologic doses results in a high concentration of cytokines in the circulation and often in suboptimal levels in tissues at the site of tumors. In contrast, cytokine gene transfer allows the localized expression of the cytokine at the targeted sites, avoiding deleterious side effects and resembling the paracrine mode of action of cytokines, which are produced in high amounts at the site of tumors and act on the immune system by providing transient signals between cells to generate effector responses.

Ahmed *et al.* first investigated whether the constitutive expression of IL-28A at the tumor site may affect the tumorigenicity of B16 melanoma cells, which are responsive to type III IFNs and classified as a low immunogenicity [14]. This study provided initial evidence that the tumorigenicity of B16 cells producing IL-28A in immunocompetent mice is highly impaired or completely abolished, and that the inhibition of tumor establishment is dependent on the amount of IL-28A released by the genetically modified tumor cells [14]. Whereas 50% of mice injected with B16 clone producing 100 to 150 ng of IL-28A for 24 hours per 10^6 cells developed tumors, 100% of animals injected with B16 clone releasing 1 to 5 ng of IL-28A developed tumors. When B16 clone, which produced IL-28A but was resistant to the antiproliferative effect of IL-28A, was used to examine whether the antitumor effect of IL-28A was due to direct action on B16 cells or mediated by a host response, type III IFN-unresponsive B16 clone expressing IL-28A displayed reduced tumorigenicity and repressed the growth of parental B16 cells *in vivo* to a level comparable to IL-28A-responsive B16 cells, providing evidence that host-defense mechanisms play a major role in mediating type III IFN-induced antitumor activity *in vivo* [14]. In this tumor model, about 10% mice, which rejected B16 melanoma cells producing IL-28A, survived the subsequent parental B16 tumor challenge, suggesting the failure of development of a strong long-lasting immune memory [14]. Taken together with the findings that tumor-infiltrating immune cells were not observed in tumor tissues from B16 cells secreting IL-28A and mouse primary lymphocytes and macrophages are unresponsive to type III IFNs, it was proposed as one of the possible mechanisms that IL-28A produced by genetically modified B16 cells could first act on neighboring keratinocytes and other tumor stromal cells, and could inhibit their tumor-supportive function, leading to the reduced tumorigenicity in the B16 melanoma tumor model [14].

The antitumor therapeutic potential of type III IFN gene transfer into experimental tumors was further evaluated in animal models by another research group using various approaches, comprising both the use of genetically modified cells and *in vivo* delivery of type III IFN gene via injection of naked plasmid DNA. To examine the antitumor potency of type III IFNs *in vivo,* Sato *et al.* transfected B16/F0 mouse melanoma cells with IL-28A cDNA, which resulted in *in vitro* growth inhibition and increased caspase-3 and caspase-7 activity [47]. Transduction of IL-28A increased $p21^{Waf1/Cip1}$ levels and decreased phosphorylation of Rb (Ser^{780}), suggesting a mechanism for the observed cell arrest. In addition, B16/F0 cells producing IL-28A did not form pulmonary metastasis when injected into C57BL/6 mice. Histological examination of the lungs revealed cellular infiltrates and NK cells were demonstrated to be responsible for the major part of antitumor effect of type III IFN [47]. Moreover, the biological effects of ectopic IL-28A, secreted by the injected tumor cells, on the host's immune response have been thoroughly investigated. Targeting of Colon 26 liver metastatic lesions by hydrodynamic gene delivery of plasmid DNA encoding mouse IL-28A led to marked reduction of liver metastatic foci along with survival advantages [47]. By studying the *in vivo* turnover of different lymphocyte subsets in mice injected with IL-28 plasmid DNA, the number of NK cells and NKT cells in the liver markedly increased [47]. In contrast, B16 lung metastases were not successfully treated by hydrodynamic injection of IL-28A expression plasmid, indicating that the local delivery of type III IFN to target sites is necessary for the control of metastatic tumor growth, and that type III IFN-induced systemic cytotoxic T cell (CTL) response is relatively weak in this tumor model [47].

Despite the type III IFN-resistant phenotype, successful induction of antitumor response following type III IFN IL-28A gene transfer was subsequently confirmed in the MCA205 tumor model [46]. We observed that *in vivo* growth of MCA205 producing IL-28A was efficiently inhibited by an IL-28A-elicited host-mediated immune response [46]. In this tumor model, the tumorigenic behavior of MCA205 cells producing either type I IFN IFN-α or type III IFN IL-28A was compared after subcutaneous injection. IFN-α-secreting MCA205 (MCA205IFN-α) cells were rejected efficiently compared to IL-28A-producing MCA205 (MCA205IL-28) cells, which exhibited only a delay of tumor growth [46]. This finding implicated that the potency of the antitumor activity of IL-28A might be slightly lower than that of IFN-α although MCA205IL-28 cells secreted approximately 3-fold less cytokine than did MCA205IFN-α cells [43]. IFN-α in contrast to IL-28A displayed direct biological effects on MCA205 cells, including enhancement of the MHC class I antigen expression, suggesting that IFN-α, but not IL-28A, can directly influence the immunogenicity of MCA205 cells.

In regard to the cellular antitumor mechanisms of IL-28A, the findings in mice selectively depleted of various immune cell populations indicated that CD8 T cells play an important role in IL-28A-mediated antitumor immunity in the MCA205 tumor model because the protective effect was partially abolished in CD8 T cell-depleted animals [46]. This finding is in clear contrast with the result obtained in the B16 melanoma tumor model, in which depletion of CD8 T cells had no consequence on the tumor growth rate [47]. Additionally, in this tumor model, local secretion of IL-28A by tumor cells induced more powerful tumor-specific cytotoxic T cells against parental MCA205 cells [46]. This is consistent with the observed dense infiltration of CD8 T cells into tumor tissues from MCA205IL-28 cells. However, primary mouse CD8 T cells are not expressing IL-28R on the cell surface and are found to be unresponsive to IL-28A treatment [46]. This characteristic of type III IFNs is in clear contrast with that of type I IFNs, which can directly act on T cells [80]. On the contrary, the expression of mRNA for IL-28R is clearly detected in Con A-stimulated mouse T cells, suggesting that the activated mouse CD8 T cells might possess the ability to respond to type III IFNs [46]. However, IL-28 does not have ability to directly enhance the cytotoxic activity of CTLs [46]. A recent report by Jordan *et al.* indicated that type III IFN IL-29 influences the cytokine production by Con A-stimulated human T cells, which is isolated from peripheral blood mononuclear cells [81]. IL-28A also displayed the biological function to induce chemokine secretion by mouse lung fibroblasts [46]. Taken together, one possible mechanism, by which IL-28A elicits CD8 T cell responses, is proposed to be that IL-28A first stimulates CD8 T cells indirectly through induction of other cytokines and chemokines by surrounding cells including stromal fibroblasts and keratinocytes, and subsequently acts on activated T cells directly [46]. Therefore, the detailed mechanisms that underlie this CD8 T cell-dependent antitumor action by type III IFNs remain to be elucidated and will require further experimental analyses.

A slower growth rate of MCA205IL-28 tumors in CD4 T cell-depleted mice was consistently observed, implicating that CD4 T cells rather inhibit IL-28A-induced antitumor response [46]. Both CD4 T cells and CD8 T cells have been described to be important for the efficient induction of antitumor cellular immunity [84, 85]. This unexpected finding that CD4 T cells are not required for the antitumor activity of IL-28A is not in agreement with the notion that CD4 T cell help is necessary for the full activation of naive CD8 T cells [86]. However, a similar inhibitory effect of CD4 T cells has been previously reported in IL-12- or IL-23-transduced CT26 tumor model [87, 88]. These findings may be possibly explained by taking into account the $CD4^+CD25^+$ T regulatory cells [89]. With regard to the relation between type III IFNs and $CD4^+CD25^+$ T regulatory cells, Mennechet *et al.* reported that IL-28A promotes the generation of partially mature DCs, which display a tolerogenic phenotype [90]. Namely, type III IFN-matured DCs with the ability to migrate lymph nodes express high levels of MHC class I and II but low levels of co-stimulatory molecules [90]. These type III IFN-treated DCs specifically induced IL-2-dependent proliferation of a $CD4^+CD25^+Foxp3^+$ T regulatory cell population in culture, which is thought, in general, to result in suppression of the antitumor immune response [89]. Therefore, type III IFN-treated DCs can stimulate the proliferation of pre-existing $CD4^+CD25^+$ T regulatory cells in the presence of IL-2 and inhibit efficient antitumor immunity. Of particular interest, these findings provide another important evidence that type I IFNs and type III IFNs can exert distinct biological effects on DC differentiation, phenotype and function.

The finding that, in the MCA205 tumor model, IL-28A-elicited antitumor response was partially abrogated in NK cell-depleted mice strongly implied that NK cells play an important role in the antitumor activity of IL-28A [46]. This finding is consistent with the result demonstrated by Sato *et al.* using the tumor model of B16 melanoma [47]. However, the surprising finding is that IL-28A is unable to directly enhance NK cell cytolytic activity both *in vitro* and *in vivo* [46]. This biological feature of type III IFNs on NK cells is in sharp contrast to type I IFNs, which markedly promote NK cell-mediated cytotoxicity in culture and *in vivo* [91]. In addition, IL-28A does not have capability to directly stimulate the growth of NK cells in culture [46]. On the other hand, IL-28A administration into SCID mice significantly expanded splenic NK cells depending on the dose of injection, and expression of IL-28A in the liver increased the number of hepatic NK cells [46, 47]. In the case of type I IFNs, exposure to type I IFNs is closely associated with NK cell blastogenesis and proliferation, but not IFN-γ expression *in vivo* [92]. Immunoregulatory effect of type I IFNs to elicit the expression of IL-15 in mouse cell populations has been proposed to contribute to the induction of NK cell proliferation [93]. In contrast, the detailed mechanisms for type III IFN-induced proliferation of NK cells *in vivo* remain largely unknown [46, 47]. Nonetheless, type III IFNs appear to augment NK cell-mediated *in vivo* antitumor activity via increasing the total number of NK cells [46]. Another possible explanation of underlying mechanisms is that IL-28A, like IL-21 [94], could enhance the cytolytic activity of NK cells previously activated by stimulators such as other cytokines and chemokines, but could not induce cytotoxic activity in resting NK cells. Recently, Abushahba *et al.* reported that DCs are involved in type III IFN-elicited NK cell activation [95]. DCs stimulated by type III IFNs secreted more amounts of bioactive IL-12, which subsequently activated NK cells [95]. Thus, there is a possibility that type III IFN activates NK cells indirectly via stimulation of DCs.

Polymorphonuclear neutrophils contribute, in some way, to the suppression of tumor growth in the MCA205 tumor model as shown by the fact that treatment with a monoclonal antibody (mAb) against Gr-1 partially abrogated IL-28A-elicited tumor growth suppression [46]. Polymorphonuclear neutrophils can be frequently involved in the generation of CD8 T cell-mediated antitumor responses [96]. Notably, evidence that polymorphonuclear neutrophils may be important for the induction of an antitumor immunity has already been suggested [96], and a specific role for polymorphonuclear neutrophils in the development of CD8 T cell-mediated antitumor responses was also demonstrated [97]. However, little is known about the biological effects of type III IFNs on this cell population. Especially, the direct biological activity of type III IFN on polymorphonuclear neutrophils remains largely to be elucidated. In contrast, type III IFNs are able to positively regulate expression of several chemokines, which activates polymorphonuclear neutrophils. This was first demonstrated in the human in culture systems using peripheral mononuclear cells [82]. Indeed, type III IFN IL-29 induces IL-8 secretion from human peripheral mononuclear cells, especially macrophages, suggesting that type III IFNs at least have capabilities to stimulate polymorphonuclear neutrophils indirectly via induction of chemokines including IL-8 [82].

The fact that MCA205IL-28 cells were more tumorigenic in IFN-γ KO mice than in syngeneic immunocompetent mice indicated that IFN-γ is involved in IL-28A-mediated antitumor responses [46]. Type II IFN IFN-γ is a pleiotropic cytokine that can act on both tumor cells and host immunity [98, 99]. IFN-γ directly inhibits proliferation of some tumor cells and indirectly suppresses tumor growth *in vivo* by activating NK cells and macrophages and inducing angiostatic chemokines such as MIG and IP-10 with consequent inhibition of tumor angiogenesis [100]. Nevertheless, abrogation of IFN-γ could not completely attenuate the antitumor action of IL-28A, indicating that IFN-γ-independent pathways are also involved in IL-28A-mediated antitumor activity [46]. In contrast, based on the finding obtained from the animals treated with neutralizing anti-IL-12 p40 mAb, IL-12 is not involved in type III IFN-mediated antitumor activity [46]. Now, little is known about the relation between type III IFNs and IL-12 expression. On the other hand, in contrast to the IFN-γ promotion of IL-12 expression, type I IFNs can negatively regulate IL-12 expression in DCs and monocytes [101, 102]. Although type III IFNs display overlapping biological activities with type I IFNs, type III IFNs may have ability to up-regulate IL-12 expression by human macrophages and mouse DCs, in contrast to type I IFNs [95, 103]. Now, further analyses are needed to determine the relation between type III IFNs and IL-12 expression. In addition, other cytokines including IL-17 and IL-23 are not required for IL-28A-induced antitumor activity [46].

IFN-γ is partially involved in type III IFN-mediated antitumor action, whereas a wide range of doses of IL-28A exert no direct effects on the release of IFN-γ by NK cells and CD8 T cells stimulated with or without anti-mouse CD3 mAb in culture [46]. In contrast, IL-28A induces IFN-γ release by primary CD4 T cells stimulated with anti-mouse CD3 mAb or co-stimulated with anti-mouse CD3 mAb plus anti-mouse CD28 mAb [48]. This biological effect of IL-28A on IFN-γ secretion appears to be dose-dependent [48]. In addition, this ability of IL-28A to induce IFN-γ secretion by CD4 T cells is T-bet dependent [48]. However, in contrast to IL-12, daily administration of IL-28A into C57BL/6 mice for 3 consecutive days could not induce measurable serum IFN-γ levels *in vivo* [46]. Therefore, the pathway from type III IFNs to IFN-γ expression in the mouse remains to be elucidated.

Abushaba *et al.* recently reported that, using BNL hepatoma line which was resistant to IL-28A treatment due to the lack of IL-28R expression, IL-28A secreted by tumor cells reduced the tumorigenicity and retarded the growth kinetics [95]. In this tumor model, NK cells were predominant effector cells activated indirectly by IL-28A. In addition, the enhanced cytotoxicity against BNL cells mediated by IL-28A was largely dependent on IL-12 produced by DCs and subsequently produced IFN-γ by NK cells [95]. In fact, both myeloid and plasmacytoid DCs responded well to type III IFNs and secreted IL-12 [95]. Therefore, further analyses are needed to elucidate the precise role of IL-12 and IFN-γ in type III IFN-induced antitumor immune responses.

In human systems, with regard to the induction of IFN-γ secretion, a recent report by Jordan *et al.* described that type III IFN IL-29 treatment induced a modest elevation of released IFN-γ in T cells, following stimulation with Con A or in a mixed-lymphocyte reaction (MLR) [81]. Thus, there is a readily accessible and functional pathway from type III IFNs to IFN-γ expression in humans that does not appear to be fully operational in the mouse system. In the case of type I IFNs, there are positive effects on human T cell IFN-γ expression following stimulation with particular molecules including polyI:C [104]. Furthermore, Liu *et al.* demonstrated that, in humans, monocyte-derived macrophages activated by TLR responded to IL-29 stimulation and secreted IL-12 and TNF-α, whereas monocyte and monocyte-derived DCs did not due to the lack of surface IL-28R expression [103]. Monocyte-derived macrophages stimulated with IL-29 responded well to IFN-γ stimulation, and produced significantly more IL-12 through up-regulated IFN-γR1 expression, whereas this activity was not found in IL-28A and IL-28B [103]. In clear contrast, monocyte-derived macrophages stimulated with IFN-α down-regulated surface IFN-γR1 expression [103].

Combination therapy with local production of IL-28A by genetically modified tumor cells and systemic administration of IL-12 protein has a synergistic antitumor effect without apparent deleterious side effects, suggesting possible advantages in this combined therapy [46]. IL-28A secretion or administration of IL-12 rejected none, whereas the combination of two manipulations resulted in rejection of MCA205 cells in 40% of mice and dramatically delayed tumor growth in the remainder [46]. The presence of protective antitumor immunity in the surviving mice indicates that the effectiveness of this combination strategy extends beyond initial rejection of MCA205IL-28 cells to the development of protective long-lasting immunity, which is specific for the initial MCA205 tumor [46]. Studies with lymphocyte subset ablation and using IFN-γ KO mice indicated that rejection of MCA205 tumor cells brought about by the synergistic effects of IL-28A and IL-12 is mediated by systemic antitumor response that is dependent on the presence of both NK cells and CD8 T cells, but not CD4 T cells, and involves IFN-γ [46]. As mentioned above, type III IFNs themselves appear to have, if any, a limited capability to stimulate IFN-γ secretion in mouse systems, whereas type III IFN significantly enhances IL-12-mediated IFN-γ secretion by CD4 T cells stimulated with anti-mouse CD3 mAb *in vitro*, and increases serum IFN-γ concentration and the total number of spleen cells as compared with IL-12 alone in C57BL/6 mice [46, 48]. This biological effect of type III IFN on IL-12-induced IFN-γ expression is common with type I IFN. It has been reported that there is a modest type I IFN effect on IL-12 induction of IFN-γ production by mouse cells in culture [105]. Thus, the enhancement of the antitumor effect by combination therapy of type III IFN IL-28A and IL-12 appears to be, at least in part, dependent on increased IFN-γ production [46].

A surprising finding was that the enhancement of the antitumor effect of IL-28A by systemic treatment with IL-12 protein is found even in IFN-γ KO mice [46]. This finding provides evidence that IL-12 is able to enhance antitumor action of type III IFN through IFN-γ-independent pathways [46]. Of interest, there have been lots of reports describing that antitumor effect of systemic administration of IL-12 protein into mice is largely abrogated in IFN-γ KO mice [106]. On the contrary, in IFN-γ KO mice, IL-12 produced by genetically modified tumor cells is able to induce production of other mediators, instead of IFN-γ, including GM-CSF by both CD4 T cells and CD8 T cells and IL-15 by non-lymphoid cells, which are critically involved in IL-12-induced antitumor activity in IFN-γ KO mice in the C26 tumor model [107, 108]. Thus, IL-12-elicited enhancement of type III IFN-mediated antitumor activity may be due to an indirect effect via the mediators including GM-CSF and IL-15, which are induced by IL-12 in IFN-γ KO mice. In addition, type I IFNs have a biological action to up-regulate expression of the heterodimeric high-affinity receptor for IL-12 comprised of ß1 and ß2 chains [109, 110], and to enhance the biological effects of IL-12. Thus, it was proposed that, like type I IFNs, type III IFNs may enhance IL-12-mediated biological effects on NK cells and T cells via up-regulation of IL-12 receptor expression, leading to augmentation of the antitumor activity.

7. Clinical application of type III IFNs

From *in vitro* and *in vivo* studies using human and murine tumor cells, it has become clear that antitumor effects of type III IFN are less effective compared with those of type I IFN. Therefore, the clinical usage of type III IFNs as anticancer drugs may be relatively limiting. However, one of the suggested benefits of potentially applying type III IFNs to the treatment of cancer is the restricted expression of its specific receptor subunit IL-28R. In this situation, the weaker magnitude of the activity of type III IFNs as compared with that of type I IFNs is anticipated to avoid causing the severe adverse side effects or to reduce the toxicity often observed in patients treated with type I IFNs such as fever, fatigue, hematological toxicity, anorexia, and depression. Actually, animal studies and clinical trials to treat patients with chronic hepatitis C virus (HCV) infection have displayed very few toxic side effects in response to Peg-IFN-λ1 administration at concentrations that elicit comparable antiviral effects as observed with Peg-IFN-α treatment. Additionally, type III IFNs cooperate with type I IFNs to inhibit *in vitro* and *in vivo* NSCLC tumor growth additively via, at least in part, enhanced $p21^{Waf1/Cip1}$ expression and induction of apoptosis [60]. Therefore, although the cooperative antitumor activity of type III IFN and type I IFN against various histological types of tumors has not been fully evaluated, our findings raise the possibility that the interferon combination therapy of type III IFN and type I IFN may not only surpass the therapeutic outcome of IFN-α monotherapy, but also reduce the side effects by decreasing the daily dose of IFN-α.

8. Conclusions and perspectives

Since the discovery of the type III IFN and IL-28R systems in 2003, this novel cytokine family has been demonstrated to have multiple biological actions, which have some similarities with those of type I IFNs. In this chapter, we have reviewed recent studies, describing the potential of type III IFNs in the treatment of cancer. A lot of reports investigating the antitumor activity of type III IFNs in *in vitro* and *in vivo* studies provided clear evidence that type III IFN has multiple biological activities to elicit direct and indirect antitumor activities. However, to date much more remains to be elucidated, not only in terms of mechanisms responsible for the antitumor responses observed in mouse tumor models but also, if any, in terms of adverse effects. The exploitation of recent findings on the antitumor action of type III IFNs will require more detailed information about the biological activities against various cell types. Especially, the biological actions of type III IFNs against different lymphoid subpopulations, including NK cells, T cells, macrophages and DCs, have to be fully clarified. In addition, only few selected points which are specifically important in tumor therapy with type III IFNs, taking into consideration not only type III IFN monotherapy but also combination therapy of type III IFN and chemotherapeutic agent or of type III IFN and type I IFN, which may cooperate for the generation of long-lasting control of tumor growth will be emphasized. Furthermore, separate attention should be paid to the role of endogenous type III IFN in the natural immune control of tumor growth using recently generated IL-28R gene knockout mice [111]. At present, the potential of type III IFNs in a clinical application to cancer therapy is unknown. Further studies will provide a better understanding of whether subtle differences in gene expression induced by type III IFNs relative to type I IFNs may reduce the adverse side effects and increase the efficacy typically seen in type I IFN cancer therapy.

9. References

[1] Isaacs, A., and Lindenmann, J. 1987, J. Interferon Res., 7, 429.
[2] Weissmann, C., and Weber, H. 1986, Prog. Nucleic Acid. Res. Mol. Biol., 33, 251.
[3] Pestka, S., Langer, J.A., Zoon, K.C., and Samuel, C.E. 1987, Annu. Rev. Biochem., 56, 727.

[4] Pestka, S., Krause, C.D., and Walter, M.R. 2004, Immunol. Rev., 202, 8.
[5] Roberts, R.M., Liu, L., Guo, Q., Leaman, D., and Bixby, J. 1998, 18, 805.
[6] LaFleur, D.W., Nardelli, B., Tsareva, T., Mather, D., Feng, P., Semenuk, M., Taylor, K., Buergin, M., Chinchilla, D., Roshke, V., Chen, G., Ruben, S.M., Pitha, P.M., Coleman, T.A., and Moore, P.A. 2001, J. Biol. Chem., 276, 39765.
[7] Peng, F.W., Duan, Z.J., Zheng, L.S., Xie, Z.P., Gao, H.C., Zhang, H., Li, W.P., and Hou, Y.D. 2007, Protein Expr. Purif., 53, 356.
[8] Adolf, G.R. 1990, Virology, 175, 410.
[9] Belardelli, F., Ferrantini, M., Proietti, E., and Kirkwood, J.M. 2002, Cytokine Growth Factor Rev., 13, 119.
[10] Pfeffer, L.M., Dinarello, C.A., Herberman, R.B., Williams, B.R., Borden, E.C., Bordens, R., Walter, M.R., Nagabhushan, T.L., Trotta, P.P., and Pestka, S. 1998, Cancer Res., 58, 2489.
[11] Belardelli, F., and Gresser, I. 1996, Immunol. Today, 17, 369.
[12] Kotenko, S.V., Gallagher, G., Baurin, V.V., Lewis-Antes, A., Shen, M., Shah, N.K., Langer, J.A., Sheikh, F., Dickensheets, H., and Donnelly, R.P. 2003, Nat. Immunol., 4, 69.
[13] Sheppard, P., Kindsvogel, W., Xu, W., Henderson, K., Schlutsmeyer, S., Whitmore, T.E., Kuestner, R., Garrigues, U., Birks, C., Roraback, J., Ostrander, C., Dong, D., Shin, J., Presnell, S., Fox, B., Haldeman, B., Cooper, E., Taft, D., Gilbert, T., Grant, F.J., Tackett, M., Krivan, W., McKnight, G., Clegg, C., Foster, D., and Klucher, K.M. 2003, Nat. Immunol., 4, 63.
[14] Lasfar, A., Lewis-Antes, A., Smirnov, S.V., Anantha, S., Abushahba, W., Tian, B., Reuhl, K., Dickensheets, H., Sheikh, F., Donnelly, R.P., Raveche, E., and Kotenko, S.V. 2006, Cancer Res., 66, 4468.
[15] Onoguchi, K., Yoneyama, M., Takemura, A., Akira, S., Taniguchi, T., Namiki, H., and Fujita, T. 2007, J. Biol. Chem., 282, 7576.
[16] Ank, N., West, H., Bartholdy, C., Eriksson, K., Thomsen, A.R., and Paludan, S.R. 2006, J. Virol., 80, 4501.
[17] Coccia, E.M., Severa, M., Giacomini, E., Monneron, D., Remoli, M.E., Julkunen, I., Cella, M., Lande, R., and Uzé, G. 2004, Eur. J. Immunol., 34, 796.
[18] Tissari, J., Sirén, J., Meri, S., Julkunen, I., and Matikainen, S. 2005, J. Immunol., 174, 4289.
[19] Sirén, J., Pirhonen, J., Julkunen, I., and Matikainen, S. 2005, J. Immunol., 174, 1932.
[20] Ank, N., Iversen, M.B., Bartholdy, C., Staeheli, P., Hartmann, R., Jensen, U.B., Dagnaes-Hansen, F., Thomsen, A.R., Chen, Z., Haugen, H., Klucher, K., and Paludan, S.R. 2008, J. Immunol., 180, 2474.
[21] Langer, J.A., Cutrone, E.C., and Kotenko, S. 2004, Cytokine Growth Factor Rev., 15, 33.
[22] Dumoutier, L., Lejeune, D., Hor, S., Fickenscher, H., and Renauld, J.C. 2003, Biochem. J., 370, 391.
[23] Dumoutier, L., Tounsi, A., Michiels, T., Sommereyns, C., Kotenko, S.V., and Renauld, J.C. 2004, J. Biol. Chem., 279, 32269.
[24] Brand, S., Beigel, F., Olszak, T., Zitzmann, K., Eichhorst, S.T., Otte, J.M., Diebold, J., Diepolder, H., Adler, B., Auernhammer, C.J., Göke, B., and Dambacher, J. 2005, Am. J. Physiol. Gastrointest. Liver Physiol., 289, G960.
[25] Osterlund, P.I., Pietilä, T.E., Veckman, V., Kotenko, S.V., and Julkunen, I. 2007, J. Immunol., 179, 3434.

[26] Zhou, Z., Hamming, O.J., Ank, N., Paludan, S.R., Nielsen, A.L., and Hartmann, R. 2007, J. Virol., 81, 7749.
[27] Sirén, J., Pirhonen, J., Julkunen, I., and Matikainen, S. 2005, J. Immunol., 15, 1932.
[28] Osterlund, P., Veckman, V., Sirén, J., Klucher, K.M., Hiscott, J., Matikainen, S., and Julkunen, I. 2005, J. Virol., 79, 9608.
[29] Matikainen, S., Sirén, J., Tissari, J., Veckman, V., Pirhonen, J., Severa, M., Sun, Q., Lin, R., Meri, S., Uzé, G., Hiscott, J., and Julkunen, I. 2006, J. Virol., 80, 3515.
[30] Davidson, S., Kaiko, G., Loh, Z., Lalwani, A., Zhang, V., Spann, K., Foo, S.Y., Hansbro, N., Uematsu, S., Akira, S., Matthaei, K.I., Rosenberg, H.F., Foster, P.S., and Phipps, S. 2011, J. Immunol., 186, 5938.
[31] Wang, J., Oberley-Deegan, R., Wang, S., Nikrad, M., Funk, C.J., Hartshorn, K.L., and Mason, R.J. 2009, J. Immunol., 182, 1296.
[32] Coccia, E.M., Severa, M., Giacomini, E., Monneron, D., Remoli, M.E., Julkunen, I., Cella, M., Lande, R., and Uzé, G. 2004, Eur. J. Immunol., 34, 796.
[33] Tissari, J., Sirén, J, Meri, S., Julkunen, I., and Matikainen, S. 2005, J. Immunol., 174, 4289.
[34] Kotenko, S.V., Krause, C.D., Izotova, L.S., Pollack, B.P., Wu, W., and Pestka, S. 1997, EMBO J., 16, 5894.
[35] Xie, M.H., Aggarwal, S., Ho, W.H., Foster, J., Zhang, Z., Stinson, J., Wood, W.I., Goddard, A.D., and Gurney, A.L. 2000, J. Biol. Chem., 275, 31335.
[36] Kotenko, S.V., Izotova, L.S., Mirochnitchenko, O.V., Esterova, E., Dickensheets, H., Donnelly, R.P., and Pestka, S. 2001, J. Biol. Chem., 276, 2725.
[37] Sheikh, F., Baurin, V.V., Lewis-Antes, A., Shah, N.K., Smirnov, S.V., Anantha, S., Dickensheets, H., Dumoutier, L., Renauld, J.C., Zdanov, A., Donnelly, R.P., and Kotenko, S.V. 2004, J. Immunol., 172, 2006.
[38] Langer, J.A., Cutrone, E.C., and Kotenko, S.V. 2004, Cytokine Growth Factor Rev., 15, 33.
[39] Donnelly, R.P., Sheikh, F., Kotenko, S.V., and Dickensheets, H. 2004, J. Leukoc. Biol., 76, 314.
[40] Yoon, S.I., Logsdon, N.J., Sheikh, F., Donnelly, R.P., and Walter, M.R. 2006, J. Biol. Chem., 281, 35088.
[41] Wolk, K., and Sabat, R. 2006, Cytokine Growth Factor Rev., 17, 367.
[42] Gibbs, V.C., and Pennica, D. 1997, Gene, 186, 97.
[43] Sommereyns, C., Paul, S., Staeheli, P., and Michiels, T. 2008, PLoS Pathog., 4, e1000017.
[44] Brand, S., Beigel, F., Olszak, T., Zitzmann, K., Eichhorst, S.T., Otte, J.M., Diebold, J., Diepolder, H., Adler, B., Auernhammer, C.J., Göke, B., and Dambacher, J. 2005, Am. J. Physiol. Gastrointest. Liver Physiol., 289, G960.
[45] Meager, A., Visvalingam, K., Dilger, P., Bryan, D., and Wadhwa, M. 2005, Cytokine, 31, 109.
[46] Numasaki, M., Tagawa, M., Iwata, F., Suzuki, T., Nakamura, A., Okada, M., Iwakura, Y., Aiba, S., and Yamaya, M. 2007, J. Immunol., 178, 5086.
[47] Sato, A., Ohtsuki, M., Hata, M., Kobayashi, E., and Murakami, T. 2006, J. Immunol., 176, 7686.
[48] Siebler, J., Wirtz, S., Weigmann, B., Atreya, I., Schmitt, E., Kreft, A., Galle, P.R., and Neurath, M.F. 2007, Gastroenterology, 132, 358.
[49] Pestka, S., Krause, C.D., and Walter, M.R. 2004, Immunol. Rev., 202, 8.
[50] Walter, M.R. 2004, Adv. Protein Chem., 68, 171.

[51] Brand, S., Zitzmann, K., Dambacher, J., Beigel, F., Olszak, T., Vlotides, G., Eichhorst, S.T., Göke, B., Diepolder, H., and Auernhammer, C.J. 2005, Biochem. Biophys. Res. Commun., 331, 543.
[52] Zitzmann, K., Brand, S., Baehs, S., Göke, B., Meinecke, J., Spöttl, G., Meyer, H., and Auernhammer, C.J. 2006, Biochem. Biophys. Res. Commun., 344, 1334.
[53] Pfeffer, L.M., Dinarello, C.A., Herberman, R.B., Williams, B.R., Borden, E.C., Bordens, R., Walter, M.R., Nagabhushan, T.L., Trotta, P.P., and Pestka, S. 1998, Cancer Res., 58, 2489.
[54] Bracci, L., Proietti, E., and Belardelli, F. 2007, Ann. N. Y. Acad. Sci., 1112, 256.
[55] Ferrantini, M., Capone, I., and Belardelli, F. 2007, Biochimie, 89, 884.
[56] Li, Q., Kawamura, K., Ma, G., Iwata, F., Numasaki, M., Suzuki, N., Shimada, H., and Tagawa, M. 2010, Eur. J. Cancer, 46, 180.
[57] Doyle, S.E., Schreckhise, H., Khuu-Duong, K., Henderson, K., Rosler, R., Storey, H., Yao, L., Liu, H., Barahmand-pour, F., Sivakumar, P., Chan, C., Birks, C., Foster, D., Clegg, C.H., Wietzke-Braun, P., Mihm, S., and Klucher, K.M. 2006, Hepatology, 44, 896.
[58] Marcello, T., Grakoui, A., Barba-Spaeth, G., Machlin, E.S., Kotenko, S.V., MacDonald, M.R., and Rice, C.M. 2006, Gastroenterology, 131, 1887.
[59] Guenterberg, K.D., Grignol, V.P., Raig, E.T., Zimmerer, J.M., Chen, A.N., Blaskovits, F.M., Young, G.S., Nuovo, G.J., Mundy, B.L., Lesinski, G.B., and Carson, W.E. 3rd. 2010, Mol. Cancer Ther., 9, 510.
[60] Fujie, H., Tanaka, T., Tagawa, M., Kaijun, N., Watanabe, M., Suzuki, T., Nakayama, K., and Numasaki, M. 2011, Cancer Sci., 102, 1977.
[61] Chin, Y.E., Kitagawa, M., Su, W.C., You, Z.H., Iwamoto, Y., and Fu, X.Y. 1996, Science, 272, 719.
[62] Sangfelt, O., Erickson, S., Einhorn, S., and Grandér, D. 1997, Oncogene, 14, 415.
[63] Sangfelt, O., Erickson, S., Castro, J., Heiden, T., Gustafsson, A., Einhorn, S., and Grandér, D. 1999, Oncogene, 18, 2798.
[64] Iwase, S., Furukawa, Y., Kikuchi, J., Nagai, M., Terui, Y., Nakamura, M., and Yamada, H. 1997, J. Biol. Chem., 272, 12406.
[65] Maher, S.G., Sheikh, F., Scarzello, A.J., Romero-Weaver, A.L., Baker, D.P., Donnelly, R.P., and Gamero A.M. 2008, Cancer Biol. Ther., 7, 1109.
[66] Li, W., Lewis-Antes, A., Huang, J., Balan, M., and Kotenko, S.V. 2008, Cell Prolif., 41, 960.
[67] Lesinski, G.B., Raig, E.T., Guenterberg, K., Brown, L., Go, M.R., Shah, N.N., Lewis, A., Quimper, M., Hade, E., Young, G., Chaudhury, A.R., Ladner, K.J., Guttridge, D.C., Bouchard, P., and Carson, W.E. 3rd. 2008, Cancer Res., 68, 8351.
[68] Fidler, I.J. 2000, J. Natl. Cancer Inst., 28, 10.
[69] Heyns, A.D., Eldor, A., Vlodavsky, I., Kaiser, N., Fridman, R., and Panet, A. 1985, Exp. Cell Res., 161, 297.
[70] Ruszczak, Z., Detmar, M., Imcke, E., and Orfanos, C.E. 1990, J. Invest. Dermatol., 95, 693.
[71] Hicks, C., Breit, S.N., and Penny, R. 1989, Cell Biol., 67, 271.
[72] Brouty-Boyé, D., and Zetter, B.R. 1980, Science, 208, 516.
[73] von Marschall, Z., Scholz, A., Cramer, T., Schäfer, G., Schirner, M., Oberg, K., Wiedenmann, B., Höcker, M., and Rosewicz, S. 2003, J. Natl. Cancer Inst., 95, 437.
[74] Dinney, C.P., Bielenberg, D.R., Perrotte, P., Reich, R., Eve, B.Y., Bucana, C.D., and Fidler, I.J. 1998, Cancer Res., 58, 808.

[75] Singh, R.K., Gutman, M., Llansa, N., and Fidler, I.J. 1996, J. Interferon Cytokine Res., 16, 577.
[76] Fabra, A., Nakajima, M., Bucana, C.D., and Fidler, I.J. 1992, Differentiation, 52, 101.
[77] Ezekowitz, R.A., Mulliken, J.B., and Folkman, J. 1992, N. Engl. J. Med., 326, 1456.
[78] Real, F.X., Oettgen, H.F., and Krown, S.E. 1986, J. Clin. Oncol., 4, 544.
[79] Legha, S.S. 1997, Semin. Oncol., 24(1 Suppl 4), S39.
[80] Stadler, W.M., Kuzel, T.M., Raghavan, D., Levine, E., Vogelzang, N.J., Roth, B., and Dorr, F.A. 1997, Eur. J. Cancer, 33 Suppl 1, S23.
[81] Jordan, W.J., Eskdale, J., Boniotto, M., Rodia, M., Kellner, D., and Gallagher, G. 2007, Genes Immun., 8, 13.
[82] Pekarek, V., Srinivas, S., Eskdale, J., and Gallagher, G. 2007, Genes Immun., 8, 177.
[83] Tough, D.F., Borrow, P., and Sprent, J. 1996, Science, 272, 1947.
[84] Marrack, P., Kappler, J., and Mitchell, T. 1999, J. Exp. Med., 189, 521.
[85] Hung, K., Hayashi, R., Lafond-Walker, A., Lowenstein, C., Pardoll, D., and Levitsky, H. 1998, J. Exp. Med., 188, 2357.
[86] Segal, B.M., Glass, D.D., and Shevach, E.M. 2002, J. Immunol., 168, 1.
[87] Clarke, S.R. 2000, J. Leukoc. Biol., 67, 607.
[88] Lo, C.H., Lee, S.C., Wu, P.Y., Pan, W.Y., Su, J., Cheng, C.W., Roffler, S.R., Chiang, B.L., Lee, C.N., Wu, C.W., and Tao, M.H. 2003, J. Immunol., 171, 600.
[89] Martinotti, A., Stoppacciaro, A., Vagliani, M., Melani, C., Spreafico, F., Wysocka, M., Parmiani, G., Trinchieri, G., and Colombo, M.P. 1995, Eur. J. Immunol., 25, 137.
[90] Sutmuller, R.P., van Duivenvoorde, L.M., van Elsas, A., Schumacher, T.N., Wildenberg, M.E., Allison, J.P., Toes, R.E., Offringa, R., and Melief, C.J. 2001, J. Exp. Med., 194, 823.
[91] Mennechet, F.J., and Uzé, G. 2006, Blood, 107, 4417.
[92] Orange, J.S., and Biron, C.A. 1996, J. Immunol., 156, 4746.
[93] Biron, C.A., Nguyen, K.B., Pien, G.C., Cousens, L.P., and Salazar-Mather, T.P. 1999, Annu. Rev. Immunol., 17, 189.
[94] Kasaian, M.T., Whitters, M.J., Carter, L.L., Lowe, L.D., Jussif, J.M., Deng, B., Johnson, K.A., Witek, J.S., Senices, M., Konz, R.F., Wurster, A.L., Donaldson, D.D., Collins, M., Young, D.A., and Grusby, M.J. 2002, Immunity, 16, 559.
[95] Abushahba, W., Balan, M., Castaneda, I., Yuan, Y., Reuhl, K., Raveche, E., Torre, A.D.L., Lazfar, A., and Kotenko, S.V. 2010, Cancer Immnol. Immunother., 59, 1059.
[96] Stoppacciaro, A., Melani, C., Parenza, M., Mastracchio, A., Bassi, C., Baroni, C., Parmiani, G., and Colombo, M.P. 1993, J. Exp. Med., 178, 151.
[97] Boehm, U., Klamp, T., Groot, M., and Howard, J.C. 1997, Annu. Rev. Immunol., 15, 749.
[98] Dighe, A.S., Richards, E., Old, L.J., and Schreiber, R.D. 1994, Immunity, 1, 447.
[99] Angiolillo, A.L., Sgadari, C., Taub, D.D., Liao, F., Farber, J.M., Maheshwari, S., Kleinman, H.K., Reaman, G.H., and Tosato, G. 1995, J. Exp. Med., 182, 155.
[100] Addison, C.L., Arenberg, D.A., Morris, S.B., Xue, Y.Y., Burdick, M.D., Mulligan, M.S., Iannettoni, M.D., and Strieter, R.M. 2000, Gene Ther., 11, 247.
[101] Cousens, L.P., Orange, J.S., Su, H.C, and Biron, C.A. 1997, Proc. Natl. Acad. Sci. U S A., 94, 634.
[102] McRae, B.L., Semnani, R.T., Hayes, M.P., and van Seventer, G.A. 1998, J. Immunol., 160, 4298.
[103] Liu, B.-S., Janssen, H.L.A., and Boonstra, A. 2010, Blood, 117, 2385.

[104] Sareneva, T., Matikainen, S., Kurimoto, M., and Julkunen, I. 1998, J. Immunol., 160, 6032.

[105] Wenner, C.A., Güler, M.L., Macatonia, S.E., O'Garra, A., and Murphy, K.M. 1996, J. Immunol., 156, 1442.

[106] Mu, J., Zou, J.P., Yamamoto, N., Tsutsui, T., Tai, X.G., Kobayashi, M., Herrmann, S., Fujiwara, H., and Hamaoka, T. 1995, Cancer Res., 55, 4404.

[107] Gri, G., Chiodoni, C., Gallo, E., Stoppacciaro, A., Liew, F.Y., and Colombo, M.P. 2002, Cancer Res., 62, 4390.

[108] Zilocchi, C., Stoppacciaro, A., Chiodoni, C., Parenza, M., Terrazzini, N., and Colombo, M.P. 1998, J. Exp. Med., 188, 133.

[109] Rogge, L., Barberis-Maino, L., Biffi, M., Passini, N., Presky, D.H., Gubler, U., and Sinigaglia, F. 1997, J. Exp. Med., 185, 825.

[110] Rogge, L., D'Ambrosio, D., Biffi, M., Penna, G., Minetti, L.J., Presky, D.H., Adorini, L., and Sinigaglia, F. 1998, J. Immunol., 161, 6567.

[111] Ank, N., Iversen, M.B., Bartholdy, C., Staeheli, P., Hartmann, R., Jensen, U.B., Dagnaes-Hansen, F., Thomsen, A.R., Chen, Z., Haugen, H., Klucher, K., and Paludan, S.R. 2008, J. Immunol., 180, 2474.

10

Interleukin 12: Stumbling Blocks and Stepping Stones to Effective Anti-Tumor Therapy

Hollie J. Pegram[1], Alena A. Chekmasova[1],
Gavin H. Imperato[1] and Renier J. Brentjens[1,2,3,*]
[1]*Department of Medicine, Memorial Sloan-Kettering Cancer Center,*
[2]*Center for Cell Engineering, Memorial Sloan-Kettering Cancer Center,*
[3]*Molecular Pharmacology and Chemistry Program,*
Memorial Sloan-Kettering Cancer Center,
USA

1. Introduction

Interleukin-12 (IL-12) is a heterodimeric pro-inflammatory cytokine long recognized to have properties capable of mediating immune effector functions in a manner compatible to enhancing endogenous anti-tumor immune responses. For this reason the cytokine has garnered significant interest from investigators in the field of immune mediated anti-cancer therapies. While the exact mechanisms whereby IL-12 mediates pro-inflammatory endogenous anti-tumor responses remains to be fully elucidated, pre-clinical murine tumor models demonstrate unequivocal anti-tumor benefit mediated by IL-12 (1-5). Preclinical studies demonstrate that the mechanisms of IL-12 mediated anti-tumor endogenous immune responses seen in these models are likely to be complex and multifactorial. Beyond the ability of IL-12 to induce an inflammatory Th1 $CD4^+$ T cell response, studies have demonstrated the ability of IL-12 to enhance CD8+ T cell cytoxicity. Additionally, preclinical studies have shown IL-12 to recruit and activate innate cytotoxic NK cells and modulate a pro-inflammatory macrophage phenotype. Further, studies have shown that T cell secretion of IFNγ mediated by IL-12 may reverse T cell anergy and confer effector T cell resistance to immune suppressive Tregs. The ability of IL-12 to activate the adaptive as well as the innate immune systems, but also further modulate the otherwise immune-hostile tumor microenvironment, suggests that the cytokine may serve as a potent immunotherapeutic agent. Significantly, pre-clinical murine tumor models have largely validated these predictions. These promising pre-clinical studies consequently spurred on a series of clinical trials treating patients with a variety of tumors with intravenous infusions of recombinant IL-12. Unfortunately, these studies have yielded only modest tumor responses in the context of associated severe and unforeseen toxicities. The IL-12 related toxicities seen in these early clinical trials served to markedly dampen enthusiasm for this cytokine as a potential anti-tumor therapeutic reagent in the clinical setting. However, subsequent clinical trials conducted utilizing direct infusion of IL-12 into accessible tumor sites has resulted in

---

* Corresponding Author

promising anti-tumor responses in the absence of toxicities induced by systemic infusion seen in earlier studies. Thus, based on these clinical trials, the potent anti-tumor effects of IL-12 can best be harnessed by restricting its administration directly into the tumor microenvironment. Therefore, optimal utilization of the anti-tumor efficacy of IL-12 may be realized utilizing novel approaches whereby the cytokine is delivered directly to the site of the tumor with limited systemic distribution to avoid previously observed toxicities. In this chapter, we review the biology of IL-12 and the predicted mechanisms whereby this cytokine may mediate anti-tumor endogenous immune responses. We further discuss pre-clinical studies to support the utilization of IL-12 in cancer therapy as well as clinical trial data, which, in part, have tempered enthusiasm for IL-12 as an effective anti-tumor reagent in the clinical setting due to associated toxicities. Finally, we present and discuss previously published approaches to overcome systemic toxicity through targeted delivery of IL-12 directly into the tumor microenvironment.

2. Basic biology and immune stimulatory effects of IL-12

IL-12 is biologically functional as a heterodimeric molecule consisting of an α and β chain, where covalently-linked p35 and p40 subunits together form the active molecule, IL-12p70 (6-8). The p35 subunit is expressed ubiquitously but only phagocytic cells produce the p40 subunit, therefore functional IL-12p70 is only produced by activated antigen-presenting cells (APCs), neutrophils and macrophages (9). The IL-12 receptor (IL-12R) is composed of two subunits, β1 and β2, and is expressed predominantly on dendritic cells (DCs), T cells and natural killer (NK) cells. The IL-12R mediates signal transduction through the Janus kinases (JAKs) but these pathways will not be discussed here (10).

Initially, IL-12 was described as "Natural killer-stimulating factor" and "cytotoxic lymphocyte maturation factor" and has since been reported to have important effects on the generation of an adaptive immune response (6, 11). It is a potent activator of NK cells, with IL-12 stimulation resulting in enhanced NK cell mediated cytotoxicity (9). The effects of IL-12 on T cells include enhanced cytotoxicity and $CD4^+$ T cell differentiation into type-1 helper T cells (Th1) (12-14). It has also been demonstrated that IL-12 could provide "signal 3" for T cell activation, where signal 2 provides co-stimulation and signal 3 upregulates the expression of the lytic protein Granzyme B, leading to increased cytotoxic effector function and overcoming tolerance (15, 16). IL-12 also mediates significant effects on T cell proliferation. In a murine model of adoptive transfer, OT-1 T cells were inoculated into an irradiated syngeneic mouse and exhibited increased homeostatic proliferation when supported with injection of IL-12 (17). Further studies have demonstrated that T cell expansion was augmented with IL-12 as a result of decreased apoptosis. This was found to be due to decreased Fas expression, increased expression of anti-apoptotic FLIP proteins and inhibition of caspase activation (18). Additionally, it has been reported that IL-12 is important in the fate of $CD8^+$ T cells where IL-12 promotes differentiation into functional effector cells and inhibits memory T cell formation (19).

An additional, but no less important outcome following IL-12 production is the induction of Interferon (IFN)-γ from B, T and NK cells (20-22). IL-12 has positive feedback loops whereby IL-12 stimulates DCs to produce more IL-12, thereby stimulating IFNγ production resulting in additional IL-12 produced by monocytes (23, 24). This IFNγ is able to further activate innate and adaptive immune systems as well as influencing the tumor microenvironment, as discussed below. Many of these IL-12 mediated anti-tumor effects are abrogated upon neutralization of IFNγ thereby demonstrating the importance of this pro-inflammatory cytokine in IL-12 mediated immune stimulation (3, 4, 25).

3. IL-12 in the tumor microenvironment

The wide-ranging effects of IL-12 have profound impacts upon the tumor microenvironment; acting directly on tumor cells, influencing the surrounding tumor stroma/structure, and modulating infiltrating immune cells. These effects, detailed below, mediate the recruitment of lymphocytes, activation of tumor infiltrating lymphocytes, as well as direct effects on tumor cells to decrease angiogenesis which combine to result in tumor eradication or inhibition.

Direct effects of IL-12 on tumor cells may include the ability of IL-12 to up-regulate expression of molecules that induce immune recognition and death of tumor cells. It has been documented that adenoviral mediated expression of IL-12 in human osteosarcoma cells or chemo-resistant breast cancer cells increased expression of Fas, and subsequent apoptosis of tumor cells (26). This was postulated to be a function of the IL-12R β1 chain activating NF-κB, a signaling effect that is thought to be absent in lymphocytes ensuring that IL-12 stimulation of T and NK cells does not result in Fas up-regulation or apoptosis. In a mouse model of mammary adenocarcinoma, it was demonstrated that IL-12 induced IFNγ led to increased surface MHC expression on tumor cells (2), increasing the presentation of tumor-associated antigens to the immune system and resulting in increased edogenous anti-tumor immune responses.

IL-12 is widely reported to increase IFNγ expression, which is responsible for mediating effects directly on the tumor cells, including upregulation of inducible nitric oxide synthase (iNOS) and indolamine 2,3-dioxygenase (IDO) genes, as well as increased MHC expression. Utilizing a murine model of fibrosarcoma, systemic injection of IL-12 was found to induce IFNγ, which in turn mediated increased expression of IDO and iNOS mRNA by tumor cells (3). The products of these genes may slow the growth of tumor cells. IDO is thought to influence tumor growth through the deprivation of tryptophan (27). This was also demonstrated in a study employing a murine model of spontaneous breast cancer treated with systemic IL-12 injection (1).

An important tumor microenvironment modulatory effect by IL-12 is the inhibition of angiogenesis. Folkman and others have elegantly demonstrated the anti-angiogenic role of IL-12 against fibroblast growth factor-induced corneal neo-vascularization. This effect was abrogated upon neutralization of IFN-γ and a downstream effector, IP-10, implicating the latter as the mediator of this effect (28-31). IL-12 has further been shown to mediate down-regulation of pro-angiogenic gene vascular endothelial growth factor (*VEGF*)-*C*, as well as the pro-angiogenic proteins, VEGF and basic fibroblast growth factor (BFGF) on tumor cells and supporting fibroblast cells (32, 33). There is also evidence to suggest that NK cells and $CD8^+$ T cells may contribute to the IL-12 mediated anti-angiogenic effect in some models (34, 35). Cytotoxic T and NK cells were shown to directly lyse epithelial cells, therefore contributing to inhibition of neo-vascularization. It is likely that both secreted factors, such as IP-10 from fibroblasts, as well as direct effects mediated by T and NK cells contribute to the overall anti-angiogenic effects of IL-12.

IL-12 may directly increase the expression of lymphocyte adhesion molecules within tumors, thereby increasing the infiltration of immune effectors into the tumor. For example, treatment of a poorly immunogeneic mammary adenocarcinoma with IL-12 resulted in increased vascular cell adhesion molecule (VCAM)-1 expression within tumors (2). This result was also reported in a murine model of breast cancer (1). In addition, a recent report documented IL-12 mediated activation of lympoid-tissue inducer (LTi) cells, which led to the up-regulation of adhesion molecules and increased leukocyte infiltration (36). Utilizing a murine model of melanoma, it was found that LTi cells expressing the NK cell receptor NKp46, were responsible for up-regulating both VCAM-1 and inter-cellular adhesion molecule (ICAM)-1 within the tumor microenvironment. Up-regulated expression of VCAM-1 has been demonstrated to increase the migration of lymphocytes, therefore allowing increased lymphocytic infiltration into IL-12 treated tumors (37).

A consequence of increased expression of adhesion molecules is the increased infiltration of tumors with immune effector cells, as reported in several studies wherein solid tumors were treated with IL-12. In murine models of mammary adenocarcinoma, lung alveolar carcinoma, fibrosarcoma and spontaneous breast cancer, tumor masses were infiltrated with lymphocytes following systemic IL-12 treatment (1-4, 25, 38). Infiltrating cells were NK cells, $CD8^+$ T cells, $CD4^+$ T cells, and macrophages, depending on the model utilized. Infiltration of lymphocytes is highly important for IL-12 mediated tumor regression, as depletion of CD4 or CD8 T cells prior to treatment abrogated the anti-tumor response in several murine models (2, 4, 5).

IL-12 has further been shown to mediate activation of tumor infiltrating lymphocytes (TILs). In the context of minimal residual disease following transplant in a murine model of lymphoma, IL-12 treatment was shown to activate splenocytes, as noted by up-regulation of CD25 (39). Subsequent studies have demonstrated that IL-12 therapy mediates substantial increase in Granzyme B expression, increased proportion of IFNγ secreting $CD8^+$ T cells, and greater levels of IFNγ secretion in previously quiescent tumor infiltrating $CD8^+$ T cells (38). A recent report has identified the specificity of endogenous T cells activated by IL-12 in a murine model of melanoma (40). This study demonstrated that IL-12 therapy stimulated a protective $CD8^+$ T cell response, where T cells were specific for multiple tumor associated stromal antigens. Other cells activated in response to IL-12 include B cells, as demonstrated by an increase in tumor-reactive antibodies following IL-12 treatment (2). However, the clinical relevance of these tumor reactive antibodies currently remain unclear.

IL-12 may reverse the anergic state of T cells present within the tumor microenvironment. In elegant studies, primary human lung biopsy samples were transplanted into SCID mice and treated with intra-tumoral injection of IL-12 microbeads (41-43). IL-12 therapy was found to mediate regression of tumors, which was dependent on the reactivation of $CD4^+$ T cells within the tumor. These cells were stimulated to proliferate, secrete IFNγ, and mediate complete eradication of the tumor. Additionally, anergy induced in murine $CD4^+$ T cells by regulatory T cells can be overcome with the addition of IL-12 (44). The authors demonstrate that IL-12 mediates effects on the $CD4^+$ effector T cell allowing proliferation and IFNγ secretion despite the presence of suppressive Tregs.

IL-12 has further been demonstrated to impact regulatory cell populations present in the tumor microenvironment. Using a murine model of lung carcinoma, it was demonstrated that IL-12 microsphere therapy resulted in a reduction of $CD4^+$ $CD25^+$ suppressor T cells (38). This study reported an IFNγ dependent induction of apoptosis in the suppressive T cell subset. Relieving tumor resident T cells of suppressive factors may allow the generation of effective endogenous anti-tumor responses. Recent reports have demonstrated that IL-12 can also inhibit the expansion of regulatory T cells (45). IL-12 was found to inhibit the expansion of Tregs *in vitro* and *in vivo* in a murine model of lymphoma. Inhibition of Treg expansion was shown to occur in a IFNγ dependent fashion as IL-12 did not effect Treg expansion in IFNγ receptor deficient mice.

Tumor-associated macrophages (TAMs) play a major role in promoting tumor growth and metastasis and in suppressing the antitumor immune response. Such local immune dysfunction is recognized as one of the major barriers to cancer immunotherapy (46). Macrophages are also functionally plastic, meaning that they can convert between functional states (47). In particular, it has been reported that TAMs can be converted from a M2 suppressive phenotype to an M1 inflammatory phenotype following treatment of tumor-bearing mice with IL-12 containing microspheres (48, 49). Moreover, tumor lesions treated with tumor targeted T cells engineered to secrete IL-12 were infiltrated with activated M1 type of macrophages that were not found in tumors upon T cell therapy without IL-12. The accumulation of activated macrophages was critical to the antitumor immune response as depletion of these macrophages abolished the anti-tumor response (50).

4. Preclinical studies investigating the anti-tumor therapeutic potential of IL-12

Early studies investigating the utilization of IL-12 as an anti-cancer therapeutic agent provided encouraging results, conveying the anti-tumor potential of this powerful cytokine. Intra-tumoral and systemic administration of this cytokine demonstrated marked tumor regression in several murine models of cancer. These include a poorly immunogenic mammary adenocarcinoma, lung alveolar carcinoma, fibrosaroma, spontaneous breast cancer, ovarian carcinoma, lymphoma, renal cell carcinoma, as well as a model of pulmonary metastasis of melanoma (1-5, 38, 39, 51). IL-12 was shown to mediate disease eradication in primary tumors, as well as eradication of metastasis following surgical removal of primary tumors (2). Additionally, using a murine model of minimal residual lymphoma disease following transplant, IL-12 was shown to eradicate disease following transplant without affecting lympho-hematopoietic recovery (39). Significantly, IL-12 exerts anti-tumor effects and mediates tumor regression in models of early, intermediate and late stage disease, illustrating the efficacy of IL-12 anti-cancer therapy even in the setting of advanced disease (51). These studies provided rational for the use of this cytokine in cancer therapy and several clinical approaches to utilize IL-12 in cancer therapy have been developed as discussed below.

Other therapeutic strategies to deliver IL-12 to the tumor microenvironment include the sustained release of cytokine using nanoparticles. Anti-tumor efficacy has been demonstrated in a murine model of mammary carcinoma, wherein IL-12 microsphere treatment was found to result in NK cell mediated anti-tumor effects (52). Combination therapy involving IL-12 and TNFα receptor microspheres was found to lead to superior anti-tumor function with the recruitment of $CD8^+$ T cells. Additional studies of IL-12 microsphere treatment utilized a combination of IL-12 and GM-CSF, which mediated regression of lung alveolar carcinomas in a murine model (38, 53). This study reported IL-12 mediated effects including reactivation of tumor resident T cells as well as predicted apoptosis of regulatory T cells. The anti-tumor efficacy of polymer-mediated IL-12 delivery has also been tested in murine models of malignant glioma and disseminated ovarian cancer (54, 55). These studies validate the nanoparticle mediated delivery approach, demonstrating a sustained release and therapeutic efficacy, whilst contributing to the understanding of the mechanisms of IL-12 mediated anti-tumor efficacy.

As an alternative approach to systemic infusion of IL-12, specific delivery of IL-12 directly into the tumor site may be achieved through gene therapy strategies. One such approach utilizes adenoviral vector mediated delivery of the IL-12 gene with subsequent expression and secretion of IL-12 by the infected cell. In this manner, direct intra-tumoral injection of adenovirus encoding the IL-12 gene resulted in anti-tumor responses in murine models of melanoma, laryngeal squamous cell carcinoma, glioma, renal cell carcinoma and bladder cancer (40, 56-59). Other models utilizing combinations of adenovirus and other chemotherapies have also demonstrated encouraging results. It was shown that a combination of cyclophosphamide and intra-tumoral injection of adenoviral gene transfer of IL-12 resulted in tumor eradication in a murine model of colorectal cancer (60). Additional strategies to further improve the safety of this response involve the utilization of organ specific, drug inducible adenoviral vectors. One study reported the use of a liver-specific, mifepristone-inducible adenoviral vector encoding IL-12 for the treatment of colorectal cancer liver metastasis (61). This system allowed for controlled and long term expression of the vector following systemic infusion, and was enhanced by additional treatment with the chemotherapeutic agent oxaliplatin (62). Other strategies testing drug inducible IL-12 expression have yielded similar results, confirming the ability to tightly control IL-12 production *in vivo* (63).

Additional viral vector based strategies include the utilization of other oncolytic viruses, which preferentially infect and lyse tumor cells. Intra-tumoral injection of a vesicular stomatitis virus carrying an IL-12 transgene was demonstrated to reduce tumor volume in a murine model of squamous cell carcinoma (64). This reduction in tumor volume correlated to an increased survival of treated tumor bearing mice.

Other delivery strategies include electroporation, where a voltage is applied to a cell membrane, allowing entry of plasmid DNA into a cell. To achieve this *in vivo*, studies have injected plasmids encoding the IL-12 gene intra-tumorally, followed by *in vivo* electroporation to allow for the introduction and expression of the gene into and by the regional cells (65). Utilizing a murine model of melanoma, it was found that electroporation of the IL-12 gene into the tumor resulted in tumor eradication in 47% of mice (65). This study also demonstrated the ability of IL-12 to stimulate an endogenous anti-tumor immune response as surviving mice were resistant to tumor re-challenge. Therapy resulted in increased levels of IL-12 and IFNγ in the tumor, increased lymphocyte infiltration and reduction in vascularity. These findings are consistent with previously documented effects of IL-12. This approach has similarly been successfully applied to a murine model of fibrosarcoma (66).

Other novel strategies to target IL-12 to the tumor site include anchoring IL-12 to a tumor-specific protein. One group utilized a single chain variable fragment (scFv) from an antibody specific to erbB2 anchored to IL-12 to specifically deliver IL-12 to $erbB2^+$ murine bladder cancers (67). This approach resulted in increased survival but failed to completely eradicate established disease. Similarly, investigators linked a IL-13Rα3 protein to IL-12 as a means of targeting murine melanoma (68). This group chose IL-13Rα3 as it can be a negative regulator of tumors that utilize IL-13 as a pro-tumorigenic factor. This therapy led to a significant NK T cell mediated inhibition of tumor growth *in vivo*.

Indeed, combinations of these treatment modalities have also yielded encouraging results in preclinical testing. Intra-tumoral injection of adenovirus encoding IL-12 and 4-1BBL combined with DC injection was found to mediate marked inhibition of tumor growth in a murine model of melanoma (69). Another study demonstrated the intra-tumoral injection of IL-12 encoding plasmid followed by DC vaccination led to the suppression of primary hepatocellular carcinoma and metastases (70). Significantly, utilization of this combined immune based therapy approach to augment surgical resection of primary tumor yielded superior results, leading to long term survival and resistance to tumor re-challenge in murine models of ovarian cancer, prostate cancer and hepatocellular carcinoma (51); (71); (72). Combination of IL-12 gene therapy with IL-27 gene therapy, or retinoic acid based therapies have also been described, with encouraging responses against systemic tumors (73, 74).

5. Clinical trials: Toxicity tempers the potential of IL-12 as an anti-cancer agent

Previous pre-clinical studies demonstrating the anti-tumor efficacy of IL-12 warranted the translation of this therapeutic agent to the clinical setting. A number of tumors were targeted in these trials, with modest, mixed responses. The first published trial of systemically administered IL-12 was a phase I dose escalation trial of intravenous (i.v.) administered recombinant human interleukin 12 (rhIL-12) (75). Cohorts of four to six patients with advanced solid tumor malignancies received escalating doses (3-1000 ng/kg/day) of rhIL-12 by bolus i.v. injection once and then, after a 2-week rest period, once daily for five days every 3 weeks. Forty patients were enrolled on this study including 20 with renal cell carcinomas, 12 with melanoma, and 5 with colon cancer. One melanoma patient experienced a complete regression of metastatic disease for a period of four weeks, while a second patient with renal cell carcinoma experienced a partial response that was ongoing at 22 months. Toxicities observed in this trial were fever, chills, fatigue, nausea, vomiting, and headache. Routine laboratory findings reported abnormalities including anemia, neutropenia, lymphopenia, hyperglycemia, thrombocytopenia, and hypoalbuminemia. Dose limiting toxicities included oral stomatitis and elevated transaminases. The maximum tolerated dose (MTD) (500 ng/kg) was associated with asymptomatic hepatic function test abnormalities in three patients and one on study death due to *Clostridia perfringens* septicemia. Lymphopenia was observed at all dose levels, with recovery occurring within several days of completing treatment without rebound lymphocytosis (75). These adverse events were hypothesized to be related to administration of recombinant human IL-12 and so the immune effects of this therapy were interrogated. Consistent with pre-clinical data, IL-12 was shown to up-regulate IFNγ, in a dose-dependent fashion. Additionally, a single 500 ng/kg dose of rhIL-12 was shown to increase NK cell cytolytic activity and T cell proliferation, as determined by studies on peripheral blood samples collected pre and post treatment (76). In a subsequent Phase II study of 17 patients investigators observed unexpected toxicities related to the dosing schedule of IL-12 administration (77). On this study, 12 out of 17 patients required hospitalization and two patients died. Two patients deaths occurred during the phase II study were determined to be related to IL-12 administration. Postmortem examination of these two patients showed hemorrhagic ulceration in the large intestine (patient 1) and necrotizing aspiration pheumonia and diffuse hemorrhagic colitis (patient 2). The constitutional, cardiac, renal, hematopoietic, hepatic and neurologic toxicities observed in the phase II were similar to those dose-limiting toxicities observed on phase I studies with IL-12. These toxicities resulted in the suspension of IL-12 trials by the Food and Drug Administration (FDA). Significantly, investigators subsequently determined that a single IL-12 infused loading dose given two weeks prior to consecutive treatments (as done in the initial trial) abrogated these observed toxicities.

A subsequent study by Gollob and colleagues (78), the authors describe two patients with renal cell carcinoma treated with twice-weekly intravenous rhIL-12 during a phase I trial. A cycle of therapy lasted 6 weeks. The patients had grade 4 neutropenia and grade 3 hemolytic anemias. The severe neutropenia was associated with bone marrow agranulocytosis and a preponderance of large granular lymphocytes in the peripheral blood, whereas the hemolytic anemia was associated with splenomegaly. Both patients had stable disease 4 months after the IL-12 treatment was stopped with persisted agranulocytosis and hemolytic anemia.

Additionally, thirty-four patients with measurable metastatic, recurrent or inoperable cervical carcinoma were enrolled on phase I clinical trial to investigate the anti-tumor effect of i.v administrated IL-12 at 250 ng/kg daily up to 21 days. Over half of these patients had received prior cisplatin-based chemotherapy. The most common serious toxicities were hematologic or hepatic, and all were reversible. The median survival was 6.5 months. This was the first clinical trial to demonstrate induction of cell-mediated immune (CMI) responses to specific antigens (HPV16 E4, E6, and E7 peptides) following treatment with IL-12 in women with cervical cancer. However, this improvement in immune response was not associated with enhanced objective response or survival (79).

Pharmacokinetic advantages of intraperitoneal (i.p.) rhIL-12 infusion, tumor response to i.p. delivery of cytokines, as well as its potential anti-angiogenic effect provided the rationale for further evaluation of rhIL-12 in patients with refractory or relapsed ovarian or peritoneal carcinoma. In this study (80) rhIL-12 was administered to 29 previously treated patients with peritoneal carcinomatosis from Müllerian carcinomas, gastrointestinal tract carcinomas and peritoneal mesothelioma in a phase I trial. rhIL-12 doses were dose escalated between patients from 3 to 600 ng/kg weekly up to 6 months. Three or more patients at each level received weekly i.p. injections of rhIL-12. Dose-limiting toxicity (grade 3 elevated transaminase levels) occurred in 50% of treated patients at the 600 ng/kg dose. More frequent, but less severe, toxicities included fever, fatigue, abdominal pain, and nausea. Ten patients received 300 ng/kg with acceptable frequency and severity of side effects. Two patients (one with ovarian cancer and one with mesothelioma) had no remaining disease at laparoscopy. Eight patients had stable disease and 19 patients had progressive disease. Cytokines including IL-1α, IL-2, IL-10, TNFα, and IFNγ were determined in serum and peritoneal fluid samples during therapy. Immunobiological effects included peritoneal tumor cell apoptosis, decreased tumor cell expression of BFGF and VEGF, elevated IFNγ levels and IP-10 transcripts in peritoneal exudate, and increased proportions of peritoneal $CD3^+$ T cells relative to $CD14^+$ monocytes (80). In a subsequent phase II trial thirty-four patients with ovarian carcinoma or primary peritoneal carcinoma were treated i.p. with rIL-12 (300 ng/kg weekly) (81). 12 patients completed this second phase were evaluated for response. There were no treatment related deaths, peritonitis or significant catheter related complications. Toxicities included grade 4 neutropenia (1), grade 3 fatigue (4), headache (2), myalgia (2), non-neutropenic fever (1), drug fever (1), back pain (1), and dizziness (1). Two patients had stable disease (SD) and 9 had progressive disease (PD). The authors concluded that rIL-12 can safely be administered by i.p. scheduled to patients after first line chemotherapy for ovarian/peritoneal carcinoma. Future i.p. therapies with rhIL-12 will require better understanding and control of pleiotropic effects of IL-12 since proteins with potential for both anti-tumor (IFNγ, IP-10) and pro-tumor growth effects (VEGF, IL-8) were detected in this study (81).

To avoid toxicities associated with systemic infusion of rIL-12, others have investigated subcutaneous administration of IL-12. Rook and colleagues initiated a phase I dose escalation trial of rhIL-12 treating 10 patients with cutaneous T-cell lymphoma (CTCL) with dose escalating regimens of subcutaneous (s.c.) 50, 100, or 300 ng/kg rhIL-12 twice weekly or intralesional injections for up to 24 weeks (82). Histological analysis of regressing skin lesions revealed increased numbers of $CD8^+$ T cells. In contrast to systemic rIL-12 infusion, sq or intralesional rIL-12 regimens were well tolerated with adverse effects limited to low-grade fevers and headaches.

Similarly, in another phase I trial, 28 patients with advanced renal cell carcinoma were treated s.c. with rhIL-12 that was administered on day 1 and followed on day 8 with repeated s.c. injections 3 times a week for 2 weeks. The MTD of the initial injection was evaluated at dose levels of 0.1, 0.5, and 1.0 μg/kg. A dose limiting toxicity (DLT) was observed at 1.0 μg/kg consisting of fever, perivasculitis of the skin, and leukopenia. Other notable toxicities were oral mucositis and transaminitis. These toxicities were more severe after the initial injection than after repeated injections at the same dose level. In this study, one patient had a partial response and seven patients had stable disease (83).

The efficacy of s.c. rhIL-12 for the treatment of patients with early mycosis fungoides (MF; stage IA-IIA) has similarly been tested in a phase I clinical trial. In this study rhIL-12 was administered subcutaneously biweekly (100 ng/kg for 2 weeks; 300 ng/kg thereafter). Ten of 23 patients (43%) achieved partial responses (PR); 7 (30%) achieved minor responses; and 5 (22%) had stable disease. The duration of PRs ranged from 3 to more than 45 weeks. Twelve patients (52%) ultimately progressed with a mean time to progression of 57 days (range, 28-805). Seventeen patients had treatment-related adverse events that were generally mild to moderate in severity including asthenia, headache, chills, fever, injection site reaction, pain, myalgia, arthralgia, transaminitis, anorexia, and sweating. One patient in PR died of hemolytic anemia, possibly exacerbated by rhIL-12 treatment (84).

Little and colleagues conducted phase II clinical trial wherein 36 patients with AIDS-associated Kaposi sarcoma requiring chemotherapy were treated with six 3-week cycles of pegylated liposomal doxorubicin (20 mg/m^2) plus interleukin-12 (300 ng/kg subcutaneously twice weekly), followed by 500 ng/kg subcutaneous IL-12 twice weekly for up to 3 years (85). Thirty patients had a major response, including 9 with a complete response, with an 83% overall response rate. Patients had elevated levels of IFNγ and IP-10 in their serum, indicative of an rIL-12 mediated immune response.

Finally, 42 previously treated patients (32 patients with relapsed or refractory non-Hodgkin's lymphoma (NHL) and 10 patients with relapsed Hodgkin's disease (HD)) were enrolled in a phase II clinical trial to evaluate the clinical activity and toxicity of rIL-12. Patients were treated with either intravenous (n = 11) or subcutaneous (n = 31) rIL-12. The patients had received a median of three prior treatment regimens, and 16 patients had undergone prior autologous stem cell transplantation. All patients were assessable for toxicity, and 39 of 42 (93%) patients were assessable for response. Six of 29 (21%) patients with NHL had a partial or complete response, whereas none of the 10 patients with HD responded to rIL-12 therapy. Furthermore, 15 patients had stable disease that lasted for up to 54 months. The most common toxicity was flu-like symptoms. Reversible grade 3 hepatic toxicity was observed in three patients requiring dose reduction (86). This study demonstrated increased numbers of peripheral blood CD8$^+$ T cells as well as decreased VEGF and BFGF in 37% of the treated patients indicative of a rIL-12 mediated immune response.

Additional methods of delivering IL-12 to the tumor site have been investigated. Ten previously untreated patients with head and neck squamous cell carcinomas (HNSCC) received direct injection of rhIL-12 in the primary tumor weekly, at two dose levels of 100 or 300 ng/kg, as neoadjuvant therapy prior to surgical resection. In this trial the histologic and immunohistopathologic effects of intratumorally (i.t) infused rhIL-12 were evaluated in the primary tumors and regional lymph nodes. In the primary tumor, the number of CD56$^+$ NK cells was increased in rhIL-12-treated patients compared with control non-rhIL-12 treated patients. After i.t. rhIL-12 treatment of HNSCC patients, significant effects were noted on B cells, with altered lymph node architecture in every IL-12-treated patient and excessive peritumoral infiltration of B cells in some patients (87, 88).

In a phase I/II clinical trial (89), plasmid DNA encoding human IL-12 was produced under good manufacturing practice (GMP) conditions and injected into lesions of nine patients with stage IV malignant melanoma previously treated with both standard and salvage chemotherapy regimens. Plasmid DNA was injected in cycles, three injections per cycle, for up to seven cycles. One cycle consisted of three injections at weekly interval, that is, on day 1, 8 and 15, followed by a resting period of about 8 days (89). Local injection site anti-tumor responses were seen in a majority of patients, with four patients exhibiting responses at distant metastases and a complete remission was achieved in one patient. Biopsies of lesions from responding patients demonstrated a predicted increase in IL-12, IFNγ and IP-10 expression analyzed by real-time polymerase chain reaction.

In a similar study, nine patients with metastatic melanoma were treated by intra-tumoral injection of a recombinant viral vector expressing human IL-12 derived from the canarypox virus (ALVAC-IL-12). Increases in IL-12 and IFNγ mRNA, were observed in ALVAC-IL-12-

injected tumors compared with saline-injected control tumors in four of the nine patients. ALVAC-IL-12-injected tumors were also characterized by increased T cell infiltration of the tumor (90). This therapy was well tolerated with no reported dose limiting toxicities. One patient achieved a complete response in the injected subcutaneous metastasis, but all patients developed neutralizing IgG antibodies to the viral vector, demonstrating a limitation to this viral delivery strategy.

Viral vectors, probably the most commonly used for gene delivery, often result in host immune response, systemic toxicity and integration into host genome. Plasmid DNA-based vectors avoid these problems but are lacking in efficient gene transfer efficiency. In vivo electroporation, which utilizes an electric charge to facilitate entry of macromolecules into the cell, can be a reproducible and highly efficient method to deliver plasmid DNA. A phase I dose escalation trial of plasmid IL-12 gene electroporation was studied in patients with metastatic melanoma. Patients received electroporation treatments on days 1, 5, and 8 during a single 39-day cycle, into metastatic melanoma lesions through a penetrating six-electrode array immediately after DNA injection. A sterile applicator containing six needle electrodes arranged in the circle was inserted into the tumor and six pulses at field strength of 1,300 Volts/cm and pulse duration of 100 μs were applied using a Medpulser DNA EPT System Generator. Twenty-four patients were treated at seven dose levels, with minimal systemic toxicity. Transient pain after electroporation was the primary adverse effect. Post-treatment biopsies showed plasmid dose proportional increases in IL-12 levels as well as marked tumor necrosis and increased lymphocytic infiltrate. Two of 19 patients with nonelectroporated distant lesions and no other systemic therapy showed complete regression of all metastases, whereas eight additional patients (42%) showed disease stabilization or partial responses (91).

A phase I trial to assess the safety and tolerability of i.p. injected human IL-12 plasmid (phIL-12) formulated with a synthetic lipopolymer, polyethyleneglycol-polyethyleneimine-cholesterol (PPC), was conducted in women with chemotherapy-resistant recurrent ovarian cancer. A total of 13 patients were enrolled in four dose-escalating cohorts and treated with 0.6, 3, 12 or 24 mg/m^2 of the formulated plasmid once every week for 4 weeks (92). This approach is attractive because of the ability of nanoparticles to transport larger amounts of genetic material than viral vectors, as well as the ability of this approach to bypass the induction of an endogenous immune response as is the case with viral vectors (93). However, nanoparticles lack the specificity required to home to sites of tumor (92). Intraperitoneal administration of this IL-12 gene bearing nanoparticle was well-tolerated, with mild to moderate fevers and abdominal pain reported for each patient. Treatment was associated with stable disease and decrease in serum cancer antigen (CA)-125 by 3% in one of the three patients in cohort-1; 36 and 86% in two of three patients in cohort-2; and 2, 11 and 16% in three of four patients in cohort-4 at the 5-week follow-up visit. There was an overall clinical response of 31% stable disease and 69% progressive disease at the 5±1 week post-treatment follow-up visits.

At present, several additional trials utilizing IL-12 as an anti-cancer therapy are currently enrolling patients. Avigan and colleagues are recruiting patients for a phase I/II trials to evaluate co-administration of a dendritic cell/tumor fusion vaccine with subcutaneously administered IL-12 to patients with stage IV breast cancer (Avigan D., Vaccination of patients with breast cancer with dendritic cell/tumor fusions and IL-12, NCT00622401).

Gajewski and colleagues are investigating the role of multipeptide vaccination with or without an admixture of intradermally or subcutaneously delivered IL-12, with subsequent daclizumab therapy in patients with metastatic melanoma (Gajewski T.F., A randomized phase II study of multipeptide vaccination with or without IL-12, then combined with regulatory T cell depletion using daclizumab in patients with metastatic melanoma, NCT01307618). A group at the National Cancer Institute is conducting a clinical trial using a novel IL-12 agent in patients with treatment-refractory solid tumors. This trial is designed to test the safety and effectiveness of experimental drug NHS-IL12 as a treatment for solid tumors that have not responded to standard treatments. The NHS-IL12 immunocytokine is composed of 2 IL-12 heterodimers, each fused to one of the V_H-chains of the NHS76 antibody, which has affinity for both single- and double-stranded DNA. Thus, NHS-IL12 targets delivery to regions of tumor necrosis where DNA has become exposed (NCT01417546). Other phase I/II study of metastatic melanoma will be conducted by Rosenberg group at NCI using lymphodepleting conditioning followed by infusion of tumor infiltrating lymphocytes genetically modified to express IL-12 (NCT01236573) (see below). These ongoing clinical trials convey the potential of this powerful immune stimulatory cytokine, while highlighting the necessity for careful dosing and more importantly, targeted delivery to reduce the risks of toxicity.

6. The promise of adoptive cell immunotherapy

Adoptive cell therapy involves the isolation, modification and expansion of endogenous immune cells, followed by the *ex vivo* expansion of and re-infusion of these cells into a tumor-bearing host. Indeed, the use of cells to deliver IL-12 to a tumor is attractive as natural immune cell features can be exploited whilst delivering IL-12 to the tumor microenvironment. One such example of this approach is the utilization of mesenchymal stem cells (MSCs) to deliver IL-12. MSCs have a widely reported ability to traffic to sites of tumor growth making them ideal delivery for IL-12 (94). Several groups have reported the use of MSCs to deliver IL-12 to tumors in murine models of glioma, renal cell carcinoma, breast cancer, melanoma, Ewing sarcoma and prostate cancer (95-99). These studies demonstrate that MSCs are successful delivery vehicles of IL-12 and the IL-12 delivered mediates anti-tumor responses in preclinical murine models involving increased IFNγ, increased infiltration of T cells and anti-angiogenic effects (95).

Antigen presenting cells (APCs) can also be utilized in cell transfer therapy. Although APCs have the endogenous capacity to produce IL-12, the hostile tumor microenvironment often suppresses this immune stimulatory response. Adoptive transfer of APCs genetically modified to continually produce IL-12 is aimed at initiating an endogenous anti-tumor immune response. The most commonly utilized APCs for IL-12 delivery are DCs. Intratumoral injection of DCs modified to express IL-12 mediated complete regression of neuroblastoma tumor in a mouse model (100). This effect was shown to correlate with increased tumor-specific splenocyte cytoxic capacity. Other groups have tested this approach in murine liver tumor models with similar encouraging responses (101). This latter study specifically demonstrated the generation of a protective immune response, which was dependent on T and NK cells. One alteration of this approach involves the pulsing of the IL-12 modified DCs with tumor lysates to increase the immune-stimulatory capacity of the injected cells. Using a model of colon cancer, mice were treated with tumor lysate pulsed,

IL-12 gene modified DCs which was found to dramatically inhibit tumor growth (102). This therapy resulted in an increase of endogenous immune tumor specific cytotoxicity and increased IFNγ levels, consistent with previously reported effects of IL-12. Injection of IL-12 gene modified macrophages was also found to inhibit tumor growth and spontaneous metastasis following prostatectomy in a murine model of prostate cancer (71). These studies support the utilization of APC mediated delivery of IL-12 to the tumor microenvironment as a method to initiate an effective endogenous anti-tumor response.

Other immune cells employed in adoptive transfer anti-cancer therapy include adaptive immune effector cells. Cytokine induced killer (CIK) cells are generation by the *ex vivo* activation and expansion of T cells, resulting in a cell population with both T and NK cell phenotypes (103). Using a preclinical, immunocompetent murine model of breast cancer, it was shown that augmentation of CIK therapy with IL-12 resulted in enhanced anti-tumor efficacy and complete remission in 75% of mice following therapy (104). This was found to be due to IL-12-mediated increased immune mediated cytotoxicity, improved homing and persistence, as well as *in vivo* proliferation of transferred CIK cells.

A similar strategy to deliver IL-12 specifically to tumor cells involves the use of tumor-specific T cells (50, 105). In an initial report, transgenic mouse T cells specific for the gp100 melanoma antigen were genetically modified to express an IL-12 transgene (105). These cells were then infused into irradiated mice bearing subcutaneous melanoma tumors. It was found that these IL-12 producing targeted T cells mediated rejection of tumor with dose responsive toxicity. When lower numbers of T cells were transferred into these mice, toxicity was absent and anti-tumor effects still eradicated advanced tumors, though effective therapy still required prior lymphodepletion. These anti-tumor effects were dependent on the IL-12 being present in the tumor microenvironment as T cells cultured *ex vivo* in IL-12 did not have similar anti-tumor activity. Consistent with previously published results, therapy was associated with $CD8^+$ T and NK cell infiltration and a reduction of Foxp3 expression within the tumor. To further improve the safety of this approach, an additional study reported control of IL-12 expression by a promoter containing binding sites for nuclear factor of activated T cells (NFAT) resulting in IL-12 production only upon T cell activation within the targeted tumor microenvironment (106). An additional report describes the isolation of murine T cells, genetically engineered *ex vivo* to express the IL-12 transgene and a chimeric antigen receptor (CAR) targeted to the carcinoembryonic antigen expressed on colon cancers (50). This study demonstrated the translational applicability of this approach, and a novel potentially clinically applicable approach to tumor targeted delivery of the IL-12 cytokine. This approach is currently being investigated in a clinical trial, as described to above. Rosenberg and colleagues are currently enrolling patients in a trial utilizing *ex vivo* expanded tumor-infiltrating lymphocytes modified to produce IL-12 for the treatment of metastatic melanoma (NCT1236573).

7. Conclusion

IL-12 is a potent mediator of anti-tumor immunity. The exact mechanisms of IL-12 mediated anti-tumor effects continue to warrant further investigation. While translation to the clinical setting has been hampered by toxicity and modest anti-tumor efficacy, localized delivery of IL-12 directly into the tumor may prove to be a successful approach in limited numbers of accessible tumors. However, it is perhaps in the setting of adoptive T cell immunotherapy utilizing IL-12 secreting, tumor specific T cells, where the full anti-tumor benefit of IL-12 therapy will be realized with tumor targeted, locally secreted cytokine. This approach will avert systemic toxicity while providing the requisite boost to the endogenous immune system to fully eradicate tumor. IL-12 remains a unique and promising cytokine with marked anti-tumor activity and warrants continued rigorous investigation in both the pre-clinical and clinical settings in order to realize the full anti-tumor potential of this reagent.

8. Competing interests statement

The authors have no competing professional, financial, or personal interests that may have affected the presentation of this manuscript.

9. References

[1] Boggio K, Nicoletti G, Di Carlo E, Cavallo F, Landuzzi L, Melani C, Giovarelli M, Rossi I, Nanni P, De Giovanni C, Bouchard P, Wolf S, Modesti A, Musiani P, Lollini PL, Colombo MP, Forni G. 1998. Interleukin 12-mediated prevention of spontaneous mammary adenocarcinomas in two lines of Her-2/neu transgenic mice. *J Exp Med* 188: 589-96

[2] Cavallo F, Di Carlo E, Butera M, Verrua R, Colombo MP, Musiani P, Forni G. 1999. Immune events associated with the cure of established tumors and spontaneous metastases by local and systemic interleukin 12. *Cancer Res* 59: 414-21

[3] Yu WG, Yamamoto N, Takenaka H, Mu J, Tai XG, Zou JP, Ogawa M, Tsutsui T, Wijesuriya R, Yoshida R, Herrmann S, Fujiwara H, Hamaoka T. 1996. Molecular mechanisms underlying IFN-gamma-mediated tumor growth inhibition induced during tumor immunotherapy with rIL-12. *Int Immunol* 8: 855-65

[4] Nastala CL, Edington HD, McKinney TG, Tahara H, Nalesnik MA, Brunda MJ, Gately MK, Wolf SF, Schreiber RD, Storkus WJ, et al. 1994. Recombinant IL-12 administration induces tumor regression in association with IFN-gamma production. *J Immunol* 153: 1697-706

[5] Brunda MJ, Luistro L, Warrier RR, Wright RB, Hubbard BR, Murphy M, Wolf SF, Gately MK. 1993. Antitumor and antimetastatic activity of interleukin 12 against murine tumors. *J Exp Med* 178: 1223-30

[6] Kobayashi M, Fitz L, Ryan M, Hewick RM, Clark SC, Chan S, Loudon R, Sherman F, Perussia B, Trinchieri G. 1989. Identification and purification of natural killer cell stimulatory factor (NKSF), a cytokine with multiple biologic effects on human lymphocytes. *J Exp Med* 170: 827-45

[7] Stern AS, Podlaski FJ, Hulmes JD, Pan YC, Quinn PM, Wolitzky AG, Familletti PC, Stremlo DL, Truitt T, Chizzonite R, et al. 1990. Purification to homogeneity and partial characterization of cytotoxic lymphocyte maturation factor from human B-lymphoblastoid cells. *Proc Natl Acad Sci U S A* 87: 6808-12

[8] Carra G, Gerosa F, Trinchieri G. 2000. Biosynthesis and posttranslational regulation of human IL-12. *J Immunol* 164: 4752-61

[9] Trinchieri G. 2003. Interleukin-12 and the regulation of innate resistance and adaptive immunity. *Nat Rev Immunol* 3: 133-46

[10] O'Shea JJ, Gadina M, Schreiber RD. 2002. Cytokine signaling in 2002: new surprises in the Jak/Stat pathway. *Cell* 109 Suppl: S121-31

[11] Wolf SF, Temple PA, Kobayashi M, Young D, Dicig M, Lowe L, Dzialo R, Fitz L, Ferenz C, Hewick RM, et al. 1991. Cloning of cDNA for natural killer cell stimulatory factor, a heterodimeric cytokine with multiple biologic effects on T and natural killer cells. *J Immunol* 146: 3074-81

[12] Hsieh CS, Macatonia SE, Tripp CS, Wolf SF, O'Garra A, Murphy KM. 1993. Development of TH1 CD4+ T cells through IL-12 produced by Listeria-induced macrophages. *Science* 260: 547-9

[13] Del Vecchio M, Bajetta E, Canova S, Lotze MT, Wesa A, Parmiani G, Anichini A. 2007. Interleukin-12: biological properties and clinical application. *Clin Cancer Res* 13: 4677-85

[14] Macgregor JN, Li Q, Chang AE, Braun TM, Hughes DP, McDonagh KT. 2006. Ex vivo culture with interleukin (IL)-12 improves CD8(+) T-cell adoptive immunotherapy for murine leukemia independent of IL-18 or IFN-gamma but requires perforin. *Cancer Res* 66: 4913-21

[15] Curtsinger JM, Lins DC, Johnson CM, Mescher MF. 2005. Signal 3 tolerant CD8 T cells degranulate in response to antigen but lack granzyme B to mediate cytolysis. *J Immunol* 175: 4392-9

[16] Curtsinger JM, Lins DC, Mescher MF. 2003. Signal 3 determines tolerance versus full activation of naive CD8 T cells: dissociating proliferation and development of effector function. *J Exp Med* 197: 1141-51

[17] Kieper WC, Prlic M, Schmidt CS, Mescher MF, Jameson SC. 2001. Il-12 enhances CD8 T cell homeostatic expansion. *J Immunol* 166: 5515-21

[18] Lee SW, Park Y, Yoo JK, Choi SY, Sung YC. 2003. Inhibition of TCR-induced CD8 T cell death by IL-12: regulation of Fas ligand and cellular FLIP expression and caspase activation by IL-12. *J Immunol* 170: 2456-60

[19] Pearce EL, Shen H. 2007. Generation of CD8 T cell memory is regulated by IL-12. *J Immunol* 179: 2074-81

[20] Micallef MJ, Ohtsuki T, Kohno K, Tanabe F, Ushio S, Namba M, Tanimoto T, Torigoe K, Fujii M, Ikeda M, Fukuda S, Kurimoto M. 1996. Interferon-gamma-inducing factor enhances T helper 1 cytokine production by stimulated human T cells: synergism with interleukin-12 for interferon-gamma production. *Eur J Immunol* 26: 1647-51

[21] Lauwerys BR, Renauld JC, Houssiau FA. 1999. Synergistic proliferation and activation of natural killer cells by interleukin 12 and interleukin 18. *Cytokine* 11: 822-30

[22] Yoshimoto T, Okamura H, Tagawa YI, Iwakura Y, Nakanishi K. 1997. Interleukin 18 together with interleukin 12 inhibits IgE production by induction of interferon-gamma production from activated B cells. *Proc Natl Acad Sci U S A* 94: 3948-53

[23] Ma X, Chow JM, Gri G, Carra G, Gerosa F, Wolf SF, Dzialo R, Trinchieri G. 1996. The interleukin 12 p40 gene promoter is primed by interferon gamma in monocytic cells. *J Exp Med* 183: 147-57

[24] Grohmann U, Belladonna ML, Bianchi R, Orabona C, Ayroldi E, Fioretti MC, Puccetti P. 1998. IL-12 acts directly on DC to promote nuclear localization of NF-kappaB and primes DC for IL-12 production. *Immunity* 9: 315-23

[25] Zou JP, Yamamoto N, Fujii T, Takenaka H, Kobayashi M, Herrmann SH, Wolf SF, Fujiwara H, Hamaoka T. 1995. Systemic administration of rIL-12 induces complete tumor regression and protective immunity: response is correlated with a striking

reversal of suppressed IFN-gamma production by anti-tumor T cells. *Int Immunol* 7: 1135-45
[26] Lafleur EA, Jia SF, Worth LL, Zhou Z, Owen-Schaub LB, Kleinerman ES. 2001. Interleukin (IL)-12 and IL-12 gene transfer up-regulate Fas expression in human osteosarcoma and breast cancer cells. *Cancer Res* 61: 4066-71
[27] Burke F, Knowles RG, East N, Balkwill FR. 1995. The role of indoleamine 2,3-dioxygenase in the anti-tumour activity of human interferon-gamma in vivo. *Int J Cancer* 60: 115-22
[28] Voest EE, Kenyon BM, O'Reilly MS, Truitt G, D'Amato RJ, Folkman J. 1995. Inhibition of angiogenesis in vivo by interleukin 12. *J Natl Cancer Inst* 87: 581-6
[29] Angiolillo AL, Sgadari C, Taub DD, Liao F, Farber JM, Maheshwari S, Kleinman HK, Reaman GH, Tosato G. 1995. Human interferon-inducible protein 10 is a potent inhibitor of angiogenesis in vivo. *J Exp Med* 182: 155-62
[30] Angiolillo AL, Sgadari C, Tosato G. 1996. A role for the interferon-inducible protein 10 in inhibition of angiogenesis by interleukin-12. *Ann N Y Acad Sci* 795: 158-67
[31] Sgadari C, Angiolillo AL, Tosato G. 1996. Inhibition of angiogenesis by interleukin-12 is mediated by the interferon-inducible protein 10. *Blood* 87: 3877-82
[32] Ferretti E, Di Carlo E, Cocco C, Ribatti D, Sorrentino C, Ognio E, Montagna D, Pistoia V, Airoldi I. 2010. Direct inhibition of human acute myeloid leukemia cell growth by IL-12. *Immunol Lett* 133: 99-105
[33] Duda DG, Sunamura M, Lozonschi L, Kodama T, Egawa S, Matsumoto G, Shimamura H, Shibuya K, Takeda K, Matsuno S. 2000. Direct in vitro evidence and in vivo analysis of the antiangiogenesis effects of interleukin 12. *Cancer Res* 60: 1111-6
[34] Yao L, Sgadari C, Furuke K, Bloom ET, Teruya-Feldstein J, Tosato G. 1999. Contribution of natural killer cells to inhibition of angiogenesis by interleukin-12. *Blood* 93: 1612-21
[35] Wigginton JM, Gruys E, Geiselhart L, Subleski J, Komschlies KL, Park JW, Wiltrout TA, Nagashima K, Back TC, Wiltrout RH. 2001. IFN-gamma and Fas/FasL are required for the antitumor and antiangiogenic effects of IL-12/pulse IL-2 therapy. *J Clin Invest* 108: 51-62
[36] Eisenring M, vom Berg J, Kristiansen G, Saller E, Becher B. 2010. IL-12 initiates tumor rejection via lymphoid tissue-inducer cells bearing the natural cytotoxicity receptor NKp46. *Nat Immunol* 11: 1030-8
[37] Ogawa M, Tsutsui T, Zou JP, Mu J, Wijesuriya R, Yu WG, Herrmann S, Kubo T, Fujiwara H, Hamaoka T. 1997. Enhanced induction of very late antigen 4/lymphocyte function-associated antigen 1-dependent T-cell migration to tumor sites following administration of interleukin 12. *Cancer Res* 57: 2216-22
[38] Kilinc MO, Aulakh KS, Nair RE, Jones SA, Alard P, Kosiewicz MM, Egilmez NK. 2006. Reversing tumor immune suppression with intratumoral IL-12: activation of tumor-associated T effector/memory cells, induction of T suppressor apoptosis, and infiltration of CD8+ T effectors. *J Immunol* 177: 6962-73
[39] Verbik DJ, Stinson WW, Brunda MJ, Kessinger A, Joshi SS. 1996. In vivo therapeutic effects of interleukin-12 against highly metastatic residual lymphoma. *Clin Exp Metastasis* 14: 219-29
[40] Zhao X, Bose A, Komita H, Taylor JL, Kawabe M, Chi N, Spokas L, Lowe DB, Goldbach C, Alber S, Watkins SC, Butterfield LH, Kalinski P, Kirkwood JM, Storkus WJ. 2011.

Intratumoral IL-12 gene therapy results in the crosspriming of Tc1 cells reactive against tumor-associated stromal antigens. *Mol Ther* 19: 805-14

[41] Broderick L, Yokota SJ, Reineke J, Mathiowitz E, Stewart CC, Barcos M, Kelleher RJ, Jr., Bankert RB. 2005. Human CD4+ effector memory T cells persisting in the microenvironment of lung cancer xenografts are activated by local delivery of IL-12 to proliferate, produce IFN-gamma, and eradicate tumor cells. *J Immunol* 174: 898-906

[42] Hess SD, Egilmez NK, Bailey N, Anderson TM, Mathiowitz E, Bernstein SH, Bankert RB. 2003. Human CD4+ T cells present within the microenvironment of human lung tumors are mobilized by the local and sustained release of IL-12 to kill tumors in situ by indirect effects of IFN-gamma. *J Immunol* 170: 400-12

[43] Broderick L, Brooks SP, Takita H, Baer AN, Bernstein JM, Bankert RB. 2006. IL-12 reverses anergy to T cell receptor triggering in human lung tumor-associated memory T cells. *Clin Immunol* 118: 159-69

[44] King IL, Segal BM. 2005. Cutting edge: IL-12 induces CD4+CD25- T cell activation in the presence of T regulatory cells. *J Immunol* 175: 641-5

[45] Cao X, Leonard K, Collins LI, Cai SF, Mayer JC, Payton JE, Walter MJ, Piwnica-Worms D, Schreiber RD, Ley TJ. 2009. Interleukin 12 stimulates IFN-gamma-mediated inhibition of tumor-induced regulatory T-cell proliferation and enhances tumor clearance. *Cancer Res* 69: 8700-9

[46] Sica A, Schioppa T, Mantovani A, Allavena P. 2006. Tumour-associated macrophages are a distinct M2 polarised population promoting tumour progression: potential targets of anti-cancer therapy. *Eur J Cancer* 42: 717-27

[47] Gordon S. 2003. Alternative activation of macrophages. *Nature Reviews Immunology* 3: 23-35

[48] Stout RD, Watkins SK, Suttles J. 2009. Functional plasticity of macrophages: in situ reprogramming of tumor-associated macrophages. *J Leukoc Biol* 86: 1105-9

[49] Watkins SK, Egilmez NK, Suttles J, Stout RD. 2007. IL-12 rapidly alters the functional profile of tumor-associated and tumor-infiltrating macrophages in vitro and in vivo. *J Immunol* 178: 1357-62

[50] Chmielewski M, Kopecky C, Hombach AA, Abken H. 2011. IL-12 Release by Engineered T Cells Expressing Chimeric Antigen Receptors Can Effectively Muster an Antigen-Independent Macrophage Response on Tumor Cells That Have Shut Down Tumor Antigen Expression. *Cancer Res* 71: 5697-706

[51] Mu J, Zou JP, Yamamoto N, Tsutsui T, Tai XG, Kobayashi M, Herrmann S, Fujiwara H, Hamaoka T. 1995. Administration of recombinant interleukin 12 prevents outgrowth of tumor cells metastasizing spontaneously to lung and lymph nodes. *Cancer Res* 55: 4404-8

[52] Sabel MS, Su G, Griffith KA, Chang AE. 2010. Intratumoral delivery of encapsulated IL-12, IL-18 and TNF-alpha in a model of metastatic breast cancer. *Breast Cancer Res Treat* 122: 325-36

[53] Hill HC, Conway TF, Jr., Sabel MS, Jong YS, Mathiowitz E, Bankert RB, Egilmez NK. 2002. Cancer immunotherapy with interleukin 12 and granulocyte-macrophage colony-stimulating factor-encapsulated microspheres: coinduction of innate and adaptive antitumor immunity and cure of disseminated disease. *Cancer Res* 62: 7254-63

[54] Fewell JG, Matar MM, Rice JS, Brunhoeber E, Slobodkin G, Pence C, Worker M, Lewis DH, Anwer K. 2009. Treatment of disseminated ovarian cancer using nonviral interleukin-12 gene therapy delivered intraperitoneally. *J Gene Med* 11: 718-28

[55] Sonabend AM, Velicu S, Ulasov IV, Han Y, Tyler B, Brem H, Matar MM, Fewell JG, Anwer K, Lesniak MS. 2008. A safety and efficacy study of local delivery of interleukin-12 transgene by PPC polymer in a model of experimental glioma. *Anticancer Drugs* 19: 133-42

[56] Tian L, Chen X, Sun Y, Liu M, Zhu D, Ren J. 2010. Growth suppression of human laryngeal squamous cell carcinoma by adenoviral-mediated interleukin-12. *J Int Med Res* 38: 994-1004

[57] Chiu TL, Lin SZ, Hsieh WH, Peng CW. 2009. AAV2-mediated interleukin-12 in the treatment of malignant brain tumors through activation of NK cells. *Int J Oncol* 35: 1361-7

[58] Chen L, Chen D, Block E, O'Donnell M, Kufe DW, Clinton SK. 1997. Eradication of murine bladder carcinoma by intratumor injection of a bicistronic adenoviral vector carrying cDNAs for the IL-12 heterodimer and its inhibition by the IL-12 p40 subunit homodimer. *J Immunol* 159: 351-9

[59] Siders WM, Wright PW, Hixon JA, Alvord WG, Back TC, Wiltrout RH, Fenton RG. 1998. T cell- and NK cell-independent inhibition of hepatic metastases by systemic administration of an IL-12-expressing recombinant adenovirus. *J Immunol* 160: 5465-74

[60] Malvicini M, Rizzo M, Alaniz L, Pinero F, Garcia M, Atorrasagasti C, Aquino JB, Rozados V, Scharovsky OG, Matar P, Mazzolini G. 2009. A novel synergistic combination of cyclophosphamide and gene transfer of interleukin-12 eradicates colorectal carcinoma in mice. *Clin Cancer Res* 15: 7256-65

[61] Gonzalez-Aparicio M, Alzuguren P, Mauleon I, Medina-Echeverz J, Hervas-Stubbs S, Mancheno U, Berraondo P, Crettaz J, Gonzalez-Aseguinolaza G, Prieto J, Hernandez-Alcoceba R. 2011. Oxaliplatin in combination with liver-specific expression of interleukin 12 reduces the immunosuppressive microenvironment of tumours and eradicates metastatic colorectal cancer in mice. *Gut* 60: 341-9

[62] Wang L, Hernandez-Alcoceba R, Shankar V, Zabala M, Kochanek S, Sangro B, Kramer MG, Prieto J, Qian C. 2004. Prolonged and inducible transgene expression in the liver using gutless adenovirus: a potential therapy for liver cancer. *Gastroenterology* 126: 278-89

[63] Komita H, Zhao X, Katakam AK, Kumar P, Kawabe M, Okada H, Braughler JM, Storkus WJ. 2009. Conditional interleukin-12 gene therapy promotes safe and effective antitumor immunity. *Cancer Gene Ther* 16: 883-91

[64] Shin EJ, Wanna GB, Choi B, Aguila D, 3rd, Ebert O, Genden EM, Woo SL. 2007. Interleukin-12 expression enhances vesicular stomatitis virus oncolytic therapy in murine squamous cell carcinoma. *Laryngoscope* 117: 210-4

[65] Lucas ML, Heller L, Coppola D, Heller R. 2002. IL-12 plasmid delivery by in vivo electroporation for the successful treatment of established subcutaneous B16.F10 melanoma. *Mol Ther* 5: 668-75

[66] Pavlin D, Cemazar M, Kamensek U, Tozon N, Pogacnik A, Sersa G. 2009. Local and systemic antitumor effect of intratumoral and peritumoral IL-12 electrogene therapy on murine sarcoma. *Cancer Biol Ther* 8: 2114-22

[67] Tsai YS, Shiau AL, Chen YF, Tsai HT, Lee HL, Tzai TS, Wu CL. 2009. Enhancement of antitumor immune response by targeted interleukin-12 electrogene transfer through antiHER2 single-chain antibody in a murine bladder tumor model. *Vaccine* 27: 5383-92
[68] Hebeler-Barbosa F, Rodrigues EG, Puccia R, Caires AC, Travassos LR. 2008. Gene Therapy against Murine Melanoma B16F10-Nex2 Using IL-13Ralpha2-Fc Chimera and Interleukin 12 in Association with a Cyclopalladated Drug. *Transl Oncol* 1: 110-20
[69] Huang JH, Zhang SN, Choi KJ, Choi IK, Kim JH, Lee MG, Kim H, Yun CO. 2010. Therapeutic and tumor-specific immunity induced by combination of dendritic cells and oncolytic adenovirus expressing IL-12 and 4-1BBL. *Mol Ther* 18: 264-74
[70] Kayashima H, Toshima T, Okano S, Taketomi A, Harada N, Yamashita Y, Tomita Y, Shirabe K, Maehara Y. 2010. Intratumoral neoadjuvant immunotherapy using IL-12 and dendritic cells is an effective strategy to control recurrence of murine hepatocellular carcinoma in immunosuppressed mice. *J Immunol* 185: 698-708
[71] Tabata K, Watanabe M, Naruishi K, Edamura K, Satoh T, Yang G, Abdel Fattah E, Wang J, Goltsov A, Floryk D, Soni SD, Kadmon D, Thompson TC. 2009. Therapeutic effects of gelatin matrix-embedded IL-12 gene-modified macrophages in a mouse model of residual prostate cancer. *Prostate Cancer Prostatic Dis* 12: 301-9
[72] Kayashima H, Toshima T, Okano S, Taketomi A, Harada N, Yamashita Y, Tomita Y, Shirabe K, Maehara Y. 2010. Intratumoral Neoadjuvant Immunotherapy Using IL-12 and Dendritic Cells Is an Effective Strategy To Control Recurrence of Murine Hepatocellular Carcinoma in Immunosuppressed Mice. *Journal of Immunology* 185: 698-708
[73] Zhu S, Lee DA, Li S. 2010. IL-12 and IL-27 sequential gene therapy via intramuscular electroporation delivery for eliminating distal aggressive tumors. *J Immunol* 184: 2348-54
[74] Charoensit P, Kawakami S, Higuchi Y, Yamashita F, Hashida M. 2010. Enhanced growth inhibition of metastatic lung tumors by intravenous injection of ATRA-cationic liposome/IL-12 pDNA complexes in mice. *Cancer Gene Ther* 17: 512-22
[75] Atkins MB, Robertson MJ, Gordon M, Lotze MT, DeCoste M, DuBois JS, Ritz J, Sandler AB, Edington HD, Garzone PD, Mier JW, Canning CM, Battiato L, Tahara H, Sherman ML. 1997. Phase I evaluation of intravenous recombinant human interleukin 12 in patients with advanced malignancies. *Clin Cancer Res* 3: 409-17
[76] Robertson MJ, Cameron C, Atkins MB, Gordon MS, Lotze MT, Sherman ML, Ritz J. 1999. Immunological effects of interleukin 12 administered by bolus intravenous injection to patients with cancer. *Clin Cancer Res* 5: 9-16
[77] Leonard JP, Sherman ML, Fisher GL, Buchanan LJ, Larsen G, Atkins MB, Sosman JA, Dutcher JP, Vogelzang NJ, Ryan JL. 1997. Effects of single-dose interleukin-12 exposure on interleukin-12-associated toxicity and interferon-gamma production. *Blood* 90: 2541-8
[78] Gollob JA, Veenstra KG, Mier JW, Atkins MB. 2001. Agranulocytosis and hemolytic anemia in patients with renal cell cancer treated with interleukin-12. *Journal of Immunotherapy* 24: 91-8
[79] Wadler S, Levy D, Frederickson HL, Falkson CI, Wang YX, Weller E, Burk R, Ho G, Kadish AS. 2004. A phase II trial of interleukin-12 in patients with advanced

cervical cancer: clinical and immunologic correlates Eastern Cooperative Oncology Group study E1E96. *Gynecologic Oncology* 92: 957-64

[80] Freedman RS, Lenzi R, Rosenblum M, Verschraegen C, Kudelka AP, Kavanagh JJ, Hicks ME, Lang EA, Nash MA, Levy LB, Garcia ME, Platsoucas CD, Abbruzzese JL. 2002. Phase I study of intraperitoneal recombinant human interleukin 12 in patients with Mullerian carcinoma, gastrointestinal primary malignancies, and mesothelioma. *Clinical Cancer Research* 8: 3686-95

[81] Lenzi R, Edwards R, June C, Seiden MV, Garcia ME, Rosenblum M, Freedman RS. 2007. Phase II study of intraperitoneal recombinant interleukin-12 (rhIL-12) in patients with peritoneal carcinomatosis (residual disease < 1 cm) associated with ovarian cancer or primary peritoneal carcinoma. *Journal of Translational Medicine* 5

[82] Rook AH, Wood GS, Yoo EK, Elenitsas R, Kao DM, Sherman ML, Witmer WK, Rockwell KA, Shane RB, Lessin SR, Vonderheid EC. 1999. Interleukin-12 therapy of cutaneous T-cell lymphoma induces lesion regression and cytotoxic T-cell responses. *Blood* 94: 902-8

[83] Portielje JEA, Kruit WHJ, Schuler M, Beck J, Lamers CHJ, Stoter G, Huber C, de Boer-Dennert M, Rakhit A, Bolhuis RLH, Waiter E. 1999. Phase I study of subcutaneously administered recombinant human interleukin 12 in patients with advanced renal cell cancer. *Clinical Cancer Research* 5: 3983-9

[84] Duvic M, Sherman ML, Wood GS, Kuzel TM, Olsen E, Foss F, Laliberte RJ, Ryan JL, Zonno K, Rook AH. 2006. A phase II open-label study of recombinant human interleukin-12 in patients with stage IA, IB, or IIA mycosis fungoides. *J Am Acad Dermatol* 55: 807-13

[85] Little RF, Aleman K, Kumar P, Wyvill KM, Pluda JM, Read-Connole E, Wang V, Pittaluga S, Catanzaro AT, Steinberg SM, Yarchoan R. 2007. Phase 2 study of pegylated liposomal doxorubicin in combination with interleukin-12 for AIDS-related Kaposi sarcoma. *Blood* 110: 4165-71

[86] Younes A, Pro B, Robertson MJ, Flinn IW, Romaguera JE, Hagemeister F, Dang NH, Fiumara P, Loyer EM, Cabanillas FF, McLaughlin PW, Rodriguez MA, Samaniego F. 2004. Phase II clinical trial of interleukin-12 in patients with relapsed and refractory non-Hodgkin's lymphoma and Hodgkin's disease. *Clin Cancer Res* 10: 5432-8

[87] van Herpen CML, van der Laak JAW, de Vries IJM, van Krieken JH, de Wilde PC, Balvers MGJ, Adema GJ, De Mulder PHM. 2005. Intratumoral recombinant human interleukin-12 administration in head and neck squamous (cell carcinoma patients modifies locoregional lymph node architecture and induces natural killer cell infiltration in the primary tumor. *Clinical Cancer Research* 11: 1899-909

[88] van Herpen CML, van der Voort R, van der Laak JAWM, Klasen IS, de Graaf AO, van Kempen LCL, de Vries IJM, Duiveman-de Boer T, Dolstra H, Torensma R, van Krieken JH, Adema GJ, De Mulder PHM. 2008. Intratumoral rhIL-12 administration in head and neck squamous cell carcinoma patients induces B cell activation. *International Journal of Cancer* 123: 2354-61

[89] Heinzerling L, Burg G, Dummer R, Maier T, Oberholzer PA, Schultz J, Elzaouk L, Pavlovic J, Moelling K. 2005. Intratumoral injection of DNA encoding human interleukin 12 into patients with metastatic melanoma: clinical efficacy. *Hum Gene Ther* 16: 35-48

[90] Triozzi PL, Strong TV, Bucy RP, Allen KO, Carlisle RR, Moore SE, Lobuglio AF, Conry RM. 2005. Intratumoral administration of a recombinant canarypox virus expressing interleukin 12 in patients with metastatic melanoma. *Hum Gene Ther* 16: 91-100

[91] Daud AI, DeConti RC, Andrews S, Urbas P, Riker AI, Sondak VK, Munster PN, Sullivan DM, Ugen KE, Messina JL, Heller R. 2008. Phase I Trial of Interleukin-12 Plasmid Electroporation in Patients With Metastatic Melanoma. *Journal of Clinical Oncology* 26: 5896-903

[92] Anwer K, Barnes MN, Fewell J, Lewis DH, Alvarez RD. 2010. Phase-I clinical trial of IL-12 plasmid/lipopolymer complexes for the treatment of recurrent ovarian cancer. *Gene Ther* 17: 360-9

[93] Hallaj-Nezhadi S, Lotfipour F, Dass C. 2010. Nanoparticle-mediated interleukin-12 cancer gene therapy. *J Pharm Pharm Sci* 13: 472-85

[94] Feng B, Chen L. 2009. Review of mesenchymal stem cells and tumors: executioner or coconspirator? *Cancer Biother Radiopharm* 24: 717-21

[95] Ryu CH, Park SH, Park SA, Kim SM, Lim JY, Jeong CH, Yoon WS, Oh WI, Sung YC, Jeun SS. 2011. Gene therapy of intracranial glioma using interleukin 12-secreting human umbilical cord blood-derived mesenchymal stem cells. *Hum Gene Ther* 22: 733-43

[96] Gao P, Ding Q, Wu Z, Jiang H, Fang Z. 2010. Therapeutic potential of human mesenchymal stem cells producing IL-12 in a mouse xenograft model of renal cell carcinoma. *Cancer Lett* 290: 157-66

[97] Eliopoulos N, Francois M, Boivin MN, Martineau D, Galipeau J. 2008. Neo-organoid of marrow mesenchymal stromal cells secreting interleukin-12 for breast cancer therapy. *Cancer Res* 68: 4810-8

[98] Wang H, Yang G, Timme TL, Fujita T, Naruishi K, Frolov A, Brenner MK, Kadmon D, Thompson TC. 2007. IL-12 gene-modified bone marrow cell therapy suppresses the development of experimental metastatic prostate cancer. *Cancer Gene Ther* 14: 819-27

[99] Duan X, Guan H, Cao Y, Kleinerman ES. 2009. Murine bone marrow-derived mesenchymal stem cells as vehicles for interleukin-12 gene delivery into Ewing sarcoma tumors. *Cancer* 115: 13-22

[100] Shimizu T, Berhanu A, Redlinger RE, Jr., Watkins S, Lotze MT, Barksdale EM, Jr. 2001. Interleukin-12 transduced dendritic cells induce regression of established murine neuroblastoma. *J Pediatr Surg* 36: 1285-92

[101] Tatsumi T, Takehara T, Yamaguchi S, Sasakawa A, Miyagi T, Jinushi M, Sakamori R, Kohga K, Uemura A, Ohkawa K, Storkus WJ, Hayashi N. 2007. Injection of IL-12 gene-transduced dendritic cells into mouse liver tumor lesions activates both innate and acquired immunity. *Gene Ther* 14: 863-71

[102] He XZ, Wang L, Zhang YY. 2008. An effective vaccine against colon cancer in mice: use of recombinant adenovirus interleukin-12 transduced dendritic cells. *World J Gastroenterol* 14: 532-40

[103] Schmidt-Wolf IG, Lefterova P, Mehta BA, Fernandez LP, Huhn D, Blume KG, Weissman IL, Negrin RS. 1993. Phenotypic characterization and identification of effector cells involved in tumor cell recognition of cytokine-induced killer cells. *Exp Hematol* 21: 1673-9

[104] Helms MW, Prescher JA, Cao YA, Schaffert S, Contag CH. 2010. IL-12 enhances efficacy and shortens enrichment time in cytokine-induced killer cell immunotherapy. *Cancer Immunol Immunother* 59: 1325-34

[105] Kerkar SP, Muranski P, Kaiser A, Boni A, Sanchez-Perez L, Yu Z, Palmer DC, Reger RN, Borman ZA, Zhang L, Morgan RA, Gattinoni L, Rosenberg SA, Trinchieri G, Restifo NP. 2010. Tumor-specific CD8+ T cells expressing interleukin-12 eradicate established cancers in lymphodepleted hosts. *Cancer Res* 70: 6725-34

[106] Zhang L, Kerkar SP, Yu Z, Zheng Z, Yang S, Restifo NP, Rosenberg SA, Morgan RA. 2011. Improving adoptive T cell therapy by targeting and controlling IL-12 expression to the tumor environment. *Mol Ther* 19: 751-9